Integrating Clinical Aromatherapy in Palliative Care

T0385214

of related interest

Women's Health Aromatherapy
A Clinically Evidence-Based Guide for Nurses, Midwives, Doulas and Therapists
Pam Conrad
ISBN 978 1 84819 425 0
eISBN 978 0 85701 378 1

Aromatherapy, Massage and Relaxation in Cancer Care
An Integrative Resource for Practitioners
Edited by Ann Carter and Dr Peter A. Mackereth
Forewords by Anne Cawthorn and Deborah Costello
ISBN 978 1 84819 281 2
eISBN 978 0 85701 228 9

Fragrance and Wellbeing
Plant Aromatics and Their Influence on the Psyche
Jennifer Peace Rhind
ISBN 978 1 84819 090 0
eISBN 978 0 85701 073 5

Integrating Clinical Aromatherapy in Palliative Care

Carol Rose

Foreword by Rhiannon Lewis

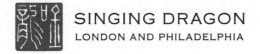

SINGING DRAGON
LONDON AND PHILADELPHIA

First published in Great Britain in 2023 by Singing Dragon,
an imprint of Jessica Kingsley Publishers
Part of John Murray Press

2

Front cover image source: Shutterstock®.
The cover image is floating chamomile flowers.

Disclaimer: The information contained in this book is not intended to replace
the services of trained medical professionals or to be a substitute for medical
advice. The complementary therapy described in this book may not be suitable for
everyone to follow. You are advised to consult a doctor before embarking on any
complementary therapy programme and on any matters relating to your health, and
in particular on any matters that may require diagnosis or medical attention.

A CIP catalogue record for this title is available from the
British Library and the Library of Congress

ISBN 978 1 83997 160 0
eISBN 978 1 83997 161 7

Printed and bound by CPI Group (UK) Ltd, Croydon, CR0 4YY

Jessica Kingsley Publishers' policy is to use papers that are natural,
renewable and recyclable products and made from wood grown in
sustainable forests. The logging and manufacturing processes are expected
to conform to the environmental regulations of the country of origin.

Singing Dragon
Carmelite House
50 Victoria Embankment
London EC4Y 0DZ

www.singingdragon.com

John Murray Press
Part of Hodder & Stoughton Limited
An Hachette UK Company

This book is dedicated to the patients with life-limiting illness and their families who continue to teach me humility and remain a constant source of inspiration.

Contents

Foreword

The fields of oncology and palliative care have long led the way in delivering a patient-centred approach to providing optimum care. For more than 30 years, therapies such as aromatherapy in these settings have contributed a complementary means of supporting the patient and their family as they navigate unknown territories in their journey with their disease. Despite this long history of aromatic integration, to date, only a handful of specialist books exist that safely and effectively guide the practitioner and healthcare professional in evidence-based aromatherapy practice for palliative care.

What Carol Rose achieves in this remarkable text shortens the gap between research and practice, amply demonstrating the value of keeping the patient front and centre in every therapeutic intervention, all the while leaning on her clinical expertise coupled with a robust evidence base. In doing so, she showcases true evidence-based practice, not only giving weight to epidemiological data but also providing emphasis on clinical judgement and the patient's personal story. Carol bridges this research-to-practice gap with flexibility, presence, humility and complete patient focus to ensure that the individual experience is seen and heard and that decisions about care are shared between the patient and practitioner.

Throughout this book, Carol effectively shares with the reader her real-world experience of accompanying those living with life-limiting disease using aromatic remedies. What is more, her contribution stands up to the evidence-based demands for rigour as well as the scrutiny of those working in the healthcare sector.

I believe *Integrating Clinical Aromatherapy in Palliative Care* is the most authoritative text to date for the specialist aromatherapy world. This is due to a combination of aligned factors that enable Carol to be best placed to write such a text. As a registered nurse, specialized in oncology and palliative care with a BSc (Hons) in Palliative Nursing, over

20 years of nursing practice, followed by a further 20 years of training and experience in clinical aromatherapy, Carol is at ease, fluent and conversant with the nursing, research, palliative care and aromatherapy worlds and where they intersect. Her skills as writer and educator have been honed over many years and her communication skills are exemplary. If you combine these factors with Carol's personal finesse of humanity, authenticity, pragmatism, caring and determination, the result is this landmark text that you hold in your hands. This is not a 'how to' book. It asks you to use your critical thinking skills and empowers you with roadmap examples of thoughtful aromatic care provision.

As Editor of the *International Journal of Clinical Aromatherapy*, over recent years, I have had the delight of publishing a number of articles written by Carol Rose, all of which have followed this same detailed, empathetic and dedicated path that stems from a place of rich experience, knowledge and the unwavering determination to keep the patient at the heart of every therapeutic encounter.

What is more, I do believe that what Carol shares in this book transcends the specialty of palliative care. Her thorough and thoughtful method is applicable across all disciplines, thereby inspiring all practitioners to take a similar sensitive yet rigorous approach with their patients.

I am deeply honoured to have been asked to contribute this foreword and leave you, the reader, the joy of discovering the contents of this extraordinary book. May it serve to further hone your knowledge and skills to improve the care you provide.

Rhiannon Lewis
International Journal of Clinical Aromatherapy
International Clinical Aromatherapy Network
September 2022

Acknowledgements

This book is the product of many who have contributed greatly throughout my life. First and foremost to the patients with life-limiting illness, their families and caregivers, I am indebted to you for your openness and resilience and for being my greatest educators.

My eternal gratitude to the aromatherapists, educators, colleagues and friends of the International Clinical Aromatherapy Network (ICAN), scientists, researchers and authors who have gone before and generously shared their time, expertise and knowledge. In equal measure, you have inspired and challenged my thinking and ultimately shaped my practice.

Thank you to all at Hospice Mid-Northland, Kerikeri, New Zealand who have supported my work. In particular, heartfelt gratitude to Jenny Coleman, Clinical Manager, whose belief and unwavering support of holistic approaches in patient care has led to a dedicated clinical aromatherapy service. Here's to the next decade!

For the road-trip where this book was first conceived, my deep appreciation to Rhiannon Lewis, whose aromatherapy expertise, vision and friendship have been invaluable. You are a shining beacon of light in the global aromatherapy community.

My sincere appreciation to those who provided expert advice and wise counsel through several manuscript drafts: Jenny Coleman, Dr Warrick Jones MD, Rhiannon Lewis and to Gill McKinnon for her generous time and eagle eyes with referencing.

Special thanks to Sarah Hamlin, Senior Commissioning Editor, Hannah Snetsinger, Senior Production Editor and all the team at Singing Dragon for their extraordinary levels of support.

For your treasured friendship and wicked sense of humour, Fi Carr, thank you for keeping me buoyant through this writing process.

To my amazing family and friends who have supported this incredible journey, I am immensely grateful for the richness you bring to my life.

To my mother, Linda, who first immersed me in a world of exotic aromatics and encouraged my decisions along this winding road. I love you dearly.

For my husband, Paul, who has been steadfast in his love, support, sage advice and endless patience. You are my love and my rock.

Special acknowledgement to the *International Journal of Clinical Aromatherapy*, as Chapters 4, 5, 6, 7, 8 and 10 are based on earlier publications. And to *Aromatika*, as sections of Chapters 1 and 15 are based on earlier publications.

Preface

My first encounter with essential oils happened in the 1980s as a newly registered nurse specializing in oncology at London's Royal Marsden Hospital. During that time, I observed patients receiving gentle hand massages using simple blends of lavender and sweet marjoram, fragrances that captured my attention. In those moments of connection, where touch was non-medicalized, a different level of communication was taking place. Patients were visibly relaxing, reassured by this compassionate form of physical touch and tangible act of caring. For me, something transformational happened as I listened to these patients speak of their restful night's sleep and tranquil dreams; a paradox given this was a busy hospital environment and they were all confronting a life-threatening diagnosis of cancer. This discovery of a different level of patient care spoke straight to my heart.

Essential oils sustained me through the subsequent years of study which had extended to a BSc (Hons) in Palliative Nursing while simultaneously working full time with patients in end-of-life care. Oncology and palliative nursing featured heavily throughout those formative years, as my work was shaped by roles involving clinical research and setting up site-specific services for cancer genetics and colorectal cancer. All the while, the balance was redressed through a love of gardening and exploring more thoroughly this world of natural therapies and how patients could benefit from these additional resources to complement their conventional medical treatments. Many of the practical aspects of aromatherapy were self-taught from the few books available at the time, while I made steady progress working with my collection of essential oils. Only after settling with my husband in New Zealand was I able to consciously rethink how to merge these unwavering passions. I qualified as an aromatherapist, specializing in those with progressive and life-limiting illness and working with them through private practice and as the lead therapist at our local community-based hospice.

The notion of putting 'pen to paper' to share my aromatherapy knowledge and clinical experience was first conceived during a road trip with Rhiannon Lewis from Provence's perfume capital, Grasse, to Nice airport. I had just completed another programme of advanced-level clinical aromatherapy study with her, and this remarkable woman showed a keen interest in my work and suggested I submit an article for the *International Journal of Clinical Aromatherapy* (*IJCA*), of which she is the Editor. Initially, I revisited cancer-related fatigue, the subject of my dissertation 20 years previously, only to discover that little in conventional medicine had changed during that time. Patients were still experiencing the same degree of distress, and yet aromatherapy research and my own clinical practice were demonstrating relaxation with sustained levels of energy in these patients. This paper became the first of a series for the *IJCA* over several consecutive years. By this time, I was teaching aromatherapy approaches in palliative care to healthcare and allied-health professionals, presenting at national and international conferences, and was honoured to become a member of the *IJCA* Editorial Advisory Board and a Fellow of ICAN. Collectively, this has led to the writing of this book.

Integrating Clinical Aromatherapy in Palliative Care presents an overview of how clinical aromatherapy can be integrated, appropriately and effectively, alongside conventional medical interventions to improve the quality of life and the care of patients with life-limiting illness. Although palliative care offers a broad remit of practice for patients with all forms of advanced disease, the majority of research-based evidence, both medical and complementary, rests with patients with advanced cancer. Therefore, the focus of this book is to evaluate the current clinical evidence of patients with life-limiting forms of cancer.

Each chapter offers in-depth insight into the common problems experienced by these patients; most importantly, from their perspective. From my personal clinical experience, I know that there is nothing as powerful as listening to the patient's story, their words, emotions and unique lived experience. It is the patient's narrative of the challenges faced when confronting their own mortality which ultimately guides our clinical practice.

The opening chapters, *Understanding the 'Tools of the Trade'* and *Principles of Practice and Methods of Application*, take a broad perspective of essential oils and botanical products to dispel the common misconception that 'natural' plant derivatives make them completely safe. This is particularly relevant to the patient with advanced cancer whose specific pathophysiology, spiritual and psychosocial factors render them vulnerable to the adverse effects of anything that has the potential to cause harm. This includes essential oils and botanical products. Emphasis is placed on essential oil safety, toxicity and storage, plus service implementation and safe methods of aromatherapy application.

Fostering Resilience in Patients with Life-Limiting Illness, *Spiritual Care in Patients with Cancer* and *The Emotional Impact of Cancer* form the foundational chapters of this book. These fundamental dimensions of humanity are frequently overshadowed by the physical symptoms that patients experience. Spiritual care, for example, is often the last chapter in palliative care books; the section where end-of-life care is discussed when death is rapidly approaching. And yet, spirituality is integral to us all. Combined with our resilience and psychosocial capacities, spirituality forms the cornerstone of our ability to cope when faced with adversity. A life-limiting diagnosis and the arduous journey that subsequently unfolds touches every element of human wholeness: spiritual, emotional, social and physical.

I invite you to take your time to delve deeply into these foundational chapters and fully absorb their detail. They are crucial to the holistic nature of aromatherapy, which seeks to unite mind, body and spirit – a contrast to conventional medicine, where illness has been compartmentalized into physical body parts, and often further separated from the spiritual and emotional dimensions of human wholeness.

The subsequent chapters relate to the common symptoms experienced by patients with advanced cancer. Successful integration of clinical aromatherapy into mainstream healthcare for these patients rests with an in-depth understanding of each symptom, including prevalence and pathophysiology, together with research-based evidence for conventional medical management, non-pharmacological approaches and clinical aromatherapy intervention. Overall, this level of understanding provides a broader perspective for practices which are relevant and appropriate, while bringing cohesion to working alongside a multi-disciplinary team.

Throughout this book, integration of clinical aromatherapy is demonstrated by means of the patient–therapist relationship; skilful communication; the judicious use of essential oils, hydrosols and other botanical products; as well as the importance of patient-centred and relationship-centred care. Clinical aromatherapy reframes symptom management to allow for greater emotional, social and spiritual expression. The aim is to redress the balance of conventional medical approaches, which tend to focus on the physical nature of symptoms and pharmacological management.

The final chapter, *The Way Forward*, is dedicated to evaluating clinical aromatherapy interventions in palliative care. This considers the potential of aromatherapy, explored within each chapter, and, at the same time, highlights the gaps which exist in clinical practice. It raises questions for clinical research and ways in which to fulfil the remit of evidence-based practice.

Integrating clinical aromatherapy is a person-centred approach which provides patients with a greater sense of control over their illness, as well as the opportunity to be more active in their care across the entire cancer trajectory. Such collaborative working serves to enrich relationships between patients, therapists and healthcare professionals.

CHAPTER 1

Aromatherapy in Palliative Care

Palliative care is a mixture of teamwork with clinical detective work to find the origins of a patient's symptoms in order to offer the best possible palliation; of attention to the psychological needs and resilience of patients and their families; honesty and truth in the face of advancing disease; and recognition that each patient is unique, a whole person who is the key member of the team looking after them. Working with, rather than doing to.

(Mannix 2017, p.24)

The evolution of palliative care is largely attributed to the lifetime work of Dame Cicely Saunders, who first introduced the concept of 'total pain' in 1964 (Saunders 1964). This seminal work revolutionized end-of-life care by emphasizing the importance of considering the patient's physical suffering within the broader context of their emotional, social and spiritual capacities. Fusing this holistic approach with conventional medicine saw the emergence of fresh, new practices, a renewed vision of the quality of life of patients with life-limiting illness and assessment of emotional and spiritual distress, all of which incorporated rigorous clinical practice, training and academic validation. These beginnings brought *terminal care* (as it was known then) into the international spotlight. The development and expansion of the hospice movement led to patient-centred care, which focused on compassion, respect and dignity of patients with life-limiting forms of cancer.

By the 1990s, the holistic principles of *terminal care* extended exponentially, emerging as *palliative care* to include patients with non-malignant diagnoses, at an earlier stage of their disease trajectory and in a variety of settings, such as hospitals and the community. Palliative care has advanced as an important integrative specialty in healthcare. Central to this advancement is the value that patients themselves place on complementary therapies.

It has been long known that patients with advanced illness seek out complementary therapies as adjuncts to their conventional medical treatments. Predominantly, this is because conventional approaches do not always provide sufficient or appropriate relief to the number and complexity of problems patients can experience. *Complementary Therapies in Cancer Care* (Kohn 1999), a pivotal report of its time, highlighted the underlying reasons. Patients spoke of the benefits of supportive approaches because they offered them touch, time and the opportunity to talk. The report also demonstrated the interest of healthcare professionals, mainly nurses, who wanted to learn more to support the choices of their patients and in doing so enrich patient care.

The results generated a UK *Directory of Complementary Therapy Services*, where over 90% of the services listed related to touch therapies, the most popular being aromatherapy, massage and reflexology (Macmillan Cancer Relief 2002). Safe integration of these top three therapies involved national guidelines for holistic aromatherapy (Tavares 2003), followed by clinical aromatherapy guidelines for specialist palliative care settings (Tavares 2011). Other initiatives, specific to integrating aromatherapy approaches within mainstream healthcare, oncology and palliative care settings, have since continued. This includes the lifetime work of aromatherapy educator Rhiannon Lewis, and the ground-breaking published works of Shirley and Len Price (2012), Dr Jane Buckle (2015) and Madeleine Kerkhof-Knapp Hayes (2015).

Despite two decades of formal intervention (originally initiated and driven by patient demand), the efficacy and relevance of complementary therapies in healthcare remains a source of debate. As reports point out, this is mostly due to the lack of evidence-based studies which conclusively support the effectiveness of such complementary therapy interventions (Sharp *et al.* 2018). Within palliative care services, measurable evidence is an obligatory requirement of funding stakeholders to ensure direct and tangible benefit to the patient. One of these services is aromatherapy, where practitioners are increasingly expected to demonstrate the therapeutic effectiveness of the interventions offered and evidence to support the cost-effectiveness of service provision.

Factors required to sustain aromatherapy services in palliative care:

- Funding of palliative care services:
  - Public
  - Charitable
  - Private
- Therapeutic effectiveness of aromatherapy interventions
- Cost-effectiveness of the service
- Evidence of improvements in patient care

Unfortunately, the bottom line is that in the absence of well-conducted clinical research to underpin evidence-based practice, the source of funded complementary therapy services hangs in the balance (Sharp *et al.* 2018). This raises several important points for aromatherapists to fulfil the complete remit of evidence-based practice.

Evidence-based practice (EBP)

Originally, EBP involved integration of the *patient's values* with *clinical experience* and the *best research-based findings*. The central placement of EBP in the Venn diagram of Figure 1.1 demonstrates that it aims to support collaborative healthcare decisions.

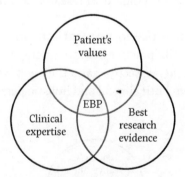

FIGURE 1.1: ORIGINAL FORM OF EBP

However, the modern interpretation of EBP within conventional healthcare has gravitated heavily towards the *best research evidence* with insufficient emphasis placed on *clinical expertise* and the *patient's values*. This is demonstrated in the EBP pyramid of Figure 1.2, where an intervention's efficacy, or performance, is evaluated under highly controlled circumstances, such as a randomized controlled trial (RCT).

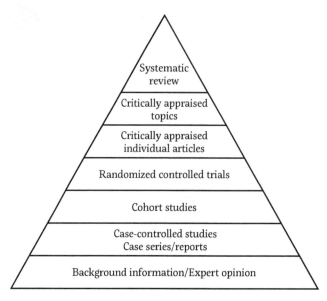

FIGURE I.2: HIERARCHY OF EBP PYRAMID IN CONVENTIONAL HEALTHCARE

Critical appraisal of research findings forms the pinnacle of this hierarchy of EBP pyramid, where current studies evaluating similar research topics are further synthesized in systematic review and meta-analysis. The overarching aim is to determine results of the highest quality which merit an unspoken 'gold standard' of research accomplishment.

Evidence-based practice in aromatherapy

By comparison, the EBP practice of aromatherapy primarily rests with the *patient's values and perspectives*, and the *knowledge and skills* of the aromatherapist, from both clinical and holistic perspectives, as shown in Figure 1.3.

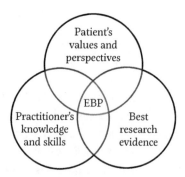

FIGURE I.3: EBP IN AROMATHERAPY

Within the context of aromatherapy in palliative care, the deficit ele-ment is *best research evidence*. Candy *et al.* (2020), in a well-designed systematic review, highlighted this very point. The team evaluated studies incorporating the most popular complementary therapies used by patients with life-limiting illness: aromatherapy, massage and reflexology (n=22). Unfortunately, the review did not include evidence to support the short-term benefits of aromatherapy and massage on quality of life, anxiety and pain, and only reflexology scored with minor benefits. Overall, the low quality of the primary research studies limited their findings. However, the authors recommend that palliative care services continue using complementary therapies, urging clinical teams to present further high-quality evidence from robustly designed studies.

The importance of integrating aromatherapy

Aromatherapy aligns seamlessly with the concept of 'integrative medi-cine', an approach which extends beyond an amalgamation of different medical interventions to encompass individualized patient care, where the focus incorporates the spiritual, emotional and social dimensions together with the physical body. Here, the values, perspectives, hopes and aspirations of the patient, their family and those closely involved in their end-of-life care are central.

The tendency within conventional medicine is to focus on the patho-physiology of disease and ways in which to achieve a cure. Even with advanced disease, where the aim of palliation is to optimize the patient's quality of life, the challenge arises among healthcare professionals with being able to see the opportunities for healing at a spiritual level, even though a biological cure is no longer possible (Steinhorn, Din and John-son 2017). While this is explored in more depth in Chapters 5 and 6, it is within these realms of spiritual and emotional care that aromatherapy can arguably make its greatest difference.

For example, where there is emotional distress such as anxiety, or existential suffering causing escalating levels of pain which appear resistant to all forms of analgesia, in these situations rarely do we see pharmacological intervention actually reaching the underlying cause of the patient's distress. The addition of other approaches which strive to restore wholeness in the patient, particularly in facilitating healing of the human spirit, cannot be overlooked. Aromatherapy is one such modality of many mind–body approaches, including massage, reflexol-ogy, mindfulness, prayer, acupuncture and music.

As holistic practitioners, qualified aromatherapists are well placed to explore the profound and 'unseen' experiences of the patient's life and its meaning. This can be achieved through a sacred space where the patient and family are assured of protected time in a relaxed environment. Skilful communication sensitively guides the conversation, in which the fragility of life can be considered, concerns may be voiced, and choices and wishes can be explored. As part of the multi-disciplinary team, aromatherapists can determine appropriate and early referral for patients and their caregivers, where spiritual and psychosocial care are central and symptom management is considered within a broader holistic context. This is a time when patients have the freedom to choose their own oils and how these will be administered to their individual requirements. From my personal clinical experience, the calm state of relaxation some patients can achieve during aromatherapy intervention, particularly through massage and essential oil inhalation, is comparable to the transcendental states of prayer and meditation. It is within this space of quietude that patients will often experience insights which reaffirm their value and self-worth, and where resilience can be strengthened by connecting with life's richness and meaning.

Despite patients seeking complementary therapies for their personal well-being and to manage distressing symptoms, the research evidence does not always support a powerful effect of such approaches. As such, if we are to sustain clinical aromatherapy services within palliative care, therapists need to consider clinical research which is relevant to our work without compromising our holistic principles of practice, or the values and perspectives of the patients. Such a notion requires cohesive partnership between patients, their families, caregivers and healthcare professionals, while simultaneously working towards a place of EBP, and this is explored throughout the subsequent chapters of this book.

CHAPTER 2

Understanding the 'Tools of the Trade'

Regardless of the strength and accuracy of a healthcare practitioner's evaluation or diagnosis, and regardless of the merits of their treatment principles and methods, the therapeutic results of these clinical skills depend entirely on the efficacy of the oils themselves.

(Holmes 2016, p.63)

Central to aromatherapy practice is the use of essential oils which may be used or combined with other plant extracts, such as hydrosols and fixed oils/macerates, all of which are natural plant derivatives. Safe integration within the clinical setting requires us to begin with a comprehensive understanding of these 'tools of the trade'. While a basic overview is provided in this chapter, readers are encouraged to take further steps through training/books to expand on this important topic that underpins all therapeutic interventions.

Core tenets

The International Organization for Standardization (2022) defines an essential oil as a 'product obtained from a natural raw material of plant origin, by steam distillation, by mechanical processes from the epicarp of citrus fruits, or by dry distillation, after separation of the aqueous phase, if any, by physical process'.

Essential oils are mixtures of secondary metabolites found in aromatic plants. They are a volatile material comprised of natural, complex and concentrated compounds derived from a single plant species. While subsequent chapters will uncover their therapeutic effectiveness and clinical use, Holmes (2016) advocates for clear guidelines when selecting essential oils for such purposes and asserts four criteria for sourcing and determining an oil's potential bioactivity:

1. Biological identity
2. Purity
3. Integrity of the oil's source material
4. Integrity of the oil's extraction process

These criteria go beyond simply establishing an oil chemical profile, determined by methods including gas chromatography and mass spectrometry (GC/MS) analysis, to provide a broader framework for practitioners procuring essential oils for clinical use.

1. Biological identity

Familiar to the aromatherapist is the International Code of Botanical Nomenclature which governs the botanical naming of all plant species (Turland *et al.* 2018). When prescribing essential oils, all documentation must include the botanical name, common name and, where necessary, the chemotype of the plant/essential oil in question.

Botanical name

The botanical name of a single plant is expressed in Latin as a two-part word. The first part identifies the genus (where the first letter is capitalized) and the second part, the species (non-capitalized). Italics identify the botanical name, and the common name generally follows in brackets (non-capitalized and non-italicized). Examples are *Lavandula angustifolia* (lavender true), *Anthemis nobilis* (roman chamomile) and *Agonis fragrans* (fragonia). Botanical naming will subsequently be used in this way throughout the book to ensure clear identification of the essential oils mentioned.

Chemotype

In some cases, there are plants of the same genus and species (that is to say with the same Latin name), which are morphologically identical and yet produce essential oils with sufficiently different chemical compositions to identify them separately. Termed *chemotype*, this is abbreviated to 'ct' and is followed by the name of the 'marker' constituent(s) identified within the essential oil's chemical profile. A common example is *Thymus vulgaris* (thyme), which produces several different chemotypes of which the main, commercially produced thyme oils include:

- *Thymus vulgaris* ct thymol
- *Thymus vulgaris* ct carvacrol
- *Thymus vulgaris* ct α-terpineol
- *Thymus vulgaris* ct geraniol
- *Thymus vulgaris* ct linalool
- *Thymus vulgaris* ct thujanol

The *Thymus vulgaris* (thyme) chemotypes are a prime example of the differences that exist between chemotype variants. Price and Price (2012) describe how thymol and carvacrol are both phenolic components of *Thymus vulgaris* which contribute to the essential oil's powerful antiseptic properties but are also irritating to the skin and mucous membranes. In contrast is the alcohol-rich chemotype, such as *Thymus vulgaris* ct linalool, dominant in the constituent linalool, with increased levels of the ester linalyl acetate. These constituents contribute to its gentle antiseptic action and safe use on the skin. The remaining alcohol-rich chemotypes of *Thymus vulgaris*, α-terpineol, geraniol and thujanol, can also be safely used via dermal application.

Specific plant part

Essential oils originate from single aromatic plant sources and are extracted from various parts of the plant, such as flowers, leaves, wood, bark, needles, grass, resin, berries, fruits, roots and seeds. Some plants produce several different essential oils, derived and extracted from varying anatomical parts of the same plant, for example bitter orange (rind, leaf and flowers), clove (bud and leaf), cinnamon (bark and leaf). These oils will each possess a unique aroma and a specific chemical profile and possibly a different therapeutic indication, even though they have been obtained from the same plant.

Terroir

Many factors affect the yield and quality of essential oil-producing plants. The French term 'terroir' encapsulates the region's climate, soil and terrain, each bringing their individual contribution to impart unique characteristics into the plant that cannot be found anywhere else in the world. *Lavandula angustifolia* (lavender true), for example, grown at altitude in Provence is renowned for its high levels of linalyl acetate (25–45%) and linalool (25–38%) (Battaglia 2018). This particular ratio is unparalleled when it comes to the sedatory action on the central nervous system (CNS), making it an oil of choice for anxiety, insomnia and stress.

2. *Purity*

Determining an oil's optimum therapeutic effectiveness requires complete certainty of its quality and assurance that it has not been altered, either naturally or by adulteration. Scientifically, this can be verified by the essential oil analyst through various forms of testing, including GC/MS analysis of an oil's chemical composition, as well as sensory inspection of its colour, aroma and consistency (organoleptics). An essential oil producer of reputable integrity will openly provide this data alongside the product.

Degradation

Natural chemical degradation of an essential oil occurs through prolonged and poor storage conditions and exposure to heat, light, humidity and oxygen. Processes of oxidation tend to accelerate in monoterpene-rich essential oils, such as citrus and pine, particularly when exposed to heat and light. Oxidized essential oils can be irritant and skin sensitizing and cause severe dermal reactions (Battaglia 2018). Minimizing oxidation requires storage of oils in dark glass bottles with as little head space of air in them as possible, thereby reducing air exposure. Refrigeration of susceptible essential oils is recommended and use within 12 months is advised (Tisserand and Young 2014).

Many clinical settings that have aromatherapy integrated within patient care have a policy in place to clearly identify details of the purchase/quality data, batch codes and expiry dates of the essential oils used in the setting. This includes procedures for ordering and maintaining turnover to ensure that essential oils are always used within their duration of shelf-life.

Contamination

Some low-level pesticide residues can transfer across into essential oils during the extraction process, particularly the expressed epicarp of citrus oils, which are among the most vulnerable. There is a trend towards recommending organically certified essential oils in clinical practice where bio-certification documentation can be requested from the oil producer. This results in a slightly more expensive oil which is unquestionable when it comes to its therapeutic use in the clinical setting.

Adulteration

Each year, there is minor seasonal variance with an essential oil's chemical composition and aroma. However, with an increasing commercial demand for standardization of chemical profiles to boost sales and profit margins, adulteration is unfortunately commonplace. Holmes (2016) details numerous processes of adulteration, the most common and profitable being the addition of 'nature-identical' synthetic chemicals designed to standardize the measurable GC/MS analysis of an oil's chemical composition. Other methods include synthetic isolates and the addition of other, less expensive essential oils, residues or oil fractions. Within aromatherapy practice, of fundamental importance is sourcing only pure, preferably organic, unadulterated essential oils that have been produced with the aromatherapy trade in mind.

3. Integrity of the oil's source material

Bioactivity and essential oil composition are also dependent on the quality of the plant material, the expertise of the grower and the skill of the distiller. Artisanal producers lovingly sowing and tending their plants, while carefully considering the seasonal time and best hours of the day to manually harvest, before sitting in vigil alongside their distillation equipment, is an art that never ceases to take my breath away when I observe it. Aromatic plants grown organically and extracted in this way, with benevolence and intent, produce essential oils of sublime quality and bioactivity that, in my opinion, cannot be matched even by the most thorough of commercial producers. The end result is an essential oil which possesses aromatic depth and smoothness and is filled with complex and subtle notes – criteria Holmes (2016) identifies as central to optimum bioactivity.

4. Integrity of the oil's extraction process

Even if all the botanical parameters are fulfilled, ultimately, the resultant oil is only as good as the extraction process.

Distillation

Common extraction processes involve hydro- or steam distillation where volatile plant constituents are vaporized using heat and water/steam, then condensed via a cooling phase to produce a distillate: a combination of oil and aqueous parts. The oil part is comprised of numerous and complex aromatic and bioactive constituents: the essential oil. The aqueous portion, known as the hydrosol (or hydrolat), contains aromatic and other water-soluble constituents at a vastly reduced concentration compared with the essential oil. Separation of the essential oil from the hydrosol is the final phase.

Hydrosols were at one stage considered by some as the by-product of essential oil distillation. However, increased knowledge of their constituents, milder fragrance and low-level concentration of active components makes them a valuable resource in aromatherapy practice. This will be illustrated in further chapters.

Cold-expression

For citrus rind-derived essential oils, cold-expression techniques are commonly used for aromatherapy practices. In this method of extraction, heat or distillation is not involved. It is a mechanical process of the rinds of the citrus fruits which results in the possibility of heavier, non-volatile components being present, some of which may cause phototoxicity.

Other extraction processes

There are several valuable texts detailing other extraction processes, including supercritical carbon dioxide extraction (Kerkhof 2018), solvent extraction and enfleurage processes (Battaglia 2018).

Organoleptic evaluation

An in-depth knowledge of essential oils is incomplete without our sensorial experience, including what we see in an oil, its colour, depth and viscosity; what we detect in its aroma, the level of smoothness and subtle notes; and what we feel when we inhale its aroma – flat and fatigued, or vibrant and alive. Central to sensorial interpretation is the language of scent. Rhind (2014, pp.148–154) has compiled a table of odour types, characteristics and common descriptors to assist with building an aroma vocabulary. Terms such as *floral, herbaceous, balsamic* and *woody* are examples of odour types, while *sweet, soft, sharp, pungent* and *dry* are characteristics which further classify an aroma. Such terminology is worth acquiring to bring us closer to the heart of an essential oil's aroma. By increasing our sensorial responses, we develop a bank of aromatic memories relevant to our clinical work, for example being able to distinguish a fresh oil from an oxidized one.

Chemical composition of an essential oil

Essential oils are complex mixtures of chemical constituents which, either singly or in combination, underpin their biological activity within the human body. Generally, an essential oil is comprised of between 20 and 200 organic compounds, the majority being in minute concentrations of less than 1% (Tisserand and Young 2014). This is demonstrated in the GC/MS analysis of *Agonis fragrans* (fragonia); see Figure 2.1.

CERTIFICATE OF ANALYSIS

Sample Name	Fragonia
Botanical Name	*Agonis fragrans*
Certification Date	November 2021
Batch Number	AF22
Part of Plant Used	Leaves
Country of Origin	Australia
Method of Analysis	Area of Normalisation Based on ISO 7609:1985

No.	Component	Result / Area %
1	alpha-pinene	25.56%
2	beta-pinene	1.49%
3	myrcene	1.91%
4	para-cymene	2.05%
5	limonene	2.29%
6	1,8 cineole	28.80%
7	gamma-terpinene	2.16%
8	linalool	10.76%
9	terpinen-4-ol	2.77%
10	alpha-terpineol	6.01%
11	myrtenol	4.22%
12	citronellol	0.98%
13	geraniol	1.42%
14	beta-caryophyllene	0.60%
15	alpha-humulene	1.03%
16	viridflorene, bicyclogermacrene	1.14%

Date of Manuf Nov 2021, Relative Density @ 20C: 0.898, Refractive Index @ 20C: +1.469, Optical Rotation @ 20C: +11.90

FIGURE 2.1: GC/MS ANALYSIS OF *AGONIS FRAGRANS* (FRAGONIA), REPRODUCED WITH KIND PERMISSION FROM ESSENTIALLY AUSTRALIA

Safe aromatherapy practice and the clinical use of essential oils rests with a clear understanding of their basic chemical composition. Organic chemistry is a complex subject which has been covered in several excellent texts.

Specific to aromatherapy is Bowles's (2003) *The Chemistry of Aromatherapeutic Oils*. For the clinical setting, Table 2.1 provides examples of a range of essential oil compounds, their main therapeutic properties and essential oil sources that are referred to in this book. These and other chemical compounds are also discussed in relevant chapters.

Table 2.1: Examples of essential oil compounds, sources and properties

Main chemical component	Common essential oil sources mentioned in this book *Botanical name* (common name)	Properties
Monoterpenes		
d- and l-limonene	Dominant in all citrus-rind oils, plus also: *Citrus aurantium var amara flos* (neroli) *Cupressus sempervirens* (cypress) *Canarium luzonicum* (elemi) *Piper nigrum* (black pepper) *Foeniculum vulgare* (sweet fennel) *Myrtus communis* (myrtle) *Picea mariana* (spruce black) *Agonis fragrans* (fragonia) *Litsea cubeba* (may chang)	• Olfactory stimulation with d-limonene induces physiological and psychological relaxation (Joung *et al.* 2014) • Anxiolytic minimizes symptoms of mild mood disorders and cancer pain (Bagetta *et al.* 2010) • d-limonene demonstrates a protective effect in salivary cells exposed to radiotherapy (Saiki *et al.* 2018)
α-pinene β-pinene	Dominant in all conifer oils, plus also: *Myrtus communis* (myrtle) *Pinus sylvestris* (scots pine) *Leptospermum scoparium* (manuka) *Citrus reticulata* (mandarin) *Citrus limon* (lemon) *Laurus nobilis* (laurel leaf)* *Picea mariana* (spruce black) *Boswellia carterii* (frankincense)	• Respiratory mucolytics, general tonic and stimulant (Rhind 2012; Pénoël and Franchomme 1990 cited in Bowles 2003) • *α-pinene, neuropathic analgesic (Baudoux, Blanchard and Malotaux 2006) • (+)-α-pinene, (+)-β-pinene antimicrobial and antifungal, particularly to *Candida albicans* (Rivas da Silva *et al.* 2012)

para-cymene	*Coriandrum sativum* (coriander seed) *Melaleuca alternifolia* (tea tree) *Canarium luzonicum* (elemi) *Origanum majorana* (sweet marjoram) *Boswellia carterii* (frankincense) *Zingiber cassumunar* (plai)	• Antibacterial properties (Dhifi *et al.* 2016) • Analgesic properties most likely related to rubefacient effect where dermal application increases localized blood flow (Bowles 2003)
Monoterpene alcohols		
linalool	*Lavandula angustifolia* (lavender true)* *Citrus aurantium var amara flos* (neroli) *Lavandula latifolia* (spike lavender) *Citrus bergamia* (bergamot)* *Coriandrum sativum* (coriander seed) *Agonis fragrans* (fragonia) *Mentha citrata* (bergamot-mint) *Citrus aurantium var amara fol.* (petitgrain) *Thymus vulgaris ct linalool* (thyme ct linalool) *Cananga odorata* (ylang ylang) *Pelargonium graveolens* (geranium) *Origanum majorana* (sweet marjoram) *Litsea cubeba* (may chang)	• Anti-nociceptive (Wang and Heinbockel 2018) • Antispasmodic (Bowles 2003) • *Potentiates gamma-aminobutyric acid (GABA) receptor responses in the CNS typically causing anxiolytic, sedative and anti-convulsant effects (Tisserand and Young 2014) • l-linalool antispasmodic effect (Lis-Balchin and Hart 1999) • l-linalool anti-inflammatory (Holmes 2019) • l-linalool sedative effect (Bowles 2003; Linck *et al.* 2010)
terpinen-4-ol	*Melaleuca alternifolia* (tea tree)* *Origanum majorana* (sweet marjoram) *Kunzea ambigua* (kunzea) *Zingiber cassumunar* (plai)**	• Anti-fungal (Yu *et al.* 2015) • *Antimicrobial (Carson and Riley 1995) • Analgesic (Rhind 2012) • **Anti-inflammatory (Holmes 2019)
α-terpineol	*Melaleuca alternifolia* (tea tree)	• Important synergistic influence on the antimicrobial effects of tea tree oil (Carson and Riley 1995)

cont.

Monoterpene alcohols		
menthol	*Mentha x piperita* (peppermint) *Mentha arvensis* (cornmint)	• Anti-nociceptive (Wang and Heinbockel 2018) • Localized anaesthesia by cooling (Pénoël and Franchomme 1990 cited in Bowles 2003) • Activates TRPM8 channels (Horvath and Acs 2015) • Enhances sensation of improved airflow (Burrow, Eccles and Jones 2009) • Anti-emetic potential through partial antagonism of 5-HT3 receptors (Heimes, Hauk and Verspohl 2011)
geraniol	*Cymbopogon martinii* (palmarosa) *Pelargonium graveolens* (geranium) *Rosa damascena* (rose) *Coriandrum sativum* (coriander seed)	• Analgesic (Bowles 2003; Rhind 2012)
Terpenoid esters		
linalyl acetate	*Lavandula angustifolia* (lavender true) *Citrus bergamia* (bergamot) *Salvia sclarea* (clary sage) *Citrus aurantium var amara flos* (neroli) *Origanum majorana* (sweet marjoram) *Mentha citrata* (bergamot-mint)	• Antispasmodic and sedative (Bowles 2003) • Antinociceptive (Bagetta *et al.* 2010; Baudoux *et al.* 2006; Harris 2016)
isobutyl angelate and amyl-angelate	*Anthemis nobilis* (roman chamomile)	• Antispasmodic and sedative (Bowles 2003) • Analgesic, antispasmodic, anti-inflammatory (Baudoux *et al.* 2006)
bornyl acetate	*Picea mariana* (spruce black)	• Anti-inflammatory effect on respiratory mucosa (Chen *et al.* 2014)

benzyl benzoate	*Cananga odorata* (ylang ylang)	• Anxiolytic effect with possible action on serotenergic and dopamine pathways (Zhang *et al.* 2016) • Antispasmodic, relaxant and anti-inflammatory (Baudoux 2007)
Monoterpene aldehydes		
citral (geranial/neral)	*Cymbopogon citratus* (lemongrass) *Melissa officinalis* (melissa) *Litsea cubeba* (may chang)	• Sedative, anti-infectious, anti-fungal, anti-inflammatory (Rhind 2012)
β-citronellal	*Melissa officinalis* (melissa)*	• *Potentiates GABA receptor responses in the CNS (Aoshima and Hamamoto 1999) • Anti-infectious, anti-fungal, anti-inflammatory (Rhind 2012)
Monoterpene ketones		
italidone	*Helichrysum italicum* (helichrysum)	• Wound regeneration, anti-haematomal effects (Bowles 2003)
menthone	*Mentha x piperita* (peppermint)	• Mucolytic (Bowles 2003)
Monoterpene oxides		
1,8-cineole (ether oxide)	*Elettaria cardamomum* (cardamom) *Eucalyptus globulus* (blue gum eucalyptus) *Eucalyptus radiata* (narrow-leaf eucalyptus) *Myrtus communis* (myrtle) *Lavandula latifolia* (spike lavender) *Salvia rosmarinus ct cineole* (rosemary ct cineole) *Agonis fragrans* (fragonia) *Ocimum tenuiflorum* (holy basil)	• Skin penetration enhancer (see Table 2.2) • Anti-nociceptive and smooth muscle relaxant (Ferreira-da-Silva *et al.* 2015) • Neuropathic analgesic (Baudoux *et al.* 2006) • Anti-fungal (Yu *et al.* 2015) • Expectorant and anti-inflammatory (Bowles 2003) • Anti-inflammatory effect in respiratory diseases (Juergens 2014)

cont.

Sesquiterpenes		
chamazulene (sesquiterpene-derived azulene)	*Matricaria recutita* (german chamomile) *Achillea millefolium ct chamazulene* (yarrow ct chamazulene)	• Anti-inflammatory (Bowles 2003)
β-caryophyllene	*Copaifera balsam* (copaiba balsam) *Cananga odorata* (ylang ylang) *Pelargonium graveolens* (geranium) *Piper nigrum* (black pepper) *Helichrysum italicum* (helichrysum) *Melissa officinalis* (melissa)	• Analgesic, anti-inflammatory and antispasmodic properties (Baudoux *et al.* 2006; Harris 2016; Johnson, Rodriguez and Allred 2020) • Exerts a selective effect on CB2-receptor (Johnson *et al.* 2020)
Sesquiterpene alcohols		
α-bisabolol	*Matricaria recutita* (german chamomile) *Santalum spicatum* (sandalwood)	• Anti-nociceptive effect (Alves *et al.* 2010) • Analgesic, anti-irritant and anti-inflammatory effects (Tomic *et al.* 2014; Wang and Heinbockel 2018)
α-santolol β-santalol	*Santalum spicatum* (sandalwood)	• Anti-viral, anti-inflammatory (Bowles 2003)
Phenols		
carvacrol	*Thymus vulgaris ct carvacrol* (thyme ct carvacrol) *Thymus vulgaris ct thymol* (thyme ct thymol) *Satureja hortensis* (summer savory) *Syzygium aromaticum* (clovebud)	• Analgesic activity (Wang and Heinbockel 2018) • Potent antibacterial, antimicrobial and anti-fungal (Buckle 2015) • Rubefacient (Bowles 2003)
thymol	*Thymus vulgaris ct thymol* (thyme ct thymol) *Thymus vulgaris ct carvacrol* (thyme ct carvacrol)	• Anti-nociceptive (Wang and Heinbockel 2018) • Antibacterial, antimicrobial and anti-fungal (Buckle 2015) • Rubefacient (Bowles 2003)

Phenylpropanoid methyl ethers		
methyl chavicol	*Artemisia dracunculus* (tarragon)	• Antispasmodic (Baudoux *et al.* 2006; Harris 2016)
eugenol (also a phenylpropanoid phenol)	*Syzygium aromaticum* (clovebud) *Ocimum tenuiflorum* (holy basil) *Piper nigrum* (black pepper)	• Analgesic rubefacient (Harris 2016) • Anti-nociceptive (Wang and Heinbockel 2018)
Phenylpropanoid aldehydes		
cinnamaldehyde	*Cinnamomum verum* (cinnamon bark)	• Antibacterial, anti-viral (Bowles 2003) • Anti-fungal (Rhind 2012)

The concept of synergy

It is evident from the examples in Table 2.1 that essential oils are comprised of a number of complex chemical constituents, each with their own biological action in the human body. Understanding the basic chemistry lays an important foundation for practitioners to recognize the therapeutic differences of essential oils and the importance of *the whole.*

Conventional medicine relies on pharmacology, which isolates the active principle, discarding nature's careful formulation of other trace constituents on the basis that these are superfluous in treating the intended target area. In aromatherapy, if we discard the trace constituents, we risk compromising the subtle yet powerful effect of synergy, where the overall therapeutic effect is greater than the sum of its parts. Synergy applies to the whole essential oil, which is more effective than its individual chemical components. This view is upheld by Mills (1991), who asserts that 'at no time must the view of the whole be lost'.

Routes of entry

It is widely acknowledged that essential oils enter/impact the body via two main routes of administration: inhalation and dermal application. Other routes, such as ingestion, rectal and vaginal application, may require specialist qualification as a medical herbalist or medical practitioner trained in aromatic medicine (this is dependent on the country where the therapist resides). Several aromatherapy authors provide exceptional accounts of essential oil absorption, metabolism and excretion, including Bowles (2003), Rhind (2012), Price and Price (2012) and Tisserand and Young (2014). Appropriate to palliative care are inhalation and dermal routes, which form the focus of this section.

Inhalation

The volatility of essential oils makes entry into the body via inhalation both rapid and straightforward. Essential oil vapours are carried via the nose, along the trachea into the finer bronchioles of the lungs to reach the alveoli. The lipophilic nature of essential oils facilitates diffusion across the vast respiratory mucosa into the circulatory system. This direct interface makes inhalation a valuable therapeutic option for respiratory symptoms, such as breathlessness (see Chapter 10), where both local and systemic effects may be desirable.

Absorption also occurs via the nasal epithelium, which is thin and well vascularized, enabling rapid access into the bloodstream.

Additionally, the olfactory pathway supports delivery of sensory information directly to the limbic system and associated brain structures. This functional aspect of essential oil inhalation produces physiological and psychological responses in the amygdala, hypothalamus and hippocampus. These structures of the limbic system are responsible for mood, emotions and regulation of the autonomic nervous system. Furthermore, unlike other senses, essential oil inhalation bypasses the thalamus, allowing for rapid signal processing at speeds between 150 and 200ms (Olofsson 2014). Within palliative care, where spiritual and emotional issues are often foremost for the patient and family, utilizing the olfactory pathway is an important option in situations requiring fast-acting effects on the limbic system. This is discussed further in subsequent chapters. Methods of inhalation are outlined in Chapter 3.

Dermal application

Within aromatherapy, the skin is recognized as a principal interface for essential oils to be absorbed into the body. However, the concentrated chemical composition of an essential oil precludes them from being applied to the skin undiluted. Prior to application, dilution of essential oils in a suitable excipient is required (see Chapters 3 and 12).

Dermal absorption begins with the stratum corneum, the skin's outer layer, and is also thought to occur via the sebum-lined hair follicles (Bowles 2003). Layers of keratinized cells function as a primary barrier within the stratum corneum, limiting the rate of constituent absorption, which is variable and largely dependent on an oil's chemical composition. However, this simplistic explanation does not account for evaporation. Occlusion of areas where essential oil blends have been applied minimizes the evaporation processes while simultaneously increasing the rate of absorption. This can be achieved with drapes during whole or part body massage, or for specific management, such as joint pain, compresses and cling-wrap are useful occlusives. Other factors which optimize dermal absorption are warmth, hydration and health of the skin.

For patients with life-limiting illness, the dermal route is invaluable on several counts, primarily through relaxation massage, which, in itself, possesses several local and systemic benefits, as it:

- initiates a general relaxation response throughout the body
- increases lymphatic flow to eliminate waste products and stimulates vascular flow, which brings oxygen and nutrients to the area
- enhances range-of-movement, balance and co-ordination
- decreases pain intensity and discomfort, by releasing muscle tension
- enhances sleep quality
- eases respiratory function through slower, calmer and focused breathing
- aids digestive function, which enhances absorption and elimination processes
- increases skin hydration via application of oils, as well as stimulates skin circulation
- can calm the CNS using rhythmic strokes, easing systems associated with psychological stress and distress to facilitate mental clarity
- offers relief from isolation and touch deprivation
- rebuilds hope and resilience.

Also, localized dermal absorption using topical application of essential oil blends or hydrosol preparations can be invaluable for skin-related symptoms. This includes pruritus, malignant wound management and skin care in the end-stage of life (see Chapter 12) or as an adjunct for the localized management of underlying pain experiences, such as neuropathic, inflammatory or somatic pain (see Chapter 9). Various methods of topical application are discussed in Chapter 3.

Metabolism and excretion

All organic substances entering the body are susceptible to metabolism and subsequent excretion. Within the palliative setting, where essential oils are predominantly delivered via inhalation and dermal routes using reduced doses, the quantity of constituents reaching the systemic circulation is likely to be minimal. Generally speaking, most metabolic transformation occurs in the liver, and the kidneys are the principal organs of excretion.

Fixed oils and macerates

In relation to aromatherapy, Parker (2014) and Price and Price (2014) have produced exceptional texts detailing a wide range of fixed oils, waxes and macerates.

Fixed oils

Alongside high-quality essential oils, fixed oils (or carrier oils) are important 'tools of the trade'. The term *fixed* simply means that the oil does not evaporate, which differentiates these oils from the volatile nature of essential oils. Fixed oils are derived from nuts, seeds and kernels with the best quality oils being cold-pressed, often under pressure, to extract the oil, which is then filtered and further refined (Parker 2014). Ensuring that production remains as close as possible to its natural source and, preferably, organically bio-certified, is important to safeguard bioactivity.

Fixed oils are largely comprised of triglycerides (TAG) of fatty acids and glycerol. The TAG profile for each fixed oil ultimately influences the characteristics of the overall oil. There are a variety of fatty acid forms, including saturated and unsaturated, monosaturated and polysaturated fatty acids.

Plant-based fixed oils rich in saturated fatty acids include cocoa and shea butters, which are solid oils with low melting points. These are renowned for being slow to absorb, and leave a greasy feeling. Even in a solid state they never feel dry to the touch, making them a useful ingredient for protective skin and lip balms.

By comparison, unsaturated fatty acids are less stable, more fluid and prone to oxidation. Therefore storage follows the same principles as that of an essential oil. Fixed oils of *Olea europaea* (olive), *Prunus amygdalus dulcis* (sweet almond) and *Persia gratissima* (avocado) are predominantly rich in monounsaturated fatty acids. Polyunsaturated fatty acid rich oils, include *Oenothera biennis* (evening primrose) and *Vitis vinifera* (grapeseed).

Waxes

Waxes do not contain triglycerides or glycerol molecules, differentiating them from a fixed oil and contributing to their hydrophobic nature, making waxes useful when moisture retention or waterproofing is required. A prime example is *Simmondsia chinensis* (jojoba), which is discussed in Chapter 12 related to skin management.

Macerates

Macerated oils are a form of oily extract where a fixed oil, such as *Olea europaea* (olive), is used as the solvent/extraction medium for another plant that has medicinal properties. One method is to steep clean dry and chopped plant material in a warm vegetable oil. Oil-soluble elements from the plant material are thereby gradually extracted, including the volatile components and plant pigments. The result is a macerated oil with additional therapeutic properties from the plant. Methods of maceration are described by Price and Price (2014, pp.15–16) and are used to produce oils such as *Hypericum perforatum* (St John's wort) and *Calendula officinalis* (marigold).

An array of fixed oils and macerates are suitable for aromatherapy massage or for topical and clinical applications in patients with life-limiting illness. These are discussed in relation to specific symptoms where a fixed oil, wax or macerate can therapeutically contribute.

Toxicity, safety and storage

Generally, essential oils are extremely safe when selected and administered appropriately and possess far fewer potential adverse effects than most prescribed pharmacology. However, an essential oil is an isolated plant extract, not a whole plant, with high concentration and a lipophilic nature which facilitates its absorption and distribution in the body. In addition to its known beneficial properties, there is potential with any therapeutic use of an essential oil for toxicity, adverse effects and interactions to occur. Safe integration requires knowledge of this scale of possibility.

Essential oil toxicity, safety and storage is an extensive topic whose evidence-base is covered comprehensively in the seminal publication *Essential Oil Safety* by Tisserand and Young (2014). Derived from their work, the following summary will consider these aspects in the context of palliative care.

Toxicity

Otherwise known as 'poisoning', toxicity represents the level at which a substance causes functional impairment. Toxicity can develop locally or systemically, and can be reversible although in severe cases may cause irreversible damage which, if extensive, causes death. Toxicity is related to the dose, frequency of use of a substance and the individual's sensitivity. Tisserand and Young (2014) assert that differences in metabolic and eliminative capacity, as well as drug interactions, contribute to toxic susceptibility, making infants, those taking prescription medications, pregnant women, the elderly and those with life-threatening illnesses more at risk. It is understood that this also includes patients with life-limiting illness, where deterioration in normal organ and system function is inevitable.

Toxicity of mixtures

As discussed, single essential oils are complex mixtures of constituents whose concentration varies with location, batch, source and species. In clinical practice, two or more essential oils are often mixed together, which has the potential to increase the risk of toxicity, particularly if the oils contain the same constituents, or ones which possess similar toxicity. This needs to be considered when formulating a blend to determine safe maximum doses.

Oral toxicity

Ingestion of essential oils is reported as the most frequent cause of toxic effects, where oils are ingested in amounts exceeding typical therapeutic doses. Toxicity can be acute and lead to organ damage or significant neurological consequences, and, rarely, even death. Chronic toxicity, where lower doses of essential oils are taken for long periods of time, can cause gradual deterioration of organ function. In their intensive investigation, Tisserand and Young (2014) report that hepatotoxicity (liver), neurotoxicity (central nervous system) and nephrotoxicity (kidneys) are all consequences of essential oil ingestion of high volume and concentration.

In patients with life-limiting illness, oral ingestion of essential oils is precluded because patients are often frail and elderly, prescribed poly-pharmacy is common and continuous deterioration of systemic function is evident. Furthermore, while ingestion of essential oils poses the biggest risk for toxicity, inappropriate undiluted or high-dose and long-term exposure via inhalation or skin application can also result in toxicity.

Inhalation toxicity

While inhalation is unlikely to produce toxic reactions, caution is required when using essential oil vapours with anyone who is a known asthmatic or has other respiratory pathology, or anyone with hyper-reactivity to fragrances. This is discussed further in Chapter 10, *Breathlessness in Patients with Life-Limiting Illness*.

Adverse skin reactions

In relation to adverse skin reactions, Tisserand and Young (2014) succinctly describe this as contact dermatitis with three principal variants relevant to essential oils: irritant contact dermatitis (ICD), allergic contact dermatitis (ACD) and photosensitization. These dermal reactions are unique to the individual and difficult to predict and therefore careful consideration of skin safety is required when employing the dermal route.

Irritant contact dermatitis

Even when diluted, single essential oil constituents, whole essential oils, or combinations can irritate the skin. Although ICD is not considered an allergic reaction, Tisserand and Young (2014) describe it as a complex event, triggered by a disruption to the epidermal barrier which leads to a cascade of inflammatory cytokines and chemokines being released from skin cells. Characteristically, ICD appears quickly after the first exposure, manifesting as localized reddening of the skin, sometimes forming a wheal or, in severe cases, blistering or burns (Buckle 2015).

Essential oils containing large amounts of phenolic constituents, carvacrol or thymol are most likely to induce ICD, for example *Origanum vulgare* (oregano) and *Thymus vulgaris ct thymol* (thyme ct thymol). Aldehyde constituents are also considered skin irritants in high doses, most notably, cinnamaldehyde found in *Cinnamomum verum* (cinnamon bark). Although these constituents are known dermal irritants, it does not necessarily mean they will induce ICD in every individual. Conversely, essential oils that are considered non-irritating to the skin may in fact cause irritation in a person with sensitivities. Therefore, conducting a thorough assessment is fundamental before proceeding with skin application (see section *Safe administration of essential oils and fixed oils*).

Allergic contact dermatitis

With regard to essential oil skin application, ACD clinically presents as a red rash or in darker pigmented skins, as a much darker area. These visible signs occur as a result of an immune response generating the release of substances, such as histamine, into the dermal layers of the skin, causing tissue damage.

While there are four classifications of allergic skin reactions, Tisserand and Young (2014) report that only type 1 (immediate hypersensitivity) and type 4 (delayed hypersensitivity) can be induced by essential oils. Readers are referred to the authors' succinct account of the physiological processes which occur immediately with type 1 exposure. However, a delayed response happens in type 4, where little or no visible signs are evident with the first contact but a significant inflammatory reaction can occur with subsequent exposure (this type 4 is the most common reaction seen with essential oils and fragrance ingredients). In these situations, essential oil use must be stopped immediately and dermal rescue applied (see section *Safe administration of essential oils and fixed oils*) or seek urgent medical assistance for those experiencing more severe allergic reactions.

Photosensitization

Phototoxins exist mainly in the expressed epicarp of citrus, such as essential oils of *Citrus bergamia* (bergamot), *Citrus limon* (lemon), *Citrus aurantiifolia* (lime) and *Citrus paradisi* (grapefruit). When an essential oil containing furanocoumarins is applied dermally at a concentration sufficient to elicit the response, subsequent exposure of the treated areas of skin to UV light causes these constituents to become activated. Consequently, inflammatory processes generate an erythemic response, typically 36–72 hours after exposure, which clinically presents as inflamed, painful, sunburn-like skin, sometimes with blistering.

Tisserand and Young (2014) caution that even at a 1% concentration, which further reduces furanocoumarins from less than 3% to less than 0.03%, phototoxic effects can still occur. The authors report that the furanocoumarin content of *Citrus reticulata* (mandarin) is insufficient to cause phototoxic reactions and expressed *Citrus sinensis* (sweet orange) is not phototoxic. Specific warnings must be discussed with the patient in advance of use and clearly identified in the labelling to avoid exposing the treated skin to UV light (sunbed/strong sunlight) for up to 12 hours.

Safe practice

Although some essential oils have the potential to interact with prescribed pharmacology, this primarily relates to oral ingestion, as discussed previously. Essential oil inhalation and skin application are deemed the safest routes for patients with life-limiting illness, where blood levels of essential oil constituents will be relatively low, thereby minimizing drug interactions. However, these patients often present with other medical conditions, which require vigilance when using essential oils. A number are summarized in Table 2.2.

Table 2.2: Summary of essential oil interactions with existing medical conditions/related pharmacology

Medical condition or specific medication	Possible interaction	Examples of essential oil or constituents
Anti-depressant drugs	Monoamine oxidase inhibitors (MAOIs) Oral ingestion of essential oils increases the potential interaction of some constituents, e.g. eugenol with MAOIs	Contraindicated are eugenol-rich essential oils including: *Syzygium aromaticum* (clove bud, leaf, stem) *Cinnamomum verum* (cinnamon leaf) (Buckle 2015)
Blood pressure	Hypertension Hypotension	Tisserand and Young (2014) were unable to identify any quality evidence to establish whether essential oils exert an adverse physiological effect on the regulation of human blood pressure. Therefore, no contraindications for essential oil use are reported
Diabetes medication: Glibenclamide Tolbutamide Metformin	Constituents of some essential oils influence blood glucose levels and may induce hyperglycaemia or hypoglycaemia when taken orally	Examples include: *Cinnamomum verum* (cinnamon bark) *Foeniculum vulgarae* (sweet fennel) *Melissa officinalis* (melissa) *Myrtus communis* (myrtle) *Pelargonium graveolens* (geranium) (Comprehensive list via Tisserand and Young 2014, p.59) Diabetic retinopathy As per platelet aggregation (see below)

cont.

Medical condition or specific medication	Possible interaction	Examples of essential oil or constituents
Epilepsy	Oral ingestion of some essential oils can cause convulsions Medication-controlled epileptics are more vulnerable	Potential convulsant essential oils include: *Achillea millefolium* (yarrow) *Gaultheria fragrantissima* (fragrant wintergreen) *Lavandula stoechas* (spanish lavender) *Lavandula latifolia* (spike lavender) *Mentha pulegium* (pennyroyal) *Salvia rosmarinus ct verbenone, ct camphor* (rosemary ct verbenone, ct camphor) *Tanacetum vulgarae* (tansy) *Hyssopus officinalis ct pinocamphone* (hyssop ct pinocamphone) (Comprehensive list via Tisserand and Young 2014, p.134)
Platelet aggregation	Inhibition of blood clotting with increased effects of warfarin, heparin or aspirin Antagonist activity relates to some essential oils with high levels of sesquiterpenes and sequiterpenoids (Moharam *et al.* 2010) Topical methylsalicylate can inhibit systemic platelet aggregation (Tanen *et al.* 2008)	Contraindicated in any form: *Gaultheria procumbens* (wintergreen) *Betula lenta* (sweet birch) Cautionary use: *Cinnamomum verum* (cinnamon bark) *Foeniculum vulgarae* (sweet fennel) *Ocimum basilicum ct estragole* (sweet basil ct estragole) *Ocimum tenuiflorum* (holy basil) *Pogostemon cablin* (patchouli) *Syzygium aromaticum* (clovebud) *Thymus vulgaris ct carvacrol, ct thymol* (thyme ct carvacrol, ct thymol) (Comprehensive list via Tisserand and Young 2014, p.117)

Pregnancy	Oral ingestion of essential oils and application via pessary/ suppository can be excreted via the breastmilk in nursing mothers	Essential oils evidence-based FOR USE in pregnancy (Conrad 2019): *Citrus bergamia* (bergamot) *Lavandula angustifolia* (lavender true) *Citrus limon* (lemon) *Citrus aurantium var amara flos* (neroli) *Citrus aurantium var amara fol.* (petitgrain)
Route of prescribed medication in palliative care	Prescribed medication is commonly administered orally and other routes include sub-lingual, transdermal, subcutaneous, rectal Transdermal patches include oestrogen, nicotine, opioids such as fentanyl, anti-emetics such as scopolamine Topical chemotherapy such as 5-fluorouracil (5% cream)	Caution: Avoid dermal application of essential oils in close proximity to transdermal medication patches or subcutaneous infusions/lines in situ Contraindicated via dermal application where topical 5-fluorouracil cream is applied: Essential oils rich in 1,8-cineole and nerolidol. Both increase permeability of stratum corneum by 95% (Williams and Barry 1991) and 20-fold increase (Cornwell and Barry 1994) respectively

Safe administration of essential oils and fixed oils

Table 2.3 summarizes the central points for safe purchase, storage and administration.

Table 2.3: Key points for safe administration of essential oils and fixed oils

Purchasing of essential oils and fixed oils	• Purchase from a reputable essential oil producer/distributor • Choose essential oils and fixed oils with known provenance • Ensure that fixed oils are as unrefined as possible • Ensure that oils are high-quality, bio-certified organic or wild-crafted • Obtain data and bio-certification from supplier • Select oils which display the botanical and common names, chemotype where necessary, plus a batch code to ensure traceability • Purchase in quantities required. Minimize oxidation processes by decanting larger quantities into smaller bottles, label carefully and store • Label all essential oil bottles with the botanical and common name of the plant source; expiry dates; external use only; flammable

cont.

Storage of essential oils and fixed oils	• Within healthcare, store essential oils in the same way as prescribed pharmacology, in a designated locked area • Employ a system which clearly identifies oil purchase, quality data, batch codes and expiry dates • Keep away from children • Store in a cool, dark place • Essential oils are highly flammable so do not use near naked flames, cigarettes, fire or during oxygen therapy (see Chapter 10) • Store oils in dark glass bottles • Ensure that all essential oils have a dripulator/dropper insert in situ to minimize accidental ingestion by children, plus a child-resistant bottle cap • Refrigerate oils susceptible to oxidation and use within 12 months of purchase • Discard oils which have reached their expiry date. Oxidized oils can cause skin sensitization
Safe administration	• Ensure that a qualified practitioner oversees essential oil administration • Establish detailed clinical guidelines for safe administration practices • In palliative care, only administer essential oils via dermal and inhalation routes – no oil ingestion • Follow essential oil dose and dilution recommendations appropriate to the palliative care setting • Ensure a detailed assessment of the patient's health history, allergies (including nut allergies if fixed oils being used), any sensitivities to fragrance or perfumes and any family history sensitivities. This is additional to assessment of the patient's medication, other non-prescribed medication and understanding their specific priorities of concern, as outlined throughout this book • Document clearly in the patient's records a rationale for any essential oils used; the route of application; the botanical and common names of each essential oil (plus the chemotype where relevant), any base substances used, with details of the amount/dose used of each • Avoid applying any essential oils with photosensitization properties to skin exposed to sunlight • Avoid using the same essential oil blend repetitively in any application. Change the formulation regularly • Use essential oils in well-ventilated areas

Procedures for adverse reactions	**Inhalation** • Open windows and expose the patient to fresh air • Seek medical assistance if the patient complains of difficulty in breathing or shows signs of respiratory distress **Eyes** • Rinse the affected eye cautiously with water for several minutes. Remove contact lenses if in situ and continue rinsing • Seek medical advice if irritation persists **Skin** • If a reaction does occur, remove any contaminated clothing • Wash the affected skin for at least ten minutes using a mild, unperfumed soap to remove oil traces. Water alone will not clear the trace particles • Expose the skin to the air (not sunlight) to allow further evaporation of any remaining essential oil • Apply *Aloe vera* gel to the area, if needed, to soothe the skin • For reactions extending over larger areas apply oatmeal bathing/sponging as described by the Tisserand Institute (2022): 1/3–1 cup pulverized oats Muslin bag or thin sock Add the oats to the bag or sock, soak in warm water, squeezing to work in the water. Apply to irritated area using a gentle compressing action. Leave to sit on surface of skin for at least 10–15 minutes. Repeat as necessary • Seek medical attention if irritation persists

CHAPTER 3

Principles of Practice and Methods of Application

Traditionally, aromatherapy practice in the palliative care setting relates to relaxation, relief of stress and emotional support. Termed *holistic aromatherapy*, this fundamental approach rests with compassionate and skilful touch combined with essential oils blended to create a deeply relaxing experience for the individual (Tavares 2011).

The principles of holistic aromatherapy interweave closely with those of the holistic care model employed by palliative care professionals where the physical, emotional, social and spiritual aspects of the patient are central domains of clinical practice. Globally, many hospices and palliative care units have embraced holistic aromatherapy as an integral part of patient-centred care, administered by qualified therapists employed either as a member of the multi-disciplinary team (MDT) or in a voluntary capacity.

In recent decades, *clinical aromatherapy* has emerged as an advanced level of aromatherapy practice where essential oils are selected by their unique chemical composition appropriate to managing a patient's specific symptoms. Such approaches are proving valuable adjuncts for symptom management, particularly when conventional interventions have been exhausted.

Principles of aromatherapy practice in palliative care

Clinical aromatherapy approaches are dependent on a thorough understanding of the patient's symptom experience and their priorities of concern. Tailoring interventions to meet the individual's particular issues means that patients no longer receive a 'blanket approach' to care but an intervention which considers their individual strengths and specific emotional, spiritual, physical and social capacities. Collectively, these serve to optimize a feeling of well-being. This requires a cohesive interplay between holistic and clinical aromatherapy principles.

Creating a sacred space

By the time a patient is referred to the palliative care team, they have generally followed a convoluted journey (see Chapter 6). Clinical environments are habitually busy, noisy and rarely conducive to private conversation or space for contemplation. Health professionals are often pressured by time constraints, which makes personal disclosure, or opportunities for expressions of anxiety, fear or uncertainty, impossible for patients and their family.

Patients are much more likely to respond to an invitation in a quiet, well-prepared therapy room where comfortable chairs, soft furnishings and pleasing décor are supported with personal touches of flowers, music and subtle aromas. However, not everyone has the luxury of a dedicated room, and reality means adapting to the environment of a hospital ward, aged care facility or a person's home, where working spaces may be far from perfect. A clinical space can be transformed by making use of curtains and screens, a 'do not disturb' sign, re-arranging furniture to enhance space and bringing treasures from the garden, such as fresh flowers, small bunches of herbs or foliage, which can be arranged on a table close to the patient. Combining a sacred space with an unhurried approach enables the patient to feel safe to connect with their innermost concerns and allow suppressed emotions to begin to surface.

Opening the conversation

Importantly, the circumstances need to be right. Although an appointment may have been pre-arranged, the patient may not feel up to seeing anyone on the day. Being prepared for how swiftly things can change and maintaining a level of flexibility is crucial.

Allowing sufficient time for the patient to settle into the session enhances a feeling of being welcomed into a restful and unhurried space. Be led by the patient's cues because, 'when we listen attentively, we observe behaviours and emotional responses as well as attending to the language used, the tone of voice, the fluency or hesitancy of expression' (Mannix 2021, p.95). These are the important signposts which guide us.

For some patients, there may be a specific issue they want to share, while others may feel too exhausted or overburdened to converse and there are those who may feel too afraid or find difficulty putting their experiences into words. In these situations, asking the patient, 'How would you like to feel today?' swiftly frames the focus to the present, allowing the person to observe themselves in order to shape their specific wishes. In truth, this question generally raises a level of surprise in patients, more often because they have never been asked to self-explore in this way. It is a powerful starting point because it sets a tone that is completely patient-centred.

Inclusivity

While clinical experience has taught me the importance of inclusivity, it can be a fine line to tread when working alongside the patient with advanced illness. Patients can become fatigued easily, particularly if too many questions are asked, or if they are faced with an influx of choices and decisions to make. Lengthy assessments can be minimized by asking the MDT for patient details and a general update prior to the session.

Invariably within healthcare, there is a rush to 'diagnose and dispense', rather than take time to be with a person. A patient will be more receptive to the therapist or health professional who creates an opportunity for stillness and space, even in the busiest of environments. Combined with mindful observation, attentive listening, sensitive questions and accurate reflection using the patient's words collectively involves the patient. They feel acknowledged; their story is heard, which more often leads to collaborative decision-making.

Collaborative decision-making

For the most part, the patient's experience from diagnosis through to end-of-life care is complex and often fraught with high levels of emotional and spiritual distress. This is largely underpinned by a sense of disempowerment, where their normal daily routines are infiltrated by a clinical focus on their illness and its management. Within aromatherapy, the qualitative work of Dunwoody, Smyth and Davidson (2002), who investigated aromatherapy massage in patients with advanced cancer (n=11), identified collaborative decision-making as one of the most important aspects of the therapeutic relationship. Patients report an increased sense of empowerment, as well as feeling valued as an individual with specific treatment needs, rather than being 'just another cancer patient'. An effective means of reinstating a sense of control is by inviting patients to choose their own essential oils, botanical products and route of application.

Selecting essential oils

Selecting between four and six essential oils, relevant to the patient's principal concerns and taken from cues within the conversation, minimizes the burden of too much choice. This is followed by inviting the patient to quietly savour the aroma of one single essential oil at a time.

'Enjoying the aroma' was reported by patients as a key factor in the effectiveness of aromatherapy inhaler sticks to aid peaceful sleep (Dyer *et al.* 2016). Deepening the patient's connection with the essential oil is achieved by asking, 'How does the aroma make you feel?' (Lewis 2015). Once again, the patient is guided towards self-exploration and the emotions and/or the memories a single essential oil evokes. This process cannot be rushed. It requires sensitivity and the judicious use of silence to make space for the patient to process their feelings without interruption, judgement or discouragement.

Not all the selected oils need to be individually explored. Be guided by the patient's responses; two or three oils are generally ample to empower a personal choice. Some patients like to be actively involved in the creation of the blend, others do not. Be mindful of differences. Using the patient's words and phrases throughout a session demonstrates acknowledgement and respect, and further assists compliance with the intervention.

Essential oil options are discussed throughout this book as they relate to the specific symptom.

Selecting the application

Primarily, this depends on the issues being addressed and requires discussion with the patient and often the family. This determines the most appropriate applications, timing and duration of aromatherapy interventions and any additional assistance that may be required. We will now look at common applications suitable for this patient group, which are also explored further in subsequent chapters.

Aromatherapy applications
Inhalation
Tissue

This is one of the simplest methods of application, where the vapours of a single drop of essential oil on a tissue can be inhaled by the patient as required throughout the day or tucked beneath their pillow at night. The tissue needs to be replaced daily.

When inviting a patient to inhale an essential oil aroma for the first time, place a single drop on a strip of tissue, allowing a few moments for it to dry first, before suggesting the patient slowly draws the tissue closer until they become aware of the aroma. This gradual approach provides a clear indication of the person's level of odour acuity. Avoid inhalation directly from the essential oil bottle, which at full concentration and close proximity can be overwhelming.

Aromatherapy inhaler stick

Essential oils delivered via aromatherapy inhaler sticks have proved beneficial and popular in patients with cancer (Dyer *et al.* 2016; Stringer and Donald 2011). Gentle inhalation enables an olfactory effect within the first one to three cycles of breath. However, more than three breath cycles increases the essential oil exposure time to allow a deeper physiological effect, where the individual oil components are systemically absorbed (Holmes 2019). This level of therapeutic flexibility, as it relates to numbers of breath cycles, empowers the patient to control their symptom experience at any given time.

The total number of essential oil drops used in a device is dependent on the individual's situation, their level of olfactory acuity and any relevant breathing or sensitivity issues. Indications for use and total number of drops are discussed in relevant chapters.

Bioesse® aromapatch

Continuous, low-level essential oil inhalation can be achieved through these small, adhesive patches which are sited on clean, oil-free skin of the upper chest and easily concealed below the level of clothing necklines. Options are available for these commercially pre-loaded patches using single essential oils, or blank/unscented patches where a bespoke mixture of undiluted oils can be prepared and a single drop placed onto the reservoir. The patch is designed with an occlusive barrier to prevent dermal absorption of the essential oil. Depending on the situation, therapeutic effectiveness of the patch lasts between six and eight hours (Theno 2022). Where blank patches are being used, the reservoir can be topped up with the bespoke blend to extend the therapeutic effect.

Diffusion

Through clinical visits to hospices, it is apparent that essential oil diffusion has become a trend in palliative care, primarily to 'freshen' the patient's room or to create a calming, restful ambience. However, it is easy to exceed diffusion where over-exposure to concentrated essential oil vapours can induce headaches, vertigo, nausea and lethargy (Tisserand and Young 2014).

Cold-air ionic diffusion, using specific machines or the popular ultrasonic devices designed to vaporize essential oils with water into a mist, are the safest options for the palliative setting. Cleaning of diffusion systems is important to prevent bacterial and fungal growth, particularly in water-based units, which can retain moisture in the system if left unused. Policies need to be in place to ensure water-based units are thoroughly sanitised on a daily basis.

Between two and three drops of essential oil are typically added to this type of diffuser appliance, depending on the size of the room, ventilation capacity and proximity to the patient. Standard recommended diffusion times are between 30 and 60 minutes at a time, or 30 minutes on and 60 minutes off (Tisserand and Young 2014). Diffusion creates a mild to moderate olfactory effect. Cautionary use is advised with patients with breathing issues or those in end-of-life care, and this is discussed in the relevant chapters.

Rollerball applicators
A 10ml rollerball applicator is an extremely versatile option for the palliative patient. Essential oils diluted to 3% in a fixed oil, such as *Simmondsia chinensis* (jojoba), can be applied to pulse points inside the wrist or behind the ears, or just simply rolled across the chest, once or twice a day. For the person with poor dexterity or patients entering the end-stage of life, this offers a flexible, nasocutaneous low-level essential oil inhalation.

Skin application
Massage
Touch is a powerful means of communicating that you are there, you have time and that you care. Regardless of the patient's diagnosis, physical or mental state of health, touch acknowledges their worth as a human being. Often it is the simplest act of holding another person's hand which alleviates fear, anxiety, isolation or loneliness and has the potential to transform their quality of life.

Aromatherapy massage has been consistently popular in patients with cancer as a source of physical, psychological and emotional relief (Corner, Cawley and Hildebrand 1995a; Dunwoody *et al.* 2002; Fellowes, Barnes and Wilkinson 2004; Kite *et al.* 1998) as well as being a reason to seek complementary therapies (Adam and Jewell 2007). In her exceptional book *Medicine Hands*, Gayle MacDonald (2007) comprehensively explores massage specific to patients with cancer and as respite for family and caregivers. For patients with life-limiting illness, relaxation massage requires careful consideration and adjustment to suit the individual, and is the recommended form of massage.

Indications for massage
These are specific to each symptom and discussed in subsequent chapters.

Contraindications and cautions to massage
Full body massage is rarely administered to patients with life-limiting illness where energy levels can easily be depleted. It is contraindicated in the following situations:

- Infection (temperatures above 38 °C)
- Infectious diseases
- Advanced osteoporosis
- Risk of fracture from bone metastases
- Limbs or areas with existing fractures
- During chemotherapy treatment
- Fatigue
- Delirium
- Severe heart conditions such as angina

Cautions to massage – adjustments must be made to any massage sequence to avoid the following:

- Close proximity to prescribed transdermal medication patches
- Areas of damaged, irritated or broken skin
- Near or over areas of varicose veins
- Close proximity to intravenous infusion sites, port-a-cath, Hickmann lines, drains, catheters
- Areas of current or recent radiotherapy
- Recent inoculation sites (within 24 hours)
- Peripheral neuropathy or any loss of sensation to the skin or body parts
- Any areas of pain or discomfort

Adjustments

Often adjustments to the session are required which are specific to the individual. For example, massage of shorter duration and administered to particular areas of the body, such as the hands, feet, face, back, neck and shoulders, or abdomen. Between 10 and 20 minutes is sufficient to instil a deep level of relaxation and afterwards allow for a longer rest period.

Massage can also be combined with other applications, for example a warm footbath followed by a foot massage or incorporating a hand massage while the feet are soaking. Combinations are discussed as they relate to specific symptoms/situations in chapters where massage is relevant.

Fixed oils

There are numerous fixed oils that can be used as a base substance for plain oil massage or to dilute essential oils. Preferred oils are those which are more fluid and can permeate the skin layers deeply. *Prunus armeniaca* (apricot kernel) is an optimal carrier without being greasy, making it suitable for the face. Combined with *Prunus amygdalus dulcis* (sweet almond) in a 2:1 ratio, it creates a slightly richer oil for the body, while *Macadamia ternifolia* (macadamia) and *Simmondsia chinensis* (jojoba) are other useful options with good absorption. Fixed oils are selected for their individual properties which will contribute to the overall therapeutic effect required. These are further explored in chapters where fixed oils are appropriate to symptom management, particularly Chapter 12, *Skin-Related Symptoms in Palliative Care.*

Essential oil dilution

Safe skin application requires dilution of the essential oil. Typically, this is achieved through a fixed oil or another base substance and is expressed as a percentage. In a person of general good health, between the ages of 12 and 65 years old, the percentage concentration would be between 2 and 3% for a large body area, such as a full body massage. Within palliative care, where advanced disease is present, often with multiple and complex symptoms, where the patient is fragile and in deteriorating health, a guideline maximum concentration for adult aromatherapy massage would be between 0.2 and 1%. Localized, topical application requires an increased concentration and this is detailed in the related chapters.

Variations exist when calculating essential oil concentrations.

Largely this relates to the number of essential oil drops per ml which ranges between 20 and 40 drops/ml, depending on the diameter of the dripulator/dropper insert, viscosity of the essential oil, room temperature, and so on.

Table 3.1 outlines commonly used essential oil concentrations for different volumes of fixed oil which are appropriate to skin applications in palliative care. For the purpose of this book, these figures assume that 20 drops of essential oil = 1ml and, therefore, percentages described throughout are based on this calculation. However, for practitioners conducting clinical research, where replication of studies may be necessary in different settings, the use of numbers of drops of essential oil should be avoided altogether. In these situations, where reproducibility and consistency are required, oil blends must be formulated using essential oil volume or weight.

Table 3.1: Calculating essential oil concentration

Essential oil concentration required	Total number of drops (d) of essential oil(s) for different volumes of fixed oil			
	10ml	25ml	50ml	100ml
0.2%	0.2d	0.5d	1d	2d
0.5%	1d	2.5d*	5d	10d
1%	2d	5d	10d	20d
1.5%	3d	7.5d*	15d	30d
2%	4d	10d	20d	40d
5%	10d	25d	50d	100d

*0.5 drop can be rounded up or down appropriate to the situation

Other methods of skin application
Topical application
Localized skin application using a topical essential oil blend of slightly higher concentration can be invaluable for a variety of symptoms experienced by this patient group. This includes pain, pruritus and wound management (see Chapters 9 and 12 respectively) where applications, as directed by the aromatherapist, can be applied by the patient or their caregiver. Generally, larger surface areas require a concentration range between 3 and 5%, while smaller, localized areas require concentrations between 5 and 20%. Recommendations for specific symptoms/situations are made in relevant chapters.

Compresses

A compress can deliver cold or heat to a selected area of the body, depending on the circumstances of the condition being treated. A folded facecloth or light hand-towel can be soaked in plain water or a hydrosol that is therapeutically appropriate to the situation, and then squeezed out and applied directly to the patient's skin. Compresses can be wrapped around limbs or laid across the abdomen, covered with an additional dry towel and left in place for as long as the patient finds it comfortable. The therapeutic effect can be enhanced by preparing an appropriate essential oil blend which can be applied to the skin before-hand. Common issues include pain, swelling and constipation. Suitable situations for compress use are discussed in subsequent chapters.

In palliative care, compresses using warm hydrosols can also be applied to the ailing body to instil heat. Gentle, repeated compressions of warm moist towels along the limbs, chest, abdomen and back can be immensely soothing. This is particularly beneficial to the patient in end-of-life care (see Chapter 14).

Aromatic bathing

The sense of weightlessness that comes with being enveloped in a bath of water, together with improved circulation, muscle relaxation and ease of movement, can be immensely comforting for some patients, particularly those with pain. Aromatic bathing maximizes dermal absorption of essential oils, with an additional psychological effect achieved by stimulating olfaction. Essential oils appropriate to spiritual and emotional care can deepen the physical, emotional and existential experience of relaxation (see Chapters 5 and 6). The effect can be extended with a dedicated rest period afterwards.

For patients with life-limiting illness there are precautions to consider. Essential oils must be fully diluted in a fixed oil or non-perfumed Castile liquid soap before adding to the bath. The total number of essential oil drops for an adult is six to eight drops, diluted in 10ml of excipient. Oils with known skin irritant properties, such as those high in phenol or aldehyde constituents, should not be used (see Chapter 2), as well as those rich in monoterpenes (citrus) and menthol.

In a chapter dedicated to aquacare in her 2015 book, Kerkhof-Knapp Hayes advocates a shorter duration of up to ten minutes' bathing with a water temperature of between 36 and 37°C. Contraindications include cardiovascular insufficiency, low blood pressure, advanced ascites, poor temperature control (particularly hyperthermia), extensive skin damage, inflammatory conditions or increasing deterioration. Caution must be applied to those with transdermal medication patches in situ so as not to submerge them underwater.

Aromatic footbaths

The tradition of aromatic footbathing is an ancient practice in Japan. The Japanese believe that if the feet are warmed, the whole body warms, thereby creating a depth of relaxation that is considered equal to that of immersing the entire body in a hot spring. Within palliative care, where patients may be unable to bathe, receiving an aromatic footbath can be extremely relaxing and is less demanding on their energy. In fact, when it is combined with foot reflexology, Kohara *et al.* (2004) reported sustained improvements in patients' energy levels (see Chapter 7, *Cancer-Related Fatigue*).

Depending on the essential oils used, an aromatic footbath in the evening can be calming and sedating, while a morning footbath can be uplifting and energizing. Although a single drop of essential oil is all that is required in a footbath, it must be diluted in an appropriate excipient, such as 5ml of a fixed oil. A warm footbath of 10–15 minutes' duration is sufficient, with an extended rest time afterwards. The same principles apply if using a warming handbath.

Contraindications are the same as for bathing. Other cautionary measures include reducing water temperature with the elderly or anyone with altered skin sensation, poor circulatory flow (including leg oedema), peripheral neuropathy or anyone where transdermal medication patches are in situ on the limbs involved.

Aromatic anchoring

Described by Harris (2004, p.15), aromatic anchoring 'fixes the conditioned link between the aroma and the desired response' by repeating aromatics used within the session, both blend and application, over several consecutive sessions (three is ideal). Associated details of the initial session, such as music, ambience and symptom control, must also remain consistent to aid positive responses. Once aromatic anchoring has been established, and to extend the deeply relaxing effects achieved during the aromatherapy session, the essential oils can be prepared in a variety of forms for 'easy application' by the patient at home. This includes aromatherapy inhaler sticks, rollerballs, Bioesse® aromapatches or massage oil blends. Such personalized products are reported by patients and their families as being 'small but important' measures which bring 'significant comfort' (Berger, Tavares and Berger 2013).

A useful point to remember is not to combine too many interventions all at once. There is a lot to be said for the old adage 'less is more', which is of particular relevance to the palliative patient.

Documentation
Patient records
Documentation of all interactions with the patient and family is a crucial part of the therapist's role. Ideally, this should take place within 24 hours of seeing the patient. A patient's computerized records are a legal account of every clinical interaction between the patient and all members of the MDT.

Aromatherapy interventions are most suited to the patient's individualized care plan, a section generally administered under the umbrella of the clinical nursing team. A concise summary of the session is required, outlining the aromatherapy intervention(s) administered, the botanical and common names for essential oils and other botanical products, together with the total amount used, such as number of drops or millilitres. Directions for use of any ongoing preparations and instructions for monitoring the therapeutic effectiveness are also required. Importantly, document any feedback from the patient or issues of concern. If relevant, include a follow-up date/time of the next review. Collectively, this provides staff with a clear picture of the aromatherapy plan to continue monitoring and evaluating its effectiveness.

Policy and clinical guidelines
Aromatherapy services within palliative care are required to maintain records that adhere to those of the wider organization. Guidance for writing policy and procedures for aromatherapy and complementary therapies services is succinctly addressed by Carter and Mackereth (2017). More often, an overarching policy is required which is accompanied by clinical guidelines detailing the specifics of service intervention, the process of audit and evaluation. The aim of such formal documentation is to ensure safe clinical practice using a high level of professional intervention. It is structured to allow for formal evaluation which provides an overall impression of the service, highlighting areas that are meeting the clinical standards and those which may need further attention.

Integrating aromatherapy approaches within the healthcare setting requires careful consideration, detailed planning, and concise policies and documentation to guide clinical practice, using a variety of approaches. Fundamentally, the therapist's holistic and person-centred approach is central and is discussed in depth throughout the chapters of this book.

CHAPTER 4

Fostering Resilience in Patients with Life-Limiting Illness

Clinical research has recently brought the subject of resilience, a complex and often neglected aspect of patient care, into the spotlight. The focus of interest lies with exploring the complexity of the human response to the challenges of ill-health, in order to explain why some individuals are better able to cope with adversity than others.

The concept of resilience has particular relevance for patients within palliative care who are confronting their own mortality and the intense loss which accompanies a life-limiting illness. Resilience offers a means of protection, particularly against the negative impact of stress, at the same time supporting an individual's adjustment to their end-of-life care (Molina *et al.* 2014; Seiler and Jenewein 2019).

Fostering resilience primarily rests with a comprehensive understanding of the specific factors underpinning a person's innate capacity to cope and the unique combination with which each patient presents. This helps to identify those who may need additional support and enables practitioners to tailor aromatherapy interventions specific to the patient's individual strengths and needs.

Definitions of resilience

In his powerful memoirs of life in Auschwitz, Professor Viktor Frankl (1984, p.112) wrote, 'When we are no longer able to change a situation, we are challenged to change ourselves.' In the worst imaginable circumstances, his firm belief was that the human spirit can rise above any given situation. These early and striking observations of resilience are human realities which are difficult to define.

The concept of resilience has since continued to evolve, with the focus of research extending beyond the individual to other areas of human experience. This includes palliative care, where a broader outlook considers the patient, their families, staff, organizations and communities. For definitions specific to these areas, readers are referred to the exceptional collective works edited by Monroe and Oliviere (2009), *Resilience in Palliative Care.*

Resilience can be considered as an individual's ability to maintain or restore relatively stable psychological and physical functioning when confronted with stressful life events and adversity (Bonanno, Westphal and Mancini 2011). This is a view which aligns with the holistic nature of palliative care.

Resilience in the context of cancer

Resilience has predominantly been evaluated in patients receiving active forms of cancer treatment and survivors of cancer. Optimism, hope and early coping were identified as critical elements of resilience in a systematic review conducted by Molina *et al.* (2014). Opportunities for personal growth and improved quality of life were evident in many who overcame cancer and its treatment. Importantly, the authors highlight that adversity presents itself across the entire cancer trajectory, with each stage generating its own unique set of stressful challenges. However, not everyone reacts to adversity in the same way, raising questions as to whether clinical differences exist in how resilience manifests across the cancer spectrum and whether interventions to foster resilience need to be adjusted at each stage.

In a recent large-scale review, Seiler and Jenewein (2019) examined factors which promote resilience and post-traumatic growth in patients across the cancer trajectory. Currently, limited evidence is available to support a reliable relationship between socio-demographic factors and resilience in patients with cancer, in addition to disease-related variables such as the time since diagnosis and the severity of the disease itself. However, Seiler and Jenewein 2019 identified strong associations in the following four common areas:

- Personality traits
- Social circumstances
- Positive coping strategies
- Optimism, hope and spirituality

Personality traits

Anecdotal evidence has long supported the relationship of positive personality traits underpinning resilience in patients facing life-threatening illness. Research-based findings have been more specific, identifying optimism, self-esteem, positive emotions and personal control as being central to an individual's resilience (Seiler and Jenewein 2019).

Integral to positivity is laughter and the expression of positive emotions, including gratitude, interest and love, all of which have been shown to increase levels of resilience and improve quality of life (Manne *et al.* 2015; Tugade, Fredrickson and Barrett 2004). Predominantly, this has been evaluated around the time of diagnosis or during cancer treatment.

Social circumstances

Supportive, meaningful relationships, where an individual has the perception of being loved, valued and esteemed, are considered strong determinants of resilience. Specifically, Seiler and Jenewein (2019) identified sustainable relationships, which enable patients to share and process their cancer-related experiences, as an important means of support when adjusting to each stage of the cancer trajectory. Patients with this level of social support generally report higher levels of resilience and lower levels of distress (Somasundaram and Devamani 2016).

Positive coping strategies

A critical element of resilience is the ability to employ problem-focused coping strategies. Self-determination to overcome difficulties, self-efficacy, flexibility in adapting to change, positive reappraisal and social interaction are among several strategies used, where patients report less distress and experience an improved quality of life (Eicher *et al.* 2015; Seiler and Jenewein 2019).

Optimism, hope and spirituality

In patients with cancer, optimism is consistently associated with better adjustment to the disease itself, an improved sense of well-being and reduced distress, and is positively linked to resilience and hope (Seiler and Jenewein 2019). Existential strategies which foster hope are also central to building resilience in this patient group (see Chapter 5). Hope is considered a flexible experience which changes over time and is influenced by personality, relationships and social support (Li *et al.* 2016).

Resilience in the context of life-limiting illness

Few studies have evaluated resilience in those with advanced stage disease. Of those meeting entry criteria for systematic review, high levels of social and psychological support, combined with optimism, hope and spirituality, are central to increased levels of resilience in this patient group (Molina *et al.* 2014; Seiler and Jenewein 2019).

Resilience is an important area and although under-researched in patients with life-limiting illness, there are parallels to be drawn with studies evaluating quality of life in these patients. In a systematic review of qualitative data, McCaffrey *et al.* (2016) identified a broad range of domains which patients consider important to their quality of life. These are summarized in Table 4.1. Spiritual aspects were identified in all but one of the studies that met the robust selection criteria (n=24), closely followed by social and physical domains. When compared with the four common factors underpinning resilience in patients with cancer that were identified by Seiler and Jenewein (2019), several similar threads exist. Therefore, it seems reasonable that fostering resilience in patients with life-limiting illness has the potential to positively influence several important aspects of their quality of life.

Table 4.1: Patient-reported aspects important to their quality of life (McCaffrey *et al.* 2016)

Aspects	Examples
Cognitive aspects	• Mental alertness, ability to read, watch television, hold a conversation • Fearful of losing cognitive capacity
Emotional aspects	• Optimism and positive thoughts considered important to combat negativity
Aspects of healthcare	• Access, co-ordination, continuity of healthcare services
Aspects of personal autonomy	• Having choice and control • Maintaining independence contributes to normalcy • Loss of independence leads to loss of dignity and increased frustration
Physical aspects	• Physical health • Strength and ability to get around, continue activities such as gardening • Uncontrolled symptoms impair quality of life

Preparatory aspects	• Making preparations, organizing finances, wills, funeral arrangements, delegating tasks, dealing with unresolved issues, saying final farewells
Social aspects	• Relationships are critical to quality of life, including partner intimacy • Retaining social networks, role in society • Being treated with respect, feeling valued • Maintaining dignity and a sense of normalcy
Spiritual aspects	• Hope, comfort, meaning and purpose were all voiced by patients • Organized religion for some patients • Environment (indoor/outdoor) influenced quality of life • Being among nature enhanced quality of life

The holistic nature of resilience

Resilience is a complex area, largely defined by the interplay of several factors, as summarized in Table 4.1. These factors align with the holistic care model where an individual is considered an integrated whole, comprising physical, psychological, social and spiritual dimensions (see Figure 4.1). Each patient presents with a unique combination of these dimensions, relevant to their individual circumstances.

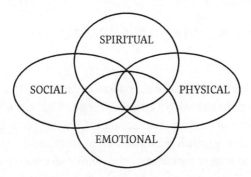

FIGURE 4.1: THE HOLISTIC CARE MODEL

Although the holistic care model is integral to the philosophies of several health disciplines, including palliative care, the deeply embedded root of the biomedical model often reduces the focus of its care to the physical element, specifically the diagnosis of disease and the physical aspects of symptoms and their management. Consequently, insufficient attention is given to a patient's social, emotional and spiritual dimensions and the inter-connectedness which exists (Youngson 2012). This is increasingly evident in patients with life-limiting illness, where studies evaluating psychological and spiritual aspects of care identified these symptoms as being frequently under-recognized by healthcare professionals and consequently undertreated (Austen *et al.* 2016; Balboni *et al.* 2009; Edwards *et al.* 2010; Epstein-Peterson *et al.* 2015; O'Connor *et al.* 2010). Furthermore, this implies a negative impact on a patient's level of resilience and quality of life.

The potential of aromatherapy

Interventions which foster resilience generally target existential and psychosocial distress. These areas are recognized aspects of successful aromatherapy intervention which are explored in Chapters 5 and 6.

Understanding the factors which underpin resilience (see Seiler and Jenewein 2019 list) helps to identify patients in need of additional support and tailor interventions to address their unique capacities. Within aromatherapy, although formal evaluation of interventions which foster resilience has not been undertaken, the following case study demonstrates the beneficial effects of integrating clinical aromatherapy approaches.

CASE STUDY 4.1: WINNIE'S EXPERIENCE

Referral

Winnie presented to the specialist palliative care team in a rapidly deteriorating state of health with a complex range of symptoms arising from advanced cancer of unconfirmed sources. Clinical concern surrounding her essential oil ingestion prompted an aromatherapy referral by the nursing team to ensure safe integration with prescribed pharmacology.

Background summary

Throughout her life, this independent, erudite 69-year-old lady had used plant-based medicine to maintain her health and well-being. Although taking prescribed opioids for pain relief and anti-emetics for nausea, her preference was to integrate natural approaches alongside her conventional regime. She felt overly drowsy with prescribed pharmacology, particularly anti-emetics, which she had stopped taking because she felt it was easier to cope with persistent nausea than intense drowsiness.

Winnie was self-medicating with essential oil ingestion. Unfortunately, this was not based on the professional advice of a qualified aromatherapist and involved:

- *Boswellia carterii* (frankincense) 2 drops undiluted, sublingually three times daily
- *Copaifera officinalis* (copaiba balsam) 2 drops undiluted, sublingually three times daily

Personal goals

Having experienced a complex pathway through the healthcare system, Winnie's priorities were to:

- be involved in all treatment decisions
- continue self-administration of essential oils
- live as well and independently as she could in the life she had left
- see her new grandchild, due to be born in a few months.

Aromatherapy intervention

Many of the extended family were present at the first home visit and space was limited. Winnie was weak with fatigue and largely confined to one room due to the limitations of her breathlessness, for which she required supplemental oxygen. Her oral mucosa was red and dry but intact.

We discussed her current ingestion of essential oils, which had been ongoing for several weeks with no alleviation of her symptoms, and further deterioration in her health had been noted. Winnie described a spiritual and cultural connection with *Boswellia carterii* (frankincense) and enjoyed the aroma of the *Copaifera officinalis* (copaiba balsam). As such, it was suggested that she continue using both essential oils but change the route of application from sublingual to topical use.

We considered other essential oils and base substances with analgesic and anti-inflammatory properties, more suited to her current pain experience relating to the right kidney. Being mindful of her deteriorating renal function, a suggestion was proposed for a topical pain-relief blend starting at a concentration of 3%, plus an aromatherapy inhaler stick formulated with her choice of essential oils from a selection designed to alleviate nausea (see Table 4.2). Winnie was willing to try this combination and agreed to stop essential oil ingestion.

Table 4.2: Winnie's aromatherapy interventions

Method of application	Botanical products used *Botanical name* (common name)	Amount used	Directions for use
Topical pain relief blend 3%	Essential oils *Boswellia carterii* (frankincense) *Copaifera officinalis* (copaiba balsam) *Kunzea ambigua* (kunzea) *Lavandula latifolia* (spike lavender) *Zingiber cassumunar* (plai)	10% 25% 30% 25% 10%	Patient-assisted Apply three times daily Review after one week
	Base substances *Calophyllum inophyllum* (tamanu) *Simmondsia chinensis* (jojoba)	40% 60%	
Aromatherapy inhaler stick 'Nausea-relief'	*Lavandula angustifolia* (lavender true) *Citrus bergamia* (bergamot) *Zingiber officinale* (*ginger*) CO_2-total extract *Simmondsia chinensis* (jojoba)	4 drops 5 drops 4 drops 1ml	Patient-directed as required At each use, inhale 4–8 breath cycles

Within 24 hours, the clinical team reported that Winnie was less restless at night, with an associated reduction in pain intensity. One week later, at the next home visit, Winnie described how she was sleeping through the night, she no longer required supplemental oxygen and the nausea was easing.

By the third visit (one week later again), her breathlessness had totally resolved and the nausea was well controlled with regular use of the aromatherapy inhaler stick. Her pain level had significantly reduced to the extent she had completely stopped her prescribed opioids. However, fatigue remained a persistent issue, which we explored.

Winnie spoke of the exhaustion she felt from no longer being independent. This was not how she had lived her life. Conversations ensued between the multi-disciplinary team (MDT) and her close family members to determine how she could achieve her goal of living more independently. With improved physical symptoms, the support of a daily carer, as well as the clinical team available via a 24-hour on-call service, Winnie was quickly able to return to independent living.

At the next aromatherapy follow-up, she attended the hospice day centre. She described how she had returned to her normal diet, was feeling physically stronger, less fatigued and sleeping well. This resulted in a further decrease in her level of pain intensity, with an associated self-reduction in the pain-relief blend to twice daily applications.

Reflection

From a patient's perspective, personal autonomy is a central aspect of palliative care (McCaffrey *et al.* 2016). In this case, autonomy was achieved by supporting Winnie's decision to integrate natural approaches within her end-of-life care and involving her in all essential oil choices and intervention options. Central to the success of this approach was the cohesive nature of the MDT. Recognizing and utilizing the strengths of each discipline, together with timely intervention, provided a structure of holistic support for this lady. This in turn fostered her resilience to the extent that she was able to return to independent living with a restored degree of 'normalcy' in the life she had left. Winnie was also able to welcome her second grandchild into the world.

In Winnie's words: 'The most important part is being listened to and being heard. It's about being supported in how I want to do things. The positivity this (hospice) team brings is allowing me to do that and to live my life well.'

CHAPTER 5

Spiritual Care in Patients with Cancer

Spirituality forms a vital dimension of our being and yet, there is a common misunderstanding that spirituality and religion are synonymous. Chochinov and Cann (2005, p.S107) explored these differences, summarizing that 'within the religious realm, spirituality aligns itself to a personal God whereas within the secular realm, it invokes a search for significance and meaning'. As such, spirituality and religion can be viewed as distinctly different but at the same time complementary. Spirituality can find its expression through religion as a particular set of beliefs, or it can be experienced through broader contexts of relationships and life experience, making it personal and unique to the individual.

The relationship between spirituality and illness

In recent years, an increasing number of studies have investigated the relationship between spirituality and illness, particularly in the area of cancer and the end-stage of life (Austen *et al.* 2016; Balboni *et al.* 2009; Delgado-Guay *et al.* 2011; Epstein-Peterson *et al.* 2015). A diagnosis of cancer is life-changing, impacting the individual physically, socially, emotionally and spiritually. Deep existential questions of meaning and purpose can be triggered more often in patients with cancer than with any other chronic illness (Cohen *et al.* 1996).

A strong sense of spirituality has been identified as crucial to a patient's ability to cope with illness (Alcorn *et al.* 2010) and is associated with an improved quality of life (Balboni *et al.* 2007). Patients consider their spirituality a source of positivity, hope and gratitude (Delgado-Guay *et al.* 2011), providing strength and comfort in times of adjustment, or in prioritizing what holds meaning and importance in their lives (Puchalski 2012).

Spiritual and religious beliefs are fundamentally important to patients with life-limiting illness, influencing their coping strategies and quality of life. While spirituality can be a source of strength for patients, it can also be a source of distress.

Spiritual distress

Puchalski (2012) advocates that spiritual distress can occur at any point within the cancer trajectory, particularly around initial diagnosis, and with recurrence of disease, but is most prevalent at the end-stage of life.

Spiritual distress does not manifest as a set of pre-determined symptoms, rather a variety of expressions of distress which are unique to each patient. For some patients, it may influence how they experience and express the physical symptoms of their disease, particularly pain. For others, spiritual distress may cause greater concern than their physical symptoms.

In a review of the qualitative research, Edwards *et al.* (2010) identified fear, insecurity and nervousness as predominant manifestations of spiritual distress. Associated increases in anxiety, depression, panic attacks, uncertainty and fear of the unknown were also reported. Spiritual suffering can be expressed through questioning the meaning of life, anger with God, or viewing illness as a punishment for life choices (Richardson 2014). Additionally, feelings of guilt, shame or an inability to trust oneself, other people or God/a higher being can result in a lack of inner peace (Speck 2011).

The concept of 'total pain'

Richardson (2014) advises that in situations where a patient is not responding adequately to recognized interventions of symptom management, consideration must be given to what else could be contributing to their distress. To assist healthcare professionals, Saunders (1967) proposed the concept of 'total pain', which comprises physical, social, emotional and spiritual components of distress (see Figure 5.1). Each patient will present with a unique combination of components which are specific to their situation.

For several decades, this concept has been well received within the palliative care community. However, a large-scale study of patients with advanced cancer (n=343) found that the majority report their spiritual needs are unmet by healthcare professionals and spiritual issues are not discussed as freely as patients desire (Balboni *et al.* 2009). Subsequent studies in the advanced disease setting report similar findings (Austen *et al.* 2016; Epstein-Peterson *et al.* 2015). This raises the crucial question of whether the concept of spirituality, by which healthcare professionals practise, actually corresponds to what spirituality means to the patient.

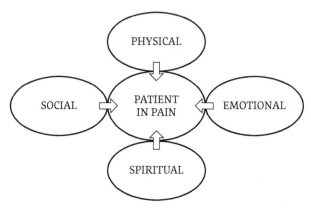

FIGURE 5.1: THE CONCEPT OF 'TOTAL PAIN' (SAUNDERS 1967)

The patient's perspective

A striking theme of the qualitative research is that the terms *spiritual* and *spirituality* do not generally form part of a patient's vocabulary. Edwards *et al.* (2010) highlight that fulfilling *relationships* are considered crucial to a patient's inner peace and spiritual wholeness. Included are relationships with self, family, friends, nature and music, together with God or a higher being. Additionally, this extends to healthcare and other allied professionals involved in the patient's care. Central to these professional relationships, patients advocate kindness, compassion, sensitivity and respect, where the emphasis is on a patient-centred approach (Edwards *et al.* 2010).

Many patients share that having a healthcare professional who is open to spiritual discussion enables them to explore the challenges they face when confronted with their own mortality (Richardson 2014). However, while most healthcare professionals recognize the importance of spiritual care, few feel equipped to address this with their patients. Lack of training, skills and confidence in spiritual matters are identified as sources of concern (Austen *et al.* 2016; Epstein-Peterson 2015). Other prohibitory factors include limited time, insufficient privacy and diminished continuity of care (Epstein-Peterson *et al.* 2015;

Richardson 2014). For many healthcare professionals, the assessment and delivery of spiritual care remains confusing. As a result, there is a risk of inadequate care where the focus is placed on religious needs rather than incorporating the wider aspects of spirituality.

Spiritual care

Spiritual care can take many forms, including recognizing spiritual distress, inviting conversation about spiritual matters, acknowledging and encouraging an individual's spiritual beliefs, and making appropriate referral to spiritual advisors and other support networks. Predominantly, the focus rests with being present with the patient, sharing their journey by listening and connecting with them as a human being, as well as assisting them to find meaning, hope and strength (Edwards *et al.* 2010). Valuable practical guidance, as proposed by Rousseau (2000a), is summarized here:

- Control physical symptoms
- Provide a supportive presence
- Encourage life review to assist the patient to recognize purpose, value and meaning
- Explore issues of guilt, remorse, forgiveness and reconciliation
- Encourage and facilitate religious expression
- Reframe goals to ones which are short term and achievable
- Encourage use of meditation, guided imagery, music, reading, poetry and art that focus on healing rather than cure

Several recommendations have been put forward in support of complementary approaches being integral to the provision of spiritual care, including aromatherapy (Adam and Jewell 2007; Puchalski 2012; Speck 2011). Although the therapeutic benefit of aromatherapy is yet to be fully evaluated in this area, its potential cannot be underestimated.

The potential of aromatherapy

The valuable contribution of aromatherapy in spiritual care is reflected in the observations of Dr Hann, a Medical Director at the Centre for Palliative Care Studies in San Diego, who states, 'When the care team is confronted with tough patients with difficult to manage pain or complex psycho-social issues, we turn to aromatherapy for help' (Schwan and Ash 2004, p.8).

Much has been written on aromatherapy interventions for the management of physical and psychosocial symptoms associated with cancer and the end-stage of life (Buckle 2015; Harris 2004; Kerkhof-Knapp Hayes 2015; Warner 2018). However, there are additional factors which may assist a deeper understanding of the spiritual dimension of care in order to effectively integrate aromatherapy interventions.

Therapeutic relationships

A principle and consistent finding of qualitative aromatherapy research is the greater emphasis patients place on the patient–therapist relationship (Berger *et al.* 2013; Corner *et al.* 1995a; Dunwoody *et al.* 2002; Kite *et al.* 1998). Further observation by Dunwoody *et al.* (2002) identified that patients did not necessarily focus on their illness with the aromatherapist, preferring to discuss their everyday concerns and fears. The benefit of being able to talk openly and freely with the aromatherapist is consistently reflected in patients' descriptions:

> 'Prior to the (aromatherapy) treatment I was so low, so stressed out, I did not want to talk about my problems, but she (the aromatherapist) let me get it all out, my emotional hang-ups and a lot of the time it wasn't even about cancer.' (Dunwoody *et al.* 2002, p.500)

> '(Being able to) open up and discuss concerns in a way that had previously been difficult in other settings.' (Kite *et al.* 1998, p.178)

> 'It (aromatherapy) put me in touch with my deeper self.' (Berger *et al.* 2013, p.1297)

Sharing these innermost troubles is a fundamental aspect of spiritual care. Building such compassionate relationships provides valuable spiritual support which patients report as being the most important aspect of their spiritual expression (Edwards *et al.* 2010). Clearly, spiritual care for patients is relational and, as such, is not an 'intervention' but an expression of the way care is delivered.

Sensitive communication

Effective and tender skills of communication, using open-ended questions, appropriate reflection and summary, combined with an ability to actively listen without imposing 'expert advice', is paramount. Spiritual discussion often utilizes the simple but important intervention of 'life review'. Sensitive exploration enables a patient to derive meaning and purpose, as well as to gain a sense of perspective of their life. As Speck (2011) observed, it can be a time where regrets and 'unfinished business' surface and, in order to achieve inner peace, this results in a need for closure. Patients will often seek forgiveness, or have a desire to forgive another; for some, the need may be to make peace with God.

Laughter, humour and the smiles of others are among the armoury a patient utilizes to uplift their spirits (Edwards *et al.* 2010). Incorporating positive approaches which facilitate hope and an ability to embrace the moment are also important (Speck 2011). Unfortunately, hope and life-limiting illness are often considered a paradox. According to Rousseau (2000b), hope plays a vital role in enabling a patient to successfully cope with their illness and thus improve their quality of life. Constructive ways in which hope can be fostered are outlined as follows:

- Adequate control of symptoms
- Fostering and developing interpersonal connectedness and relationships
- Assistance in attaining practical goals
- Exploring spiritual beliefs
- Supporting and identifying personal attributes, such as determination, courage and serenity
- Encouraging light-heartedness when appropriate
- Affirming worth by treating the patient as a valued individual
- Recalling uplifting memories with life review

Spiritual care: When should it begin?

Speaking from experience as a hospital chaplain, Rev Dr Peter Speck (2011) asserts that existential questions arise at critical points throughout a person's life, as well as during illness. This is in line with the World Health Organization's revised approach to palliative care, which recognizes that symptoms experienced at the end-stage of life have their origins at an earlier time of the disease trajectory (Sepulveda *et al.* 2002). Therefore, involvement as early as possible facilitates the development of a therapeutic relationship with the patient, to one where they can derive support and comfort throughout their cancer journey. Additionally, it permits a process of 'letting go', by allowing patients to feel supported as they take the necessary 'small steps, with time for adjustment and grief' (Edwards 2010, p.8).

Spiritual assessment

Through sensitive exploration, spiritual assessment has the potential to consider deeper levels of a patient's personal characteristics, their strengths, coping mechanisms and support networks. This represents a vital opportunity in understanding what is important to each patient and their family, as well as identifying significant areas of distress. Such information enables caring professionals to make appropriate referrals for pastoral care. For aromatherapists, it also provides insightful guidance to essential oil selection, appropriate application and timing of interventions.

For those who prefer a structured framework, Richardson (2014) explores various validated spiritual assessment tools. In reality, though, the opportunity for such discussions often presents when least expected. It is within the peaceful surrounds of an aromatherapy room, where a patient feels relaxed and listened to, that a patient may choose to share their existential concerns. Some patients can articulate their spiritual needs easily, particularly if planning their end-of-life care has been contemplated throughout the course of their illness. Others may rationalize death through their life experiences, while others derive hope and comfort from their faith or spiritual beliefs. Some patients, though, will struggle in their search for meaning and inner peace, which prevents them from being able to express these deeply personal aspects.

Personal clinical experience has taught me to sensitively explore aspects of the patient's life where they have previously experienced difficulties. Using their words, we tenderly look into what helped them to make sense of those situations, their personal attributes and where they drew strength to help them cope. This may lead to an invitation for the patient to consider the supportive skills of other members of the multi-disciplinary team (MDT), such as the family support counsellor, or if the conversation implies a formal faith, a spiritual advisor appropriate to their beliefs. Aromatherapists are well placed to make valuable contributions to all parts of this assessment process, which involves direct liaison with the MDT to ensure clear lines of communication.

Essential oils

Aromatic oils have been recognized and used within spiritual care for thousands of years. Many underpin a variety of religious rituals and ceremonies, including several which are mentioned in the Bible for their mental, spiritual and psychological healing: *Cedrus atlantica* (cedarwood), *Boswellia carterii* (frankincense), *Hyssopus officinalis* (hyssop), *Commiphora myrrha* (myrrh) and *Nardostachys jatamansi* (spikenard) (Mojay 1997). Selecting oils which have such long-standing traditions may bring comfort to many patients but particularly those who derive strength from their religious beliefs.

Psychological manifestations of spiritual distress

Patients report that feelings of fear are worse at night when negative thoughts escalate and generate insomnia. The treatment of anxiety and insomnia are central domains of aromatherapy which have been well researched in the cancer population and are explored more thoroughly in subsequent chapters.

Lavandula angustifolia (lavender true) is the most commonly studied essential oil in this area, and often unsurpassed in its treatment of anxiety and insomnia. However, in a review of the aromatherapy literature, Dobetsberger and Buchbauer (2011) propose other popular anxiolytics, as summarized below. These oils jointly reflect the calming effects of ester- and alcohol-rich essential oils on the central nervous system (CNS) and the uplifting qualities of the monoterpene-rich oils:

- *Citrus aurantium var amara flos* (neroli)
- *Anthemis nobilis* (roman chamomile)
- *Citrus sinensis* (sweet orange)
- *Citrus bergamia* (bergamot)
- *Rosa damascena* (rose)
- *Citrus limon* (lemon)
- *Santalum spicatum* (sandalwood)
- *Pelargonium graveolens* (geranium)
- *Salvia sclarea* (clary sage)

In situations where patients are experiencing severe levels of anxiety, fear and panic, personal clinical experience draws me to the deeply calming properties of *Citrus reticulata* (mandarin), *Cananga odorata* (ylang ylang), *Canarium luzonicum* (elemi), *Origanum majorana* (sweet marjoram), *Nardostachys jatamansi* (spikenard), *Boswellia carterii* (frankincense) and *Agonis fragrans* (fragonia). Additional to these, Kerkhof-Knapp Hayes (2015) recommends *Pinus sylvestris* (scots pine), *Myrtus communis* (myrtle), *Styrax benzoin* (benzoin), *Santalum spicatum* (sandalwood) and *Citrus aurantium var amara fol.* (petitgrain). Collectively, this offers a broad selection of essential oils from which the patient can make their personal choice.

Physical manifestations of spiritual distress

Integral to the alleviation of spiritual distress and interventions which foster hope (as proposed by Rousseau 2000a and 2000b respectively) is the control of physical symptoms. Clinical aromatherapy approaches, as they relate to specific symptoms, are discussed in subsequent chapters.

Patient choice

Empowering patients to choose their own essential oils and how these will be administered is paramount for effective spiritual care. For some patients, religious beliefs and customary rituals may influence their choice of oils and applications. For others, being able to select oils which hold personal meaning may enrich their comfort. Incorporating personal choice provides patients with a greater sense of control over their illness as well as the opportunity to be more active in their care. This applies across the entire cancer trajectory. Working alongside patients in this way serves to enrich the patient–therapist relationship, a view demonstrated by Dunwoody *et al.* (2002).

Aromatherapy applications
Olfaction

Odour and its complex relationship with emotion and memory, triggered by a simple sensory cue, is an area of relevance for the aromatic management of spiritual distress. 'Life review' is a key intervention of spiritual care, although some patients may find this process difficult as they struggle to derive meaning and perspective. Integrating aromas which hold significance for a patient has the potential to reconnect them with important memories of their life, enabling them to reflect and communicate more easily. According to Lewis (2015), the aroma does not necessarily need to be an essential oil. It can be anything which holds a personal, positive memory; one which induces comfort and inner peace. From my personal clinical experience, patients have drawn solace from the smell of seaweed, fresh soil, oily rags, old-fashioned sweets and specific flowers. Combining their chosen aromas with other relaxation techniques, such as visualization, progressive muscle relaxation or guided meditation, offers a deeper connection with life review.

Massage

In a small study examining aromatherapy massage versus cognitive behavioural therapy for emotional distress in this patient group (n=39), Serfaty *et al.* (2012) identified spiritual distress in 80% of the patients recruited, with a significant improvement in the way patients felt following aromatherapy massage (p<0.01). While aromatherapy massage may be beneficial for patients with an elevated performance status, massage of shorter duration or moderated to hand or foot treatments (Chang 2008; Kohara *et al.* 2004), or utilizing gentle relaxation approaches such as the M-technique (Buckle 2015) or Nursing Touch (Carr 2022), may be more comfortable for patients with symptoms of fatigue or those entering the end-stage of life.

End-of-life care

Towards the end of life, spiritual issues become more prevalent as a patient confronts the nearness of death. At this time, a patient may not be able to sustain deep existential conversations, and adjustments to sessions will be necessary. Aromatherapy specific to end-of-life care is discussed further in Chapter 14.

Spiritual distress in family and caregivers

Existential questions are not exclusive to the patient. Family, caregivers, children and friends closely involved in the care and support of their loved one frequently struggle with their own spiritual issues. Invariably, the focus of attention is predominantly on the patient, and spiritual distress in family members and caregivers often goes undetected. If left unaddressed, this can be detrimental to the individual's future health and well-being (Edwards *et al.* 2010).

Aromatherapy can be immensely beneficial in assisting the family and caregivers during all transitions of their loved one's illness, including bereavement (see Chapter 14).

Spiritual and religious differences may exist between the patient and those close to them, which can result in further distress if differing views are imposed. Sensitive communication is paramount here. Aromatherapy has the potential to create a calm, tranquil environment conducive to family members and caregivers expressing their fears, doubts and anxieties, which may help prevent spiritual needs becoming spiritual distress.

CASE STUDY 5.1: CHARLOTTE'S EXPERIENCE

Referral

Charlotte presented to the specialist palliative care team with advanced colorectal cancer and an array of physical symptoms, including breathlessness, lumbar-sacral-hip pain and fatigue. Referral for aromatherapy intervention was initiated by the family support counsellor to aid deep-level relaxation and emotional support.

Background summary

This robust, 57-year-old lady of Māori descent was new to aromatherapy but open to receiving relaxation-based therapies. During those early weekly sessions, she shared aspects of her life story and humble beginnings within a large family with many siblings. Charlotte left school without qualifications and as a teenager worked in a bar where she witnessed the detrimental effects of alcohol destroying relationships of the people within her community. Her concern was with their children left alone at home. This became a motivating factor for her to change her life and make a difference to the lives of others. Wisely, she re-invested her earnings into night school to gain qualifications.

Personal goals

Courage and determination were central to Charlotte's inner strength, together with the focus of her work, which gave her meaning and purpose, fulfilling her spiritually, emotionally and socially. Her primary goals were to:

- continue working for as long as possible
- be able to drive her pick-up truck (a source of mental relaxation).

Aromatherapy intervention

The central focus of Charlotte's aromatherapy sessions was her capacity to choose. We discussed whatever she brought to the session then, from a selection of essential oils considered beneficial for each issue (some examples are listed in Table 5.1), she would make a final choice of two or three oils.

Table 5.1: Examples of essential oils from which Charlotte could choose

Spiritual care	*Agonis fragrans* (fragonia)
	Cupressus sempervirens (cypress)
	Myrtus communis (myrtle)
	Nardostachys jatamansi (spikenard)
Emotional relaxation	*Agonis fragrans* (fragonia)
	Anthemis nobilis (roman chamomile)
	Citrus reticulata (mandarin)
	Citrus sinensis (sweet orange)
	Cupressus sempervirens (cypress)
	Lavandula angustifolia (lavender true)
Alleviate breathlessness	*Agonis fragrans* (fragonia)
	Boswellia carterii (frankincense)
	Copaifera officinalis (copaiba balsam)
	Eucalyptus radiata (narrow-leaf eucalyptus)
	Picea mariana (spruce black)
	Santalum spicatum (sandalwood)

Method of application

This varied from week to week and included massage, rollerball applicators and aromatherapy inhaler sticks, although Charlotte's preference was for slow-stroke back massage (using a dedicated massage seat) with her chosen essential oils diluted in a fixed oil to 1%.

Aromatherapy sessions

The familiarity, warmth and space of the therapy room became an opportunity for Charlotte to focus on her self-care and healing processes. It also provided a safe and trusting space where she could lower her strong persona that was customary for others. In this space she felt able to talk about her concerns, including the disease-related changes happening within her body which were outside her control; how to explain her illness to the staff she managed and the pupils she taught; and what she wanted to leave in place for her family's future.

The day came when the palliative chemotherapy she was receiving was no longer being effective and a decision was made to bring it to an end. She arrived at the therapy room in tears, knowing that she was facing the reality of her own mortality and said, 'Every last thread of hope has just been ripped away from me.' Using a single drop of *Cupressus sempervirens* (cypress) essential oil on a tissue, we gently worked together with her breath, quietly supporting inhalation of the oil vapours with focus on extended exhalation.

Although the plant is not indigenous to New Zealand, the smoky balsamic notes of its monoterpene and sesquiterpenol-rich components are renowned for their stabilizing and restorative effects (Rhind 2012). In Zeck's (2014, p.80) experience, cypress essential oil is unsurpassable for major life transitions which often involve 'a bottoming out emotionally and spiritually...(where) the past and future seem to be dynamically opposed in the present moment'.

For Charlotte, that single drop of *Cupressus sempervirens* (cypress) essential oil evoked a vivid childhood memory of crossing a stream with her siblings. It was filled with sensory descriptions, the rush of cold water around her ankles, the slime of the river stones beneath the soles of bare feet, the fresh aroma of the trees and squeals of children's laughter. In that moment, she was mindful of happier times and the close relationship with her siblings, which over the years had fallen apart. This was a poignant moment where she realized it was time for reconciliation.

The feedback from the aromatherapy session to the MDT generated a family meeting, where siblings came together to settle their differences. As the processes of forgiveness and healing took shape, this lady's family members were invited for aromatherapy sessions where they learned basic massage techniques appropriate to Charlotte's end-of-life care and helped to prepare her essential oil blends. The love and compassionate intent involved in this shared process proved to be a powerful way of restoring connectedness within this family.

Reflection

For Charlotte, hope was reinstated through family reconciliation. Optimism was rekindled through their shared stories of happier times; of re-integrating socially as a family; of knowing her family would be supported in their bereavement; of closure. Collectively, this assurance facilitated Charlotte's adjustment to her end-of-life care at home, surrounded by her family.

CASE STUDY 5.2: ROGER'S EXPERIENCE

Referral

At 71 years old, Roger was newly referred to the specialist palliative care team following a recent diagnosis of advanced colorectal cancer.

Background summary

This was Roger's first visit to the hospice day centre. He arrived alone and, outside in the car park, he promptly vomited. The clinical nurse who had gone to his aid made an immediate referral for aromatherapy intervention and suggested the use of essential oil of ginger, believing this would bring anti-emetic relief to Roger's symptom.

Aromatherapy session

Inside the therapy room, Roger sat quietly for some time clutching a vomit bowl. The lighting was lowered and a window was opened to bring movement of air into the room and the sounds of birdlife from the garden. Eventually, he began to relax into the chair, and the vomit bowl was placed to one side; he took a few sips of water and accepted the offer of a mouth-rinse, commenting on the subtle flavour of the diluted *Mentha x piperita* (peppermint) hydrosol, which he found pleasing in comparison with the over-the-counter product he had at home. When he felt composed, he said, 'Did you know I was sick in the car park?' This was our starting point.

Gently, we explored his experiences with the symptom. How each morning he would wake feeling 'queasy' and occasionally during the night when he was unable to sleep. Sensitive questioning invited him to explore the 'queasiness', where he described those initial moments of waking in the morning, when for a few seconds he felt 'normal' before the rush of reality overwhelmed him. That was when he felt 'queasy'; sometimes it would lead to him actually being sick. When asked if being sick brought him any relief, he shook his head, 'It doesn't take away the intense feeling.' Staying with his words, we invited Roger to explore this intense feeling. After several moments, he said, 'It makes me feel afraid.'

He continued to describe the fear; how he had felt afraid of this visit, particularly not having attended the day centre before which caused him to be sick in the car park. He explained how his son was arriving from overseas and his fear of whether he would be well enough to enjoy his company, knowing it would be their last fortnight together. He became tearful and slightly breathless.

Using gentle breathing techniques, we worked together, focusing his attention on longer exhalations. When his breathing started to return to normal, his attention was gradually redirected to his hands clutching his abdomen, and he was carefully guided to release his fingers and instead gently stroke the area where he felt the 'intense feeling'. As he exhaled, his hands made a complete circle to soothe his abdomen. After several rounds, he spoke of feeling more comfortable and expressed a wish to lie on the massage table.

Roger found the warmth of the table soothing and was receptive to an invitation to introduce essential oils to deepen the process of relaxation. From a small number of oils selected for the presenting issues, his final selection included *Agonis fragrans* (fragonia) and *Citrus bergamia* (bergamot) for spiritual and emotional support alongside *Santalum spicatum* (sandalwood) for breathwork.

Method of application
Fixed oils of *Prunus armeniaca* (apricot kernel) and *Prunus amygdalus dulcis* (sweet almond) in a 3:1 base substance ratio were used to dilute the essential oils to 1%.

Aromatherapy application
Slow-stroke, light-touch, abdominal massage for approximately five minutes enabled Roger to relax deeply and sleep. On wakening, he said he felt more comfortable, softer in the abdomen, but most importantly the weight of the 'intense feeling' had completely disappeared. We discussed whether he would like to continue using the oils at home. He opted for the massage blend, appreciating the notion of being able to soothe the fear himself.

Feedback of the aromatherapy session to the MDT generated interest in the approaches used. Roger returned for a further two aromatherapy sessions during his son's visit where he connected well with the combined abdominal massage and controlled breathwork. He spoke of his enjoyment with his son, fishing and revisiting quiet moments together on the beach as they had done when his son was growing up.

Reflection
There is much to learn from Roger's experience and the physical manifestation of spiritual distress. It highlights the importance of taking time to evaluate the underlying issues contributing to the presenting symptoms. All too often, it is easy to fall into the trap of rushing the process and reaching for the essential oil to match the physical symptom. The richness here came from offering Roger a quiet space with time to relax and adjust to the situation before considering his symptom holistically.

CHAPTER 6

The Emotional Impact of Cancer

Although symptoms may have been experienced for some time and a serious health issue highly suspected, in the words of Mary Wells (2008, p.111), diagnosis is 'the point at which cancer becomes a reality, and therefore represents an appropriate place to start'. For the patient and family, diagnosis can feel overwhelming. Suddenly they find themselves in an unbearable situation, their lives adversely changed, which often triggers deep emotional reactions, including shock, disbelief, confusion, stress and fear (Greer 2002; Wells 2008). Additional to this emotional turmoil, patients must assimilate information regarding their disease and treatment options, acquaint themselves with medical terminology, as well as navigate the complexities of a healthcare system.

From the point of diagnosis, the pathway of cancer is rarely predictable. Describing it as the 'cancer trajectory', Wells (2008) explains the critical stages of a patient's journey through investigations, appointments, treatments and supportive care, at the same time emphasizing that each stage is an individual experience. As such, the impact of diagnosis on a patient's emotional, social, physical and spiritual functioning makes them susceptible to psychological distress, particularly anxiety and depression.

Prevalence of anxiety and depression

The prevalence of anxiety and depression in the cancer population has long been an area of research interest (Butow *et al.* 2015; Greer 2002; Mitchell *et al.* 2011; O'Connor *et al.* 2010), although a wide variation is reported and the overall incidence, for either psychological state, remains unclear. As such, it is important to consider the individual nature of anxiety and depression.

The nature of anxiety in patients with cancer

Anxiety produces persistent increased uneasiness in response to high levels of stress, perceived danger or threat to oneself. While anxiety can arise as a normal warning to a threat, it can also manifest from other biological sources, including uncontrolled symptoms of pain, altered metabolic states, hormone-secreting tumours, symptoms of a medical condition, an adverse reaction to medication or a presenting symptom of generalized anxiety, panic or depression (MacLeod and Macfarlane 2019; Pollard and Krishnasamy 2008). Anxiety is often accompanied by fear, an unpleasant emotional response to what is about to happen or could happen, where phobias can be triggered. MacLeod and Macfarlane (2019) identify the focus of common anxieties and fears:

- Being ill
- Separation from loved ones, homes or jobs
- Becoming dependent on others (being a nuisance or burden)
- Losing control of physical faculties
- Failing to complete life goals or obligations
- Uncontrolled pain or other symptoms
- Abandonment
- Not knowing how death will occur
- 'Death anxiety' (the fear of non-being)
- Spirituality

It is estimated that between 30 and 40% of patients report moderate to severe levels of anxiety, which frequently corresponds to critical points along the cancer trajectory (Pollard and Krishnasamy 2008). Commonly, this occurs shortly after the onset of symptoms, increasing at the time of diagnosis, and can persist with significant elevation five to six years after diagnosis (Breidenbach *et al.* 2022). For some individuals, the emotional impact of diagnosis may activate a pre-existing anxiety disorder, or anxiety may also co-exist with depression.

The nature of depression in patients with cancer

Throughout the cancer trajectory, patients are at an increased risk of concurrent depression. This often manifests over a period of time, particularly when patients are emotionally depleted by prolonged and persistently high levels of stress. In fact, conclusive findings of a meta-analysis show that within the first five years after diagnosis, up to one-sixth of patients with cancer experience syndromal depression and one-third will experience adjustment disorder or major depression (Mitchell *et al.* 2011).

Evaluation of depression in this patient group is complex because there are often numerous contributory factors, including a family history of depression or suicide, personal history of alcoholism, previous psychiatric history, previous coping strategies, stage of disease, treatment type and medications (Caruso *et al.* 2017; Pollard and Krishnasamy 2008). In addition, poor social support, physical disability, uncontrolled pain, existential concerns, tumour type, metabolic states and radiotherapy are also factors leading to depression in this patient group (Noorani and Montagnini 2007).

Given the complexity of depression and the almost impossible task of differentiating its causal symptoms, researchers collectively agree that greater emphasis needs to be placed on recognizing an individual's psychological distress (Butow *et al.* 2015; Caruso *et al.* 2017; Pollard and Krishnasamy 2008). To aid healthcare professionals, MacLeod and Macfarlane (2019) identify the psychological symptoms of major depression:

- Hopelessness
- Loss of pleasure
- Morbid guilt and shame
- Worthlessness and low self-esteem
- Request for physician-assisted euthanasia
- Persisting suicidal ideation
- Lowered pain threshold
- Decreased attention and concentration
- Cognitive slowing
- Impaired memory
- Indecisiveness
- Early morning wakening
- Ruminative negative thoughts
- Nihilistic and depressive delusions
- Feeling of unreality

Conventional management of cancer-related anxiety and depression
Interventions for anxiety
Sensitive and skilled communication is deemed the most effective starting point for patients experiencing general anxiety. Combinations

of evidence-based, first-line interventions include cognitive behavioural techniques (CBT), relaxation training and guided imagery (Butow *et al.* 2015). If these are insufficient, MacLeod and Macfarlane (2019) advocate combining psychospiritual support with prescribed pharmacology.

Managing fear can be achieved by avoiding the threat, if possible. Pre-procedural information, forewarning and sensitive education at a level the patient can accommodate all help to alleviate fear (MacLeod and Macfarlane 2019). Specific behavioural desensitization may be required for those where phobias are causing heightened emotions.

Interventions for depression

Traditionally, pharmacological intervention for cancer-related depression has focused on anti-depressants, although Caruso *et al.* (2017) report that high numbers of patients do not receive adequate dosage or effective follow-up. This is attributed to the absence of international prescribing guidelines as well as other variables, such as gender, ethnicity and intensive cancer treatments, which appear to influence anti-depressant prescription.

Unfortunately, conventional pharmacological approaches may not always alleviate psychological symptoms in this patient group. Several complicating factors exist, including patients being intolerant of drug side-effects or adverse interactions with cancer-related treatments (Smith 2015); many anti-depressants taking between four and six weeks to achieve a therapeutic remission and only effective in 50–70% of cases (MacLeod and MacFarlane 2019); and if depressed, patients are more likely to be non-compliant with medical treatment recommendations (DiMatteo, Lepper and Croghan 2000).

Non-pharmacological interventions

The most widely evaluated non-pharmacological approaches include supportive psychotherapy and CBT techniques (Caruso *et al.* 2017). However, progressive trends favour integration of effective complementary therapies alongside conventional medical approaches.

Deng and Cassileth (2005) report on evidence-based complementary approaches, including mind–body interventions, relaxation techniques, guided imagery, meditation and massage therapy, all of which improved levels of anxiety, depression and other symptoms of distress in patients with cancer. Additionally, mindfulness meditation (Zimmermann, Burrell and Jordan 2018), hypnosis, progressive muscle relaxation, music therapy, Qigong, T'ai Chi, yoga, reflexology and aromatherapy also exert a beneficial psychological effect on this patient group (Satija and Bhatnagar 2017).

Aromatherapy in cancer-related anxiety and depression: Current clinical evidence

Over several decades, a significant number of studies have evaluated the effectiveness of aromatherapy interventions for psychological symptoms in patients with cancer, including Chang (2008); Corner *et al.* (1995a); Graham *et al.* (2003); Hadfield (2001); Imanishi *et al.* (2009); Kyle (2006); Louis and Kowalski (2002); Serfaty *et al.* (2012); Stringer, Swindell and Dennis (2008); and Wilkinson *et al.* (2007). However, few have met the inclusion criteria for systematic review of such complementary approaches, mainly due to small sample size and lack of methodological rigour. This may be hindering progressive integration of aromatherapy intervention within mainstream healthcare where high-quality systematic reviews are considered reliable sources of evidence to guide clinical practice.

Recent systematic reviews have been specific to aromatherapy interventions for psychological distress. Lee *et al.* (2011) evaluated 16 randomized controlled trials (RCT) using aromatherapy approaches for anxiety management. Of these, six studies were specific to patients with cancer and the authors concluded positive anxiolytic results with no adverse effects (Graham *et al.* 2003; Kyle 2006; Soden *et al.* 2004; Stringer *et al.* 2008; Wilkinson *et al.* 1999; Wilkinson *et al.* 2007).

A subsequent analysis, conducted by Sanchez-Vidana *et al.* (2017), identified a substantial increase in the number and quality of research studies evaluating the effectiveness of aromatherapy in patients with depression. Twelve RCTs met the inclusion criteria, of which four studies involved patients with cancer (Graham *et al.* 2003; Serfaty *et al.* 2012; Soden *et al.* 2004; Wilkinson *et al.* 2007). Of these, only Serfaty *et al.* (2012) reported a decrease in profile of mood scores in patients receiving a weekly, one-hour aromatherapy massage for depression.

The potential of aromatherapy

There is much to be learned from the reviews of Lee *et al.* (2011) and Sanchez-Vidana *et al.* (2017), which have made valuable contributions to evidence-based practice. However, the findings and conclusions of both reviews are mostly derived from studies evaluating interventions in the general population. A critical question is whether these are generalizable in patients with advanced cancer where the nature of anxiety and depression is complex and long-lasting. Several points require consideration.

Assessment from the patient's perspective

A vital part of emotional care is understanding the psychological impact of diagnosis, which will differ for each patient. The factors involved include how the news was delivered, the individual's perception of the disease and related treatments, personal experiences of past traumatic events, the individual's personality and their coping strategies (Fine, Carrington-Reid and Adelman 2010). Often, there is little time and space throughout their illness journey for patients to adjust to their changing situation, or for their story to be told or fully acknowledged. Consequently, the emotional effects can be intense and long-lasting. This is demonstrated in several qualitative studies, which report that communication difficulties at the time of primary diagnosis and initial treatment remain high on the agenda of patients and their families, even at the end-stage of life (Fine *et al.* 2010; Higginson, Wade and McCarthy 1990; Kirk, Kirk and Kristjanson 2004; Sampson *et al.* 2014). Central to the findings of all these studies is that patients most value:

- being treated as a person
- being given sufficient time
- being listened to
- receiving recognition that a diagnosis of cancer represents a crisis for them and their entire family
- receiving information which is honest, person-focused and explained in a way that uses language which is familiar and understandable
- receiving information which is timely and appropriate to their stage of readiness
- being included in all discussions and decision-making
- having healthcare professionals who assert their willingness to be there for the patient and family, regardless of whether the cancer progresses.

If we are to validate and support patients' choices and decisions, these points are fundamental to our clinical practice and future research initiatives.

Multi-disciplinary team (MDT) approach

The wise counsel of Wells (2008, p.109) asserts that 'the importance of recognizing the person beneath the diagnosis cannot be over emphasised' and cautions against generalizing a person's reaction to their diagnosis, its treatment and outcome. Being mindful of the nature of anxiety and depression (as outlined by MacLeod and Macfarlane 2019) enables vigilant therapists, at any clinical encounter, to recognize psychological distress as integral and highly possible in this patient group. In particular, this applies to those who are recently diagnosed, or entering another critical stage along the trajectory, or those receiving a life-limiting diagnosis. This extends to the family and caregivers, who may also be burdened with high levels of prolonged stress.

Although delivering a formal diagnosis is outside the scope of practice of qualified aromatherapists, liaising closely with the patient's MDT is paramount. It has the potential to raise an early referral for appropriate psychological assessment, particularly if patients are hesitant. Readers are referred to the work of Butow *et al.* (2015), who outline an exceptional clinical pathway which utilizes a 'stepped care' approach, managed by a central co-ordinator, with a principal focus on the patient's preference for psychological intervention. A significant advantage of this approach is the provision of education and resources to patients,which normalizes anxiety and depression within the context of their diagnosis. It allows for integration of complementary therapies of the patient's choosing throughout their illness journey, where the MDT and therapist can collaboratively monitor effective interventions and the duration required to achieve a therapeutic response for each individual patient.

Essential oils

There is an extensive range of essential oils which regulate central nervous system (CNS) activity by exerting a sense of peacefulness and calm, making them useful for the management of psychological distress. Components of terpene alcohols, esters and the monoterpene constituents limonene or citral tend to dominate the essential oil chemistry of the most recognized and reported choices for psychological care (Perry and Perry 2006; Setzer 2009). These include: *Lavandula angustifolia* (lavender true), *Citrus bergamia* (bergamot), *Citrus sinensis* (sweet orange), *Citrus limon* (lemon), *Salvia sclarea* (clary sage), *Coriandrum sativum* (coriander seed), *Pelargonium graveolens* (geranium), *Anthemis nobilis* (roman chamomile), *Origanum majorana* (sweet marjoram), *Citrus aurantium var amara flos* (neroli), *Santalum album* (sandalwood) and

Rosa damascena (rose). Additionally, there are the sedating qualities of the aldehyde-rich oils, such as *Melissa officinalis* (melissa), *Cymbopogon citratus* (lemongrass) and *Litsea cubeba* (may chang), although these often require skilled blending to tame their pungent aromas.

Many of these essential oils are listed by Kerkhof-Knapp Hayes (2015) as suitable for those with life-limiting illness and by Buckle (2015) for use within oncology settings. Personal clinical experience further advocates: *Agonis fragrans* (fragonia), *Boswellia carterii* (frankincense), *Nardostachys jatamansi* (spikenard), *Citrus reticulata* (mandarin), *Mentha citrata* (bergamot-mint) and *Canarium luzonicum* (elemi).

Furthermore, Hongratanaworakit and Buchbauer (2004) report significant reductions in pulse rate, and systolic and diastolic blood pressure in healthy subjects using inhaled forms of *Cananga odorata* (ylang ylang). Such reductions in sympathetic nervous system activity also correspond with an observed increase in levels of alertness and attentiveness. The authors describe this as 'harmonization' of the CNS, rather than relaxation/sedation. This is a useful concept for patients, particularly those experiencing severe forms of anxiety or distress causing mental fatigue.

Spiritual care

Integral to the emotional well-being of patients, their families and the healthcare professionals involved is the spiritual aspect of care. Readers are directed to Chapter 5 for essential oils specific to existential intervention.

Inclusivity

Of the studies evaluated by Lee *et al.* (2011) and Sanchez-Vidana (2017), only two invited patients to choose their oils: Serfaty *et al.* (2012) and Wilkinson (2007). Generally, such inclusivity is integral to aromatherapy sessions outside RCTs and yet it is quite possible for this to continue within clinical research environments. An excellent example of this is the large-scale, multi-centre trial conducted by Wilkinson *et al.* (2007), investigating the effects of aromatherapy massage for cancer-related anxiety and depression (n=288). Qualified aromatherapists worked alongside patients to construct individual blends from a pre-determined selection of 20 essential oils. The results showed significant improvements in levels of anxiety in the aromatherapy group, lasting for up to two weeks post-aromatherapy massage.

Aromatherapy applications

Massage

Traditionally, the psychological effects of essential oils in patients with cancer have been investigated through aromatherapy massage (Kyle 2006; Serfaty *et al*. 2012; Soden *et al*. 2004; Stringer *et al*. 2008; Wilkinson *et al*. 1999; Wilkinson *et al*. 2007). However, a striking observation of the current research is that anxiety and depression are being managed as single variables in patients with cancer, using single interventions for relatively short periods of time.

More often, anxiety and depression co-exist in this patient group, with depressive states developing over longer periods of time. Therefore, weekly massage observed over four to eight weeks may not adequately support the intense peaks of psychological distress that patients experience, or be of sufficient duration to register the onset of depression. Individual monitoring is necessary to determine effective interventions and at what point therapeutic levels are being achieved.

Inhalation

Personal clinical experience favours essential oil inhalation as the first-line aromatherapy application to manage emotional distress in this patient group. Working alongside the patient to select oils appropriate to their unique experience and personal aroma preference is crucial.

Aromatherapy inhaler sticks provide a flexible therapeutic option where patients can be directed to take four to eight breath cycles for a physiological effect, which can be deeply calming, even sedating, depending on the oils used. For an effective uplift, one to three breath cycles can be used 'as required' between regular dosing. Between 4 and 8 drops of essential oil are appropriate for emotional distress. This creates a softer aroma designed to encourage the patient to enhance nasal inhalation and, with instruction, further extend exhalation via the mouth for each breath cycle. Importantly, patients must be able to smell the aroma and the total number of drops may need adjustment to meet their level of odour acuity. Specific to patients with breathlessness, refer to the recommendations of use as outlined in Chapter 10.

Patients with reduced dexterity, memory issues or simply a personal preference also have the option of the essential oil formulation being prepared into a rollerball applicator or a Bioesse® aromapatch (see Chapter 3).

Combination approaches

Ideally, incorporating aromatic anchoring techniques (see Chapter 3) which combine essential oil inhalation with deep-level relaxation massage, or using these alongside other approaches, such as CBT, hypnosis, guided imagery or progressive muscle relaxation, can be extremely beneficial. For example, aromatic anchoring can be established by inviting the patient to use an aromatherapy inhaler stick at the end of the chosen relaxation intervention for one to three breath cycles. This anchors them in a positive, restful space of relaxation which can be further enhanced by a dedicated post-treatment rest period. Thereafter, the patient can continue using aromatherapy inhalation at home to extend the therapeutic effect. Interventions of this nature require careful monitoring of the individual to determine the most effective combinations for their unique circumstances, as well as the duration required to achieve a therapeutic response. This is highly individualized.

Working alongside our healthcare colleagues

Recognizing stress in our healthcare colleagues is as important as identifying it in the patient and their family members. Incorporating aromatherapy interventions aimed at deeper-level relaxation for staff can contribute to the relief of anticipatory anxiety and consequential distress associated with the process of disclosing difficult news or facilitating tender conversations, as well as acknowledging the emotional toll that often accompanies this level of compassionate care. Useful approaches include formulating personalized aromatherapy inhaler sticks, educating staff in simple breathing techniques, mindfulness sessions, aromatherapy massage/bathing/footbathing and emphasizing time for self-care. Conscious care of the MDT is crucial for their psychosocial and spiritual well-being in order to approach the daily demands of their work.

CASE STUDY 6.1: GAIL'S EXPERIENCE

Referral

Following a recent diagnosis of an advanced stage brain tumour, 66-year-old Gail was immediately referred to the specialist palliative care team. Integral to her care, an aromatherapy referral was made for ongoing psychosocial and spiritual support.

Background summary

In the months prior, there had been small, seemingly insignificant changes, which were associated with the stress of other minor surgical interventions. Visual disturbance combined with posterior headaches eventually prompted Gail to seek an optometrist's opinion. From there, a domino effect of specialist appointments and hospital admissions followed, until a formal diagnosis was made.

For Gail, the entire situation felt overwhelming as she struggled to process the information, the neurophysiological changes and her limited prognosis. There was a proposed plan for palliative radiotherapy, but she felt reticent about this line of treatment. The need for a decision troubled her, largely because her lifetime preference was to manage her health as naturally as possible. In the meantime, her specialist team commenced a regime of oral steroids.

Personal goals

Gail was familiar with aromatherapy, finding essential oil inhalation beneficial for the anxiety she experienced during her earlier minor surgeries. Now, her primary concerns were:

- to feel less anxious when facing new situations
- not to feel so 'flat' in the mornings (low mood exacerbated by fatigue).

Aromatherapy session

Gail arrived at the therapy room looking tired, fearful and uncertain. Her preference was for a one-on-one session and her partner would return to collect her later. She settled into the room and over a cup of herbal tea, spoke candidly of her feelings. It had only been a month since her diagnosis and already she was conscious of the changes and the struggle to mentally process information – specifically, the many questions she was asked throughout each day and the conversations she could no longer follow.

The loss of independence, particularly with being unable to drive, or get from room to room easily inside the house, coupled with the loss of freedom and spontaneity, was a source of immense distress. To Gail, this created a sense of feeling trapped.

Other priorities of concern rested with overwhelming fatigue, where she had no energy or enthusiasm despite sleeping late into the morning, which was quite out of character for her. In her words, 'I feel flat', and this was worse in the morning as she tried co-ordinating her body and mind, her thoughts and words. Even the simplest of questions, such as what she wanted for breakfast, felt like a mental marathon. Frustration escalated each time she tried to explain this to her partner and friends. Her preference was for 'stillness and calm'.

Quietly, Gail used the session to explore other areas of concern: her visual disturbance from the glare of the computer screen and television; the altered flavour of food and constant hunger (related to the oral steroid regime) and her need for solitude. An oral inspection confirmed the absence of candidiasis, although a coated tongue suggested mild dehydration. A list was created to discuss with her partner.

Gail was familiar with aromatherapy formulation and grateful of the adjustment to the session, where the oils were selected without explanation. Silently, she savoured each oil in turn, taking her time to sit in the stillness of its aroma. Old favourites and familiarity were felt with *Citrus limon* (lemon) and *Agonis fragrans* (fragonia), but the immense stillness came from *Canarium luzonicum* (elemi). In the words of Zeck (2014, p.81), 'settle yourself down and enter into the sacred well of stillness where the rhythmic influence of your quieter self resides...' It was here where Gail experienced spiritual and emotional respite.

A second aromatherapy inhaler stick was prepared to alleviate the 'flat' feeling of the mornings. A familiar aroma for Gail which evoked happy lifelong memories came with *Elettaria cardamomum* (cardamom). As a warm, stimulating oil, it is a classic treatment for nervous/mental fatigue and depression. Holmes (2019) describes its bivalent action on the CNS, making it particularly useful for Gail's escalating anxiety and consequential exhaustion, in turn followed by low energy in the morning. The complex chemistry of *Elettaria cardamomum* (cardamom) bears its stimulating oxide, 1,8-cineole, harmonized alongside calming esters. When aligned with the similar properties of *Myrtus communis* (myrtle) and Gail's favourite *Citrus limon* (lemon), it created therapeutic stimulation which was finely attuned with relaxation. Avoiding over-stimulating an exhausted CNS was a crucial factor (see Table 6.1).

Practical suggestions were relayed to her partner regarding stronger-flavoured foods/herbs/spices, regular meals with snacks, increased oral hydration, contacting the optometrist for advice regarding visual aids for photosensitivity, and to make allowance for Gail to take an afternoon trip out, or to receive friends at home for short periods.

Three days later, Gail's partner reported that she was vigilant with using the aromatherapy inhaler sticks, and they were effective, although reclarification was required as to which one to use when. Colour differences with these devices aided simplicity, with 'white for the morning' and 'pink at any other time'.

Table 6.1: Gail's aromatherapy interventions

Method of application	Botanical products used *Botanical name* (common name)	Amount used	Directions for use
Aromatherapy inhaler stick (pink) 'Stillness and calm'	*Canarium luzonicum* (elemi) *Agonis fragrans* (fragonia) *Citrus limon* (lemon) *Simmondsia chinensis* (jojoba)	3 drops 2 drops 2 drops 1ml	Patient-assisted At each use, inhale 4–8 breath cycles Use prior to new events, or in situations of increased anxiety, day/night as required
Aromatherapy inhaler stick (white) 'Uplift'	*Elettaria cardamomum* (cardamom) *Myrtus communis* (myrtle) *Citrus limon* (lemon) *Simmondsia chinensis* (jojoba)	1 drop 2 drops 2 drops 1ml	Patient-assisted At each use, inhale 1–3 breath cycles On wakening and two-hourly thereafter during the morning only

The MDT were updated with the aromatherapy interventions and follow-up. Gail continued with these essential oil blends, fulfilling her preference for natural approaches for several more weeks before prescribed anxiolytics were introduced to manage symptoms of disease progression.

Reflection

The peace and solace of the therapy room is an opportunity for quiet contemplation and can be achieved with background sounds of the garden and birdsong. The unhurried approach enabled Gail time to process her thoughts, an act that was becoming increasingly difficult.

The essence of clinical practice is to be fully present with another person and to be flexible and adaptable to their needs. In this situation, adaptation of the session involved minimizing dialogue and questions, thereby respecting the greater expression of silence. More than words, compassionate silence conveys a deep level of reverence for the person; a simple act of spiritual consolation which can establish a rich connection in that moment.

Being in silence with another is not always easy. It requires a mental shift from 'doing something for the person' to 'being with the person' (Tornoe *et al.* 2014), which demands courage and experience (Sapeta and Simoes 2018). This is an essential part of our repertoire of skills. For Gail, respecting her silence acknowledged the gravity of her sudden losses, among them mental and physical function, conversation, pleasures with food, independence and spontaneity. Her grief is explained in the insightful words of Elisabeth Kübler-Ross MD (1969, p.99): 'In preparatory grief there is little or no need for words. It's a feeling that's expressed mutually, translated in general, by a tender touch of the hand, stroking the hair or just by quietly sitting alongside.'

CHAPTER 7

Cancer-Related Fatigue

Chapters 4, 5 and 6 have provided comprehensive insight into the spiritual and psychosocial aspects of patient care and illustrated the importance of fostering resilience as a means of supporting the patient and their family's adjustment to a life-limiting form of cancer. These fundamental dimensions of human wholeness are integral to the physical aspects of symptom management and crucial to the holistic nature of aromatherapy. As such, it is important to now explore the common physical symptoms patients experience within the context of these core dimensions.

Prevalence of cancer-related fatigue (CRF)

Qualitative studies identified that CRF is consistently reported by patients as one of their most distressing symptoms, negatively impacting their daily routine and quality of life more than any other cancer-related symptom, including pain, depression and nausea (Curt *et al.* 2000). Compared with the fatigue of healthy individuals, patients differentiate CRF as being more rapid in onset, debilitating, intense and severe, with an unrelenting nature and duration (Lane 2005; Mustian *et al.* 2007). Descriptions of their experience include 'feeling listless, sluggish, faint, despondent, apathetic, tired, slack, indifferent and having paralysing fatigue' (Ahlberg *et al.* 2003, p.640), which is unrelieved by rest or sleep (Glaus 1993).

Possible causes of CRF

Despite its prevalence and the wealth of studies investigating CRF, the underlying mechanisms are largely unknown. Possible causes are categorized into physiological, treatment-related and psychological.

Physiological factors

This is arguably the most well researched, with an array of associated causes including anaemia, cachexia, tumour burden and the release of cytokines (Ahlberg *et al.* 2003). Evidence is mounting in support of immune dysfunction, abnormal cortisol levels, increased body mass index and metabolic syndrome, as other possibilities (Mitchell 2010).

Treatment-related factors

Relationships between CRF and chemotherapy, radiotherapy, biological therapies and combined treatment modalities have been consistently demonstrated (Mustian *et al.* 2007). Patients receiving chemotherapy report rising levels of fatigue which peaks, on average, four or five days after completing a treatment cycle, then gradually decreases over time, but never returns to the pre-treatment level (Hofman *et al.* 2007). Fatigue is also reported as the most common and severe symptom of radiotherapy treatment, involving a steady rise in intensity throughout the entire course (Mustian *et al.* 2007).

Regardless of which treatment is received, patients anticipate their fatigue will resolve once treatment has ceased. However, there is increasing evidence to the contrary. Hofman *et al.* (2007) cite a large-scale study of women completing curative breast cancer treatment (n=763), of which 35% report increased fatigue up to five years after treatment ended. Unfortunately, there is little known about how or why certain treatments induce fatigue, or the long-term implications it holds for patients.

Psychological factors

Emotional distress and altered mood states, including anxiety, depression, insomnia and chronic stress, are consistently associated with CRF (Ahlberg *et al.* 2003). Coping with the emotional impact of a cancer diagnosis, an uncertain future and often overwhelming amounts of information regarding the illness and related treatments impairs memory and the ability to concentrate (Cimprich 1992a). Furthermore, significant aspects of a patient's life, role, function, ability to work and family dynamics are all adversely affected by the intensity of fatigue (Curt *et al.* 2000), creating a sense of loss, impaired coping abilities (Pearce and Richardson 1996) and spiritual distress (Potter 2004).

CRF is multi-factorial, involving complex interactions within and between each of its causal categories. At clinical presentation, there is significant individual variability among patients, making it impossible to determine a single intervention which offers complete relief (Mitchell 2010).

Conventional management of CRF

Regardless of the growing interest in CRF within healthcare, patients report they are seldom asked about their fatigue experience. Mitchell (2010) attributes this to clinicians not fully appreciating the debilitating effects of fatigue and, consequently, not offering interventions. Patients, on the other hand, regard fatigue as an unavoidable symptom of their cancer and treatment, which negates any discussion. The word *fatigue* is also unfamiliar to many patients, who tend to use metaphors to describe how they feel (Lane 2005).

Pharmacological interventions

Standard clinical interventions begin with addressing underlying pathologies, such as anaemia and infection, or associated physiological dysfunction of major systems, including endocrine, cardiopulmonary, liver, renal and neurological (Mustian *et al.* 2007). Concurrent symptoms such as pain, nausea, depression, insomnia and breathlessness are typically treated using pharmacological means. However, in spite of such interventions, Mustian *et al.* (2007) report that many patients will continue to experience persistent fatigue of moderate to severe intensity. Although pharmacological options specific to the treatment of CRF are limited, a recent narrative review identified corticosteroids and methylphenidate as medications of choice in patients receiving active cancer treatments (Klasson *et al.* 2021). Further research is required to evaluate such medications in patients experiencing fatigue of advanced disease.

With or without a known clinical cause, the National Comprehensive Cancer Network of the USA (2010) guidelines advise healthcare professionals to routinely screen patients for CRF and also to consider integrative and non-pharmacological management approaches – a preference held by most patients with CRF (Mitchell 2010).

Non-pharmacological interventions

Clinicians commonly advocate rest and energy conservation strategies to patients, despite this type of fatigue being unrelieved by rest. However, Mustian *et al.* (2007) report promising results for treatment-induced fatigue, with moderate intensity exercise of between 10 and 90 minutes' duration, three to seven times per week.

A key indicator of CRF is the presence of psychological distress (Ahlberg *et al.* 2003), prompting research interest in psychosocial interventions, including individual and/or group support, education, stress-management and behavioural strategies designed to enhance coping mechanisms and fatigue management (Mustian *et al.* 2007). Favourable reports are also associated with cognitive behavioural strategies to aid sleep quality, relaxation and management of concurrent symptoms of pain and depression (Mitchell 2010).

Complementary approaches also offer encouraging results, particularly hypnosis (Montgomery *et al.* 2007); and the use of *Panax quinquefolius l.* (American ginseng) for treatment-induced fatigue in survivors of cancer (Barton *et al.* 2009), and *Panax ginseng* (Korean ginseng) for the fatigue of advanced cancer (Yennurajalingam *et al.* 2017). In a review of complementary therapies, aromatherapy was identified as being beneficial in reducing levels of fatigue (Sood *et al.* 2007), although it is not routinely advocated by clinicians. It is important to consider the clinical evidence surrounding this.

Aromatherapy in CRF: Current clinical evidence

Several studies have investigated the use of essential oils in the management of fatigue in differing health populations, including haemodialysis (Kang and Kim 2008), osteoarthritis (Kim and Kim 2009), multiple sclerosis (Bahraini 2011) and post-partum mothers (Lee 2004). All researchers reported lower levels of fatigue in the aromatherapy groups.

Specific to CRF, an updated review of complementary and alternative medicine (CAM) approaches identified that studies with a sole focus on the symptom demonstrate a greater reduction in fatigue levels than those addressing multiple symptom management (Finnegan-John, Molassiotis and Ream 2013). Currently, only two studies have evaluated aromatherapy interventions exclusive to CRF in patients with advanced disease.

In 2004, Kohara *et al.* identified significant improvements in fatigue levels in patients (n=20) receiving a three-minute foot-soak with Lavender (botanical name unspecified) essential oil, followed by a ten-minute foot reflexology using Lavender essential oil with jojoba. Importantly, the therapeutic effects of the combined foot-soak, aromatherapy and reflexology were sustained for up to four hours following treatment.

More recently, Park, Chun and Kwak (2016) investigated the effects of aromatherapy massage on fatigue levels and sleep in a group of hospice patients (n=30). This randomized study compared 17 patients who received a ten-minute hand massage using Lavender and Bergamot essential oils (botanical names unspecified), in a 1:1 ratio blended to 1% with jojoba, with 13 patients who received a ten-minute hand massage using plain jojoba. Each group received their treatment between 9pm and 10pm, for five consecutive evenings. Although no significant differences were found, levels of fatigue were lower and sleep quantity improved in the aromatherapy group.

Similar findings are reflected in other non-cancer studies where the addition of essential oils reduced levels of fatigue (Bahraini 2011; Kang and Kim 2008). This enhanced therapeutic effect with essential oils has also been observed in studies comparing aromatherapy versus plain carrier oil massage to manage other cancer-related symptoms (Chang 2008; Corner *et al.* 1995a; Soden *et al.* 2004; Wilkinson *et al.* 1999).

The potential of aromatherapy

Aromatherapy offers plausible potential in the management of CRF. However, evidence-based research is limited, as demonstrated by Finnegan-John *et al.* (2013), where studies investigating aromatherapy interventions for this patient group did not meet the review criteria. While the authors provide a valuable 'road map' for future studies (see section *Future research recommendations*), there are additional areas, specific to aromatherapy, which warrant consideration.

Collaborative decision-making

Exploring the patient's fatigue experience and working collaboratively with interventions tailored to their needs is an important aspect of patient-centred care. The patient's choice of essential oils, hydrosols and applications, as well as considering their aroma preference and odour acuity, collectively exerts a positive and sustained influence on therapeutic outcomes for these patients.

Essential oils

Essential oil of *Lavandula angustifolia* (lavender true) features prominently in most clinical studies investigating aromatherapy and fatigue, both in cancer and non-cancer populations. Blending *Lavandula angustifolia* (lavender true) with other essential oils has also been clinically effective (see Table 7.1).

Table 7.1: Evidence-based essential oil combinations with *Lavandula angustifolia* (lavender true) for CRF

Essential oils *Botanical name* (common name)	Reference
Lavandula angustifolia (lavender true) *Citrus bergamia* (bergamot)	Chang (2008) Park *et al.* (2016)
Lavandula angustifolia (lavender true) *Anthemis nobilis* (roman chamomile) *Pelargonium graveolens* (geranium)	Kang and Kim (2008)
Lavandula angustifolia (lavender true) *Anthemis nobilis* (roman chamomile) *Zingiber officinale* (ginger)	Kim and Kim (2009)

Spiritual and emotional care

Quite possibly, the greatest potential for aromatherapy in the management of CRF rests with addressing its key psychospiritual factors. Readers are referred to Chapters 5 and 6 for essential oils specific to the spiritual and emotional aspects of patient-centred care, in addition to Chapter 8 for the management of insomnia.

Hydrosols

Aromatically, the lighter fragrance of hydrosols may be preferred by patients with heightened odour acuity. Hydrosols of *Salvia rosmarinus* (rosemary) and *Mentha x piperita* (peppermint) are useful cephalics for those experiencing cognitive or memory impairment resulting from fatigue. *Citrus aurantium var amara flos* (neroli), *Rosa damascena* (rose), *Lavandula angustifolia* (lavender true), *Boswellia carterii* (frankincense) and *Melissa officinalis* (melissa) offer comfort for those seeking quality sleep and psychological relaxation (Catty 2001).

Aromatherapy applications

Massage

Massage of longer duration can be depleting for these patients, where energy conservation is vital. Emphasis is placed on shorter duration, such as the daily ten-minute sessions employed by Kohara *et al.* (2004) and Park *et al.* (2016) and a modified M-technique described by Buckle (2003).

Allowing for a longer rest period post-treatment is more effective for patients with CRF.

Inhalation

Aromatherapy inhaler sticks offer promising potential for these patients because they are portable, easy to use and require little effort. Personalized blends can be created to manage the complex nature of symptoms with which an individual may present. More than one aromatherapy inhaler stick may be required to manage variations in fatigue levels throughout the day. For example, a patient may wish to alleviate their anxiety or uplift their mood during the daytime while a second, separate aromatherapy inhaler stick may be required to aid sleep quality for use at night.

Importantly, in the study conducted by Park *et al.* (2016), several clients in the aromatherapy group were unable to smell the 1% blend, which may have had detrimental consequences to the overall trial results. Given that psychological factors are central to CRF, using essential oils at a detectable odour level is crucial. Therefore, the total number of essential oil drops is determined by working alongside the patient to blend an aroma which is both pleasing and detectable.

Showering/bathing

A few drops of essential oils placed on a ceramic dish inside a shower cubicle can be immensely beneficial for physical and psychological fatigue. This method of aromatic inhalation is a useful way to administer citrus and other monoterpene-rich essential oils such as *Picea mariana* (spruce black), *Cupressus sempervirens* (cypress) or *Pinus sylvestris* (scots pine), known for their uplifting properties. Aromatic bathing may be soothing at the end of the day, particularly for muscle tension and psychological relaxation to aid sleep quality. To minimize energy depletion, cooler water temperatures and bathing for less than 15 minutes is recommended (Kerkhof-Knapp Hayes 2015).

Other applications

Cool compresses for face, hands and feet, aromatic footbaths and roller-ball applicators are other ways in which essential oils or hydrosols can also be utilized (see Chapter 3). There is scope for using a variety of applications which will vary according to the individual's clinical presentation, fatigue level and symptom experience.

Combination approaches

CRF is multi-factorial and no single intervention is going to offer complete relief. Combining aromatherapy approaches with other non-pharmacological interventions warrants further investigation to determine whether the therapeutic effect can be enhanced and extended for these patients.

The holistic management of CRF is also covered in Case studies 4.1 and 6.1.

Future research recommendations

Currently, the emphasis in the research is on treatment-induced fatigue, which is an entirely different experience to the fatigue of advanced stage disease, or at other times across the cancer spectrum. Finnegan-John *et al.* (2013) provide a valuable 'road map' to aid general research in this area:

- Stage of disease needs to be included to determine the relationship between fatigue levels and tumour burden
- Economic impact of the intervention being studied must be included
- Chronic nature of fatigue across the cancer spectrum must be considered
- Sustained effect of the intervention being studied must be identified and reported
- Sample sizes need to be sufficient to achieve statistical relevance
- Sample characteristics need to be included to eliminate/reduce bias
- Fatigue must be the primary outcome of investigation
- Quality assurance measures of the intervention, as well as the therapist delivering the intervention, must be included
- Optimum 'dose' needs to be determined (including techniques used, frequency of application and length of course)
- Appropriate timings to deliver the intervention need to be ascertained and included
- A feasibility study prior to a large-scale trial of complementary therapy must be conducted

CHAPTER 8

Insomnia in Patients with Cancer

Sleep is a fundamental human requirement, and yet, sleep problems are extremely common in the general population with approximately 10–15% suffering insomnia associated with stress, illness, medication and ageing (Palesh *et al.* 2010). The National Sleep Foundation (2017) characterizes insomnia by its impact on a person's sleep quality and quantity. Either singly or in combination, difficulties in getting off to sleep, maintaining sleep, or returning to sleep after waking early, for three nights a week over three months or more, is classified as insomnia.

Epidemiological studies report that within the general population, women experience insomnia more frequently than men, with a higher prevalence in individuals who are separated, divorced or widowed and a further increase if unemployed or living within a low-income bracket (Ohayon 2002).

All these factors may co-exist in patients with cancer, but the prevalence of insomnia is much higher and estimated to be between 30 and 50% (Palesh *et al.* 2010). However, not all patients report sleep disturbance to their oncology teams (Engstrom *et al.* 1999), which suggests these figures may be significantly underestimated, particularly in patients with advanced disease, where a more realistic occurrence is thought to be between 45 and 95% (Mystakidou *et al.* 2009).

Characteristics of insomnia in patients with cancer

The fact that sleep disturbance in these patients affects more than double that of the general population suggests that other factors are involved. Quite possibly these relate to diagnosis, the cancer itself, treatment, or other physical and psychological issues.

Diagnosis

A large-scale survey conducted by Davidson *et al.* (2002) identified that patients with various cancer types and at different phases of treatment (n=300) experience insomnia. Importantly, 48.2% relate the onset of insomnia to within the six-month period prior to diagnosis, extending up to 18 months afterwards. The impact of such disturbed sleep is reported by patients as follows:

- Waking several times during the night (76%)
- Difficulty falling asleep (44%)
- Waking for long periods of time (35%)
- Waking too early (33%)

Cancer type and staging

Primarily, oncology-based sleep research has focused on women with breast cancer, who are prone to insomnia arising from treatment-induced menopause and depression (Fiorentino and Ancoli-Israel 2007); distress and anxiety (Cimprich 1992b); as well as fatigue (Davidson *et al.* 2002). Compared with patients with differing cancers, Davidson *et al.* (2002) identified that those with a diagnosis of lung cancer experience the most disrupted sleep. Concerns about diagnosis and a rapid decline in health contribute to the patient's increased stress and consequent insomnia. Additionally, these patients are more likely to have other related disorders, such as chronic obstructive pulmonary disease, known to disrupt nocturnal sleep and cause daytime sleepiness.

Anecdotal evidence supports the increased prevalence of insomnia in patients with advanced cancer and in the end-stage of life, although few studies have clinically investigated sleep disturbance in this area.

Treatment-related

Similar incidences of insomnia exist in patients receiving common treatments of chemotherapy, radiotherapy and surgery (Davidson *et al.* 2002), although the causal relationships are unknown. Women receiving chemotherapy for the treatment of breast cancer are at higher risk of insomnia symptoms (Savard *et al.* 2001), with sleep disturbance prior to chemotherapy cycles and persisting for up to one year after treatment completion (Kotronoulas, Wengström and Kearney 2012). For those receiving radiotherapy treatment, Miaskowski *et al.* (2011) identified significant difficulties in getting off to sleep and maintaining sleep at the onset of treatment, which increases as therapy progresses.

Circadian rhythm and inflammation

Evidence of relationships between circadian rhythm, inflammatory processes in cancer and sleep disturbance have also been described (Fiorentino and Ancoli-Israel 2007). Although outside the scope of this chapter, readers are directed to the work of Savvidis and Koutsilieris (2012), who discuss deregulation of these molecular mechanisms which can directly impact the sleep–wake cycle.

Concurrent symptoms

Insomnia can occur as a single symptom in patients with cancer, although researchers correlate sleep disturbance with fatigue, pain and psychological distress (Engstrom *et al.* 1999; Flynn *et al.* 2010). The crucial question of whether insomnia contributes to the incidence and severity of these other symptoms, or vice versa, remains unanswered. Medications used to manage concurrent symptoms, such as cortico-steroids, stimulant anti-depressants, diuretics and bronchodilators, can also interfere with sleep patterns (Hugel *et al.* 2004).

Psychological issues

Regardless of the cancer type, stage of disease or treatment, patients consistently report that insomnia affects their ability to cope with stress, their emotions and concentration (Davidson *et al.* 2002; Flynn *et al.* 2010). Their most prevalent concerns are evidenced as:

- Family and friends
- Diagnosis
- Personal health
- Physical effects of the cancer
- Upcoming doctor's appointments
- Follow-up tests
- Recurrence of disease
- Finances
- The future

Unquestionably, insomnia impacts a patient's quality of life and increases the intensity of symptoms, such as pain, anxiety and depression (Hugel *et al.* 2004). Pain and life stress are considered common predictors of insomnia in women with metastatic breast cancer, while depression is associated with the consequences of insomnia (Palesh *et al.* 2007). The key findings of these inter-relationships are summarized in Table 8.1

and offer important insight to guide clinical assessment and appropriate intervention.

Table 8.1: Predictors of sleep disturbance in women with metastatic breast cancer (Palesh *et al.* 2007)

Predictor of sleep disturbance	Baseline scores	Subsequent scores at 4, 8 and 12 months of baseline
Depression	Higher baseline scores of depression resulted in: • Decreased number of hours asleep per night • Increased problems with waking up during the night • Increased incidence of daytime sleepiness	Subsequent scores of increasing levels of depression resulted in: • Further decreases in numbers of hours asleep • Greater frequency of waking during the night • Increased problems of daytime sleepiness
Pain	Higher levels of pain at baseline resulted in: • Increased difficulty in getting to sleep • Increased problems with waking up during the night	Subsequent scores of increasing levels of pain resulted in: • Further decreases in numbers of hours asleep • Greater frequency of waking during the night
Life stress	Higher baseline scores of life stress resulted in: • Increased difficulty getting to sleep • Increased problems with daytime sleepiness	Only measured at baseline

Conventional management of insomnia in patients with cancer

Despite the prevalence and severity of insomnia in patients with cancer, there is surprisingly limited evidence to support interventions that improve sleep quality.

Pharmacological interventions

A systematic review conducted by Howell *et al.* (2014) identified an absence of randomized controlled trials involving pharmacological interventions specific to insomnia in this patient group. Consequently, clinicians are guided by pharmacology suited to primary insomnia in the general population, which consists of the benzodiazepine group recommended for short-term use, sedating anti-depressants, sedating anti-histamines and melatonin.

Considering the complexity of cancer treatment, additional pharmacology for concurrent symptoms and the disease itself (which may directly/indirectly involve the central nervous system), researchers agree that careful consideration is required when prescribing 'general' insomnia medication for these patients (Howell *et al.* 2014; Karnell and Smith 2016; Khemlani 2008). Concerns surround the lack of evidence underpinning safety and the side-effects of insomnia pharmacology which may preclude its long-term use (Howell *et al.* 2014). More often, patients feel overwhelmed by the 'polypharmacy' of cancer treatments and symptom management, making them hesitant to take further medication for their sleep-related issues (Fiorentino and Ancoli-Israel 2007). The patient's preference is to receive information emphasizing non-pharmacological approaches for sleep management (Davidson *et al.* 2007).

Non-pharmacological interventions

Cognitive behavioural therapy (CBT) features consistently in systematic reviews as an important intervention for insomnia (Garland *et al.* 2014; Page, Berger and Johnson 2006). For cancer-related insomnia, the most effective CBT interventions are aimed at improving sleep quality, efficiency and longer duration of sleep, as shown in Table 8.2 (Davidson *et al.* 2002; Savard and Morin 2001).

Table 8.2: CBT: A multi-intervention approach
(Davidson *et al.* 2002; Savard and Morin 2001)

CBT	Brief description of the intervention
Sleep hygiene (teaches good sleeping habits)	• Reduce total caffeine intake and avoid consumption later in the day • Avoid nicotine before bedtime and heavy meals within two hours of wanting to sleep • Reduce fluid intake after dinner to reduce/prevent nocturnal urination • Incorporate exercise into the day but not within four hours of bedtime • Minimize noise (earplugs may be required) • Be exposed to natural daylight for at least 30 minutes in the morning • Avoid napping • Get up in the morning at the same time each day

cont.

CBT	Brief description of the intervention
Stimulus control	• Associate the bedroom only with sleep and sex • Avoid reading or watching television in the bedroom • Go to bed only when tired • Leave the bedroom if not asleep within 15–20 minutes (repeat as necessary throughout the night) • Keep the bedroom at a comfortable temperature • Set aside a time to relax before bed and use relaxation techniques
Sleep restriction*	• Maintain a 'sleep diary' (written in the morning) • Restrict time in bed to the average estimated sleep time • Ensure that time spent in bed is not less than five hours • Keep morning wake-up time the same • Remember that sleep efficiency determines increased increments of time in bed, calculated by: Total sleep time x 100 ÷ time spent in bed = sleep efficiency
Paradoxical intention	• Seeks to remove the fear of not being able to sleep by advising the patient to remain awake

* Requires monitoring and support
Caution in those with epilepsy, parasomnias and bi-polar disorders

Certainly, the efficacy of CBT intervention looks promising, although its advantage over other non-pharmacological interventions is yet to be determined. Quality studies are lacking, particularly aromatherapy and complementary approaches, which are poorly represented in systematic reviews (Howell *et al.* 2014; Langford, Lee and Miaskowski 2012; Page *et al.* 2006). Considering that aromatherapy has been central to insomnia management for several decades, it is important to consider its clinical relevance for this patient group.

Aromatherapy in insomnia: Current clinical evidence

Between 1997 and 2011, doctoral students of Dr Jane Buckle (2015) conducted 21 studies investigating aromatherapy approaches with insomnia as an end point. Six essential oils were used, in single or various double combinations, to alleviate sleep disturbance in adults and children (see list below). Applications varied between topical, inhaled and diffusion, with essential oil of *Lavandula angustifolia* (lavender true) being the most widely researched.

- *Lavandula angustifolia* (lavender true)
- *Citrus reticulata* (mandarin)
- *Ravensara aromatica* (ravensara)
- *Origanum majorana* (sweet marjoram)
- *Anthemis nobilis* (roman chamomile)
- *Salvia sclarea* (clary sage)

An extensive review of essential oil studies concluded that single fragrance components of essential oils, as well as the oil in its entirety, directly influence the CNS, aiding relaxation, sedation and sleep (Dobetsberger and Buchbauer 2011). Linalool, a major constituent of *Lavandula angustifolia* (lavender true), potentiates gamma-aminobutyric acid (GABA) receptor responses within the CNS (Tisserand and Young 2014). The associated anxiolytic and sedating effects therefore make it useful in the management of insomnia.

Within the cancer population, aromatherapy in insomnia management has been investigated in two ways. First, as a concurrent symptom, as shown in the study conducted by Park *et al.* (2016), who considered the effects of aromatherapy hand massage with variables of fatigue and sleep in hospice-based patients. Second, within the broader context of physical and psychological evaluation, as demonstrated in studies incorporating aromatherapy massage in patients with cancer (Corner *et al.* 1995a; Serfaty *et al.* 2012; Soden *et al.* 2004; Wilkinson *et al.* 2007).

Dyer *et al.* (2016) conducted a prospective audit of patients using aromatherapy inhalation, with insomnia as the primary variable. Of the 65 patients who received aromatherapy inhaler sticks to facilitate sleep, 83% were female and 17% male, with a variety of cancer diagnoses. Patients were invited to choose from three prepared blends (summarized in Table 8.3), instructed on how to use the device and, thereafter, self-administer as often as required. Overall, 94% of patients used their chosen device to aid sleep, with 92% reporting they would continue using it.

Table 8.3: Essential oil blends for insomnia management (Dyer *et al.* 2016)

Blend	Number of patients	Essential oils used	Rating in %	
Blend A	n=33 51%	*Citrus bergamia* (bergamot) *Santalum austrocaladonicum* (sandalwood)	Excellent	10%
			Very good	47%
			Good	23%
			Fair	10%
			Poor	10%

cont.

Blend	Number of patients	Essential oils used	Rating in %	
Blend B	n=23 35%	*Boswellia carterii* (frankincense) *Citrus reticulata* (mandarin) *Lavandula angustifolia* (lavender true)	Excellent Very good Good Fair Poor	5% 27% 36% 18% 14%
Blend C Proprietary blend	n=9 14%	*Citrus sinensis* (sweet orange) *Lavandula hybrid* (lavandin) *Citrus reticulata* (mandarin) *Citrus bergamia* (bergamot) *Lavandula angustifolia* (lavender true) *Anthemis nobilis* (roman chamomile)	Excellent Very good Good Fair Poor	0% 22% 56% 22% 0%

The potential of aromatherapy

Evidence to support the most effective aromatherapy interventions, applications and timings for insomnia management in patients with advanced disease is scarce. Studies are consistently not meeting inclusion criteria for systematic reviews, commonly due to small sample sizes and weak methodology, making comparison of aromatherapy intervention difficult. Arguably, quantitative research offers little information about the personal and subjective meaning of sleep disturbance for these patients because the context within which the patient experiences insomnia is lost. To inform our clinical practice, future research initiatives need to consider issues which are specific to the patient's insomnia experience.

Assessment from the patient's perspective

For patients, insomnia is not exclusively a night-time problem, but an around-the-clock symptom affecting every part of their lives. Qualitative researchers report that patients with cancer tend to focus on the consequences of insomnia, such as daytime sleepiness, lack of sustained concentration and the impact this has on their personal and working relationships (Flynn *et al.* 2010). Unfortunately, clinicians do not routinely discuss such sleep issues with patients, preferring to focus on standard diagnostic criteria with greater emphasis on underlying causes (Araújo *et al.* 2017). In contrast, patients are reluctant to inform their clinical team of sleep disturbance, assuming it to be a temporary and normal consequence of cancer and its treatment (Davidson *et al.* 2007).

To guide clinical consultations, the National Health Service (NHS) recommends sleep assessment in six main areas (NHS Clinical Knowledge summaries: Insomnia 2010 cited in Howell *et al.* 2014):

- Explore the person's beliefs about sleep
- Ask about the impact insomnia has on the person's quality of life, daytime functioning, ability to drive, employment, relationships and mood
- Determine whether there is an underlying cause of insomnia or an associated co-morbid condition (a detailed history recommended to include life stressors, medication and physical examination)
- Take a sleep history
- Determine the duration of symptoms
- Ask the patient to complete a sleep diary (for a minimum of two weeks)

By making the patient central to the assessment, this structured approach offers detailed insight into how insomnia affects the individual's 24-hour day, over a period of time. Skilful communication facilitates space for patients to explore insomnia within its physical, emotional, social and spiritual contexts. Critical areas of concern, for example uncontrolled symptoms, can be identified and appropriately treated. However, it must be noted that terminology, such as the word *insomnia*, may not be familiar to the patient. Conscious listening and using the patient's descriptors of sleep disturbance enrich the assessment process and make it feel less prescriptive.

Qualitative interviews with patients with cancer identified consistent themes about sleep disturbance (Davidson *et al.* 2002; Flynn *et al.* 2010; Hugel *et al.* 2004). The most prevalent are:

- Psychological issues
- Difficulty with temperature regulation
- Positioning
- Restless leg syndrome (RLS)

Each theme will be considered within the context of aromatherapy intervention.

Psychological issues

These include the impact of insomnia, as reported by patients (Davidson *et al.* 2002), the worries and concerns which keep them awake at night (Davidson *et al.* 2002; Flynn *et al.* 2010), together with the inter-relationships between insomnia and psychological variables of pain, life stress and depression (Table 8.1), all offer vital clues as to what may be disturbing their sleep.

An increased frequency of sleep disturbance, long periods of time awake and waking too early are considered consequences of insomnia. Palesh *et al.* (2007) correlate these with depression, where patients struggle to get up in the morning and feel tired and fatigued throughout the day. Subsequent studies report similar experiences in patients with a variety of cancer diagnoses (Davidson *et al.* 2002; Flynn *et al.* 2010).

Essential oils containing anxiolytic and sedating properties to calm the CNS are particularly beneficial for patients experiencing difficulty getting off to sleep and maintaining sleep. To off-set daytime napping, the uplifting and revitalizing properties of monoterpene-rich essential oils would be suited to morning and daytime use. Collectively, these have been explored within the contexts of spiritual and emotional distress (Chapters 5 and 6), as well as cancer-related fatigue (Chapter 7).

A critical consideration is selecting the most appropriate method of application. While aromatherapy massage has consistently been a popular choice in these patients for deep-level psychological and physical comfort (Corner *et al.* 1995a; Dunwoody *et al.* 2002), the long-lasting effects in alleviating depression are yet to be demonstrated. Inhaled forms of essential oils, as demonstrated by Dyer *et al.* (2016) using personalized aromatherapy inhaler sticks, offer patients an opportunity to take control of their symptom management. This patient-directed approach is a flexible treatment option for those who experience repeated nocturnal disturbance and difficulties returning to sleep.

Difficulty with temperature regulation

This theme is most commonly related to hot flushes and night sweats, where the impact of sleep disturbance arises from sudden onset menopause resulting from oncology treatment protocols, although the symptom of night sweats is not exclusive to breast/ovarian cancers. Other causal possibilities include malignant pathologies of the lung, liver, bone, carcinoid and haematological cancers, as well as associated infections, hormone treatments and medications (Cancer Research UK 2022). The frequency and intensity of sweats may reduce with medication, treatment of disease or underlying infections; however, it is a symptom that requires compassionate care and understanding. For patients, nocturnal sweats can be intense, distressing and debilitating, particularly if the patient is at home and forced to repeatedly cope with complete changes of nightwear and bedlinen.

Hydrosols, applied topically through spritzers or bathing, have been a traditional mainstay for hot flushes and night sweats. For example, Dyer, Ashley and Shaw (2008) reported a reduction in the number and duration of hot flushes in 41% of women with breast cancer (n=44) who used hydrosols of *Mentha x piperita* (peppermint) combined with *Citrus aurantium var amara flos* (neroli), compared with a plain water spray.

An important consideration here is that hydrosols require refrigeration to preserve their shelf-life. Topical applications of a cold spritzer may inadvertently exacerbate the problem of hot flushes and sweats, causing the body to react by producing more heat. In these situations, Kerkhof-Knapp Hayes (2015) advocates tepid temperatures for topical interventions. Diluting smaller quantities of hydrosol in water may be more beneficial, such as 2ml per litre of water for *Mentha x piperita* (peppermint) hydrosol and 5–10ml per litre of water for *Citrus aurantium var amara flos* (neroli). Other hydrosol choices include *Rosa damascena* (rose), *Cupressus sempervirens* (cypress), *Lavandula angustifolia* (lavender true) or *Thymus vulgaris ct linalool* (thyme ct linalool). Comparing the value of cold versus tepid temperatures of hydrosol interventions for the management of hot flushes and night sweats warrants further investigation. Such a small change has the potential to radically update current management strategies.

Stress is also a precipitating factor of hot flushes and sweats. CBT relaxation techniques, including paced breathing, relaxation and hypnosis, are promising approaches being investigated (Olver 2011). Readers are referred to Chapters 5 and 6 for existential and psychological interventions, and the section *Pathological sweating* in Chapter 12 for further specific approaches.

Positioning

Not being able to find a comfortable position is a major source of sleep interruption for patients (Flynn *et al.* 2010). Often, this is related to pain, or to devices associated with their medical treatment; surgical intervention through ostomies and scars; radiotherapy-induced skin damage; or disease-related symptoms such as breathlessness in patients with lung cancer. Symptom management is of prime importance to enable restful sleep. Aromatherapists can optimize patient comfort through appropriate bolstering to aid positioning, as well as integrating effective clinical aromatherapy approaches for specific symptom management, as discussed in relevant chapters.

Restless leg syndrome (RLS)

Hashemi, Hajbagheri and Aghajani (2015) describe RLS as a neurological disorder characterized by compulsory and often involuntary movement of the legs. This can be accompanied by intensely uncomfortable sensations including pain. Generally, RLS occurs after prolonged periods of rest with exacerbation of the symptoms at night, disturbing sleep. It is relieved by activity, but only for the duration of that action.

RLS is prevalent in the general population, in renal patients undergoing haemodialysis (Hashemi *et al.* 2015), and is a contributor to sleep disturbance in patients with cancer (Flynn *et al.* 2010). The underlying cause remains elusive, resulting in pharmacological treatments to minimize symptoms. Hashemi *et al.* (2015) report a growing interest in complementary therapies, demonstrating significant improvements of RLS in patients receiving haemodialysis using aromatherapy massage with the essential oil of *Lavandula angustifolia* (lavender true).

RLS is a complex area which requires further investigation, particularly in the cancer population. From my personal clinical experience with RLS in patients with cancer and end-stage renal disease, practical recommendations include tepid aromatic footbaths, slow-stroke effleurage of the legs, CBT relaxation interventions and sleep hygiene recommendations (Table 8.2), maintaining cool temperatures within the bedroom and alleviating the weight of bedclothes using bed-frames.

Combination approaches

Insomnia in patients with cancer is complex and multi-factorial and single interventions are not necessarily going to be effective. Combination approaches are promising, for example in reducing symptoms of depression either through aromatherapy massage plus inhalation (Sanchez-Vidana *et al.* 2017) or aromatherapy massage alongside CBT (Serfaty *et al.* 2012). Further research is required which primarily investigates insomnia and uses creative combinations through a sufficient number of sessions to capture the effectiveness of aromatherapy intervention as it relates to the patient's unique experience.

CHAPTER 9

Cancer-Related Pain within Palliative Care

Commonly, pain is the presenting symptom which initially leads a patient to seek medical attention and diagnosis. Thereafter, it represents a potent symptom of the presence of cancer, or an indicator of disease progression, and is a perpetual reminder of the very real threat to life (Krishnasamy 2008).

Over the past three decades, a wealth of educational information and international guidelines have been developed to support effective pain management, most notably, the World Health Organization (WHO 1996), which uphold the concept of 'total pain', together with guidelines of the European Association for Palliative Care (EAPC) (Caraceni *et al.* 2012) and the European Society for Medical Oncology (ESMO) (Ripamonti *et al.* 2012). Although assessment and management has evolved, Van den Beuken-van Everdingen *et al.* (2016) report an increase in pain prevalence rates in patients with advanced cancer from 64% in 2007 to 66.4% in 2016. The clinical reality indicates that unrelieved cancer-related pain remains a significant problem.

Characteristics of cancer-related pain within palliative care

Researchers describe cancer-related pain as a 'complex biologic phenomenon' involving different mechanisms which are unique to each individual (Chwistek 2017). Until now, the most widely recognized pain model is the gate control theory (GCT). Described by Melzack and Wall (1965), the emphasis rests with the relationship between modulation of inputs in the spinal dorsal horns and the dynamic role of the central nervous system (CNS). Prior to this, the psychological factors of pain were dismissed as the patient's reactions to pain, rather than being an integral part of the pain process (Melzack 1999). The GCT has remained an important working model which has led modern pain researchers to consider processes of inter-connection, or 'cross talk', between the tumour and the host's immune, peripheral and central nervous systems, collectively known as 'the neuromatrix' (Chwistek 2017; Melzack 1999). Although the exact processes are not fully understood, cancer-related pain is increasingly seen as a unique entity with differences to any other pain states.

Undoubtedly, cancer-related pain has long been recognized as a subjective experience, possessing physical, psychological, social and spiritual components (Saunders 1967). While each component will be addressed individually, it is important to remain mindful that in any given patient, the mechanisms underpinning the pain of advanced cancer are multi-factorial, can vary considerably and should not be separated.

Physical component

Cancer-related pain can be attributed to several causes, including tumour infiltration or compression on organs, bones or nerves; anti-cancer treatments such as surgery, chemotherapy or radiotherapy; musculoskeletal issues related to inactivity and generalized fatigue; or a co-existing condition such as diabetic-induced peripheral neuropathy, cerebral vascular accident or vitamin B deficiency (Keefe, Abernethy and Campbell 2005; Perdue 2019). In advanced stage disease, pain pathophysiology involves nociceptive and neuropathic pathways. Both can co-exist independently, or present as a mixed pain, possessing nociceptive and neuropathic elements (Yoong and Poon 2018).

Nociceptive pain accounts for 60% of cancer-related pain (Perdue 2019) and is further categorized into somatic and visceral (Yoong and Poon 2018):

- Somatic pain can be superficial (e.g. originates in skin, subcutaneous and mucosal tissue) or deep (e.g. originates in bone, tendons, joints), which is likely to be felt as localized, superficial and sharp pain.
- Visceral pain involves the major internal organs and is likely to be felt as diffuse, deep and dull in nature.

Neuropathic pain accounts for 20% of cancer-related pain and is largely associated with injury or compression of the nerve, or dysfunction within the nervous system. It is likely to be felt as tingling, numbness, shooting, pins and needles, and may possess sensory or motor deficits which often track the nerve pathway and beyond. Moreover, in patients with advanced cancer, pain is associated with a combination of nociceptive and neuropathic involvement which implies that, overall, 40% of cancer-related pain possesses a neuropathic element (Perdue 2019).

Psychological component

For decades, the relationship between psychological distress and pain has been an area of research interest. A meta-analysis conducted by Zaza and Baine (2002) identified anxiety, depression, emotional distress, fear and worry among the psychological elements directly related to cancer pain. In patients with advanced stages, high levels of psychological distress arising from severe pain intensity were reported.

Insight into the debilitating effects of pain comes from the patient's narrative, as demonstrated in the qualitative approach employed by palliative care researchers Gibbins *et al.* (2014), who explored the views and pain experiences of patients with metastatic cancer (n=12). Patients described the incapacitating effects of pain, where they were unable to move easily or undertake everyday tasks, at its worst rendering them bed-bound. They did not separate the physical and psychosocial symptoms of their pain, where fatigue and worry featured prominently, as did their reluctance to rely on others for help.

Spiritual component

The presence of pain is a continuous reminder to patients of their disease, often confronting them with thoughts of their deteriorating health, decreasing physical ability, forced dependency, an uncertain future and their own mortality. Spirituality underpins all dimensions of patient-centred care (see Chapter 5) and even though a patient's spirituality may not be possible to fully comprehend, Puchalski (2012, p.iii52) reminds us that 'where spirituality interacts with the other domains is the area that is relevant for clinical care'.

Social component

Spirituality is integral to the patient's social experience, which is also touched by cancer and its treatment. The inclusivity that comes with a sense of belonging and shared commonalities, whether it is within a family or the broader aspects of work and community, is crucial to a patient's social well-being (Grassi, Speigel and Riba 2017) and is highly valued by patients (Zelman *et al.* 2004).

Levels of cancer-related pain also determine how family members engage with the patient. Observations from my personal clinical experience highlight how families often assume shorter and quieter interactions when the patient's pain intensity is increased, where they feel hesitant about intervening to help and simultaneously uncertain about whether they are doing the right thing. On the other hand, patients describe how difficult it is to witness the distress their pain causes their family, and how it affects their relationships (Gibbins *et al.* 2014; Zelman *et al.* 2004).

An intricate relationship exists between pain and psychosocial and spiritual distress. Neurologically, Vadivelu *et al.* (2017) describe an anatomical overlap in regions of the brain associated with the emotional and sensory features of pain and areas affected by depression. Pain and depression are highly prevalent in these patients (Laird *et al.* 2009), and the simultaneous use of anti-depressants is advocated alongside pain relief (Wang *et al.* 2011).

Conventional management of cancer-related pain

A common starting point is the WHO (1996) analgesia ladder. Designed to guide clinicians, this stepwise, sequential approach aligns the choice of analgesia with the level of pain described by the patient, not the stage of disease (see Figure 9.1).

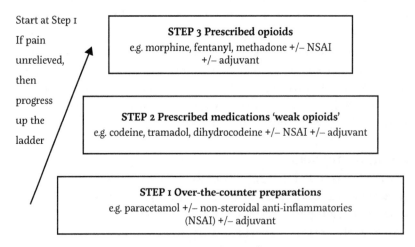

FIGURE 9.1: DIAGRAM OF THE WHO (1996) ANALGESIA LADDER

ESMO clinical recommendations (Ripamonti *et al.* 2012) advocate that analgesia must be appropriate to the patient's pain intensity, prescribed at regular around-the-clock intervals and in doses which can be administered simply and managed easily by the patient and family. Simultaneous 'rescue doses' of analgesia need to be prescribed to manage transient episodes of breakthrough pain. Adjustments are made according to the patient's response and in a stepwise fashion, i.e. if a non-opioid in Step 1 is insufficient, then a move up to the next step is required (Figure 9.1). While the WHO (1996) analgesia ladder provides a tangible foundation for pharmacological pain management, it was not designed for use in isolation. Surgery, chemotherapy and radiotherapy are other conventional approaches which offer pain relief for some patients, as do adjuvant analgesics.

Adjuvant analgesics

These are prescription medications whose primary role is not general pain management but to offer an additional analgesic effect in specific situations, for example neuropathic and bone pain. These can be used in conjunction with any step of the analgesia ladder and include tricyclic anti-depressants, anti-convulsants, corticosteroids, benzodiazepines, neuroleptics, skeletal muscle relaxants, anaesthetic agents, bisphosphonates and calcitonin (Bethann *et al.* 2018; Ripamonti *et al.* 2012).

Adverse side-effects

Unfortunately, adverse side-effects are commonplace with pain pharmacology – more so as the strength of the drug increases – and include constipation, nausea/vomiting, dry mouth and CNS toxicity. There is consensus among pain researchers that reducing the opioid dose while incorporating adjuvant analgesia alleviates the severity of side-effects (Bethann *et al.* 2018; Ripamonti *et al.* 2012). 'Opioid switching' to another opioid agonist also has potential benefit, especially in situations of CNS toxicity, where the disabling effects of hallucination, drowsiness, myoclonic jerks and confusion can be relieved. Prescribed, regular stimulant laxatives are required to alleviate opioid-induced constipation (Ripamonti *et al.* 2012).

Analgesia 'platform'

While the WHO (1996) analgesia ladder provides a pharmacological starting point for conventional pain management, Leung (2012) calls for a broader range of modalities. He proposes that each step of the analgesia ladder needs to extend horizontally, to form a much wider 'analgesia platform', where adjuvant medications and other non-pharmacological approaches can co-exist. Integrating modalities (including aromatherapy) on every platform, alongside the recommended analgesia, offers clinicians a broader range of pain-relieving options to address the patient's 'total pain' experience.

Non-pharmacological interventions

Specific to cancer pain, the role of non-pharmacological approaches has been amply debated (Cassileth and Keefe 2010; Cohen, Kahn and Gutsgell 2015; Running and Seright 2012), as well as being the subject of systematic review (Bardia *et al.* 2006; Candy *et al.* 2020; Hökkä, Kaakinen and Pölkki 2014). Studies which demonstrate encouraging data in reducing pain intensity are associated with mind–body medicine, including hypnosis, imagery and relaxation (Bardia *et al.* 2006). For patients with advanced disease, the emphasis lies with massage, where an immediate impact on pain relief was observed, although no sustained effects were reported (Hökkä *et al.* 2014).

Other modalities offering short-term benefit include acupuncture, cognitive behavioural therapy (CBT), transcutaneous electrical nerve stimulation (TENS), warm water footbathing (Hökkä *et al.* 2014) and music therapy (Gutsgell *et al.* 2013).

Phytobotanicals

With improved understanding of pain neurobiology comes a renewed and burgeoning interest in the therapeutic use of cannabis, particularly the chemotype *Cannabis sativa*, which is comprised of over 70 cannabinoids within its plant material. ElSohly and Slade (2005) describe the most abundant in *Cannabis sativa* as the terpenophenolic compounds, Δ^9-tetrahydracannabinol (THC) and cannabidiol (CBD). Differences exist in their pharmacology, whereby THC has potent psychoactive effects and CBD possesses anxiolytic and analgesic actions. These pharmacological effects are largely mediated by the endocannabinoid system (ECS), predominantly by two cannabinoid receptors, CB1 (located throughout the central and peripheral nervous systems) and CB2 (widely expressed through cells of the immune system).

In a narrative review of pre-clinical studies specific to cancer-related pain, Brown and Farquhar-Smith (2018) implicated both CB1 and CB2 receptors as possessing analgesic effects for neuropathic, inflammatory and cancer pain states. However, the results did not translate into the clinical setting. The authors attribute this to pre-clinical studies selectively targeting cannabinoid receptors with synthetics, while clinical studies, relying on phytocannabinoids, were found to have diminished agonist effects at mixed cannabinoid receptor sites.

Cannabinoids represent a promising area for cancer-related pain; however, the primary drawback is activation of CB1 receptors. In some cases, this can trigger psychosis and panic attacks, although inhibiting CB1 receptors can produce depressive or anxiety-related issues (Johnson *et al.* 2020). Further research is required in this patient group to identify the therapeutic potential of phytocannabinoids versus synthetics, and the appropriate dose, duration and route of application, while minimizing the psychoactive effects of THC.

Aromatherapy in the management of pain: Current clinical evidence

Currently, the anti-nociceptive activity of essential oils, particularly their individual components, is an area of research interest. In their review, Wang and Heinbockel (2018) evaluated the neuropharmacological activity of essential oil components. The main essential oil isolates with specific analgesic properties are summarized in Table 9.1.

Table 9.1: Examples of essential oil constituents with specific analgesic properties (Wang and Heinbockel 2018)

Essential oil constituent	Analgesic effect
1,8-cineole	Anti-nociceptive. Smooth muscle relaxant
(+)-borneol	Alleviated mechanical hyperalgesia in models of chronic inflammatory and neuropathic pain
α-bisabolol	Anti-nociceptive-like effect
carvacrol	Analgesic activity
eugenol	Local analgesic
linalool	Anti-nociceptive effect
menthol	Analgesic
methyleugenol	Anti-nociceptive
nerolidol	Anti-nociceptive. Anti-inflammatory
thymol	Anti-nociceptive

Dosoky and Setzer's (2018) review was specific to the citrus oils, examining their biological activity and safety factors in a variety of animal and human clinical studies. *Citrus bergamia* (bergamot), *Citrus aurantium var amara flos* (neroli) and *Citrus limon* (lemon) demonstrate anti-nociceptive properties in animal studies, as summarized in Table 9.2, while *Citrus sinensis* (sweet orange), *Citrus aurantium* (bitter orange), *Citrus paradisi* (grapefruit) and *Citrus junos* (yuzu) demonstrate anxiolytic, uplifting and mood-enhancing properties, positively affecting well-being.

Table 9.2: Citrus essential oils with anti-nociceptive properties (Dosoky and Setzer 2018)

Essential oil Botanical name (common name)	Mechanism(s) of analgesic action	Reference
Citrus aurantium var amara flos (neroli)	Central and peripheral anti-nociceptive action	Costa et al. (2013)
	Possesses significant anti-inflammatory activity against acute and chronic inflammation	Khodabakhsh, Shafaroodi and Asgarpanah (2015)
Citrus limon (lemon)	Neuroprotective effect attributed to radical scavenging activity	Choi et al. (2000) Campelo et al. (2011)
	Significant changes in neuro-circuitry associated with anxiety and pain after two weeks' exposure in rats	Ceccarelli et al. (2004)
	Analgesic effect induced by dopamine-related activation of anterior cingulate cortex and descending pain inhibitory system in mice	Ikeda, Taksu and Murase (2014)
Citrus bergamia (bergamot)	Chronic nociceptive and neuropathic pain through modulation of pain perception	Lauro et al. (2016) Rombolà et al. (2016) Sakurada et al. (2011)
	Components of linalool and linalyl acetate showed a peripheral anti-nociceptive effect in mice	Kuwahata et al. (2013)
	Attenuates hypothalamic-pituitary-adrenal axis by reducing corticosterone response to acute stress in mice	Saiyudthong and Mekseepralard (2011)

To determine whether pre-clinical studies are a rational basis for clinical research, Scuteri *et al.* (2021) systematically reviewed 30 studies evaluating the analgesic effect of essential oils. In acute pain models, two essential oils demonstrated significant efficacy: *Citrus bergamia* (bergamot) (Katsuyama *et al.* 2015) and *Citrus aurantium var amara flos* (neroli) (Khodabakhsh *et al.* 2015). Additionally, *Citrus bergamia* (bergamot) also demonstrated efficacy in neuropathic pain models, including situations of chronic pain (Hamamura *et al.* 2020). Conclusively, Scuteri *et al.* (2021) advocate essential oil of *Citrus bergamia* (bergamot) for consistently exhibiting the strongest analgesic effect and urge further research in the clinical setting.

Escalation of pre-clinical studies in this area is encouraging. However, Scuteri *et al.* (2021) remind us that the most potent analgesic effect comes from the 'whole' essential oil where the full range of chemical constituents are in precise ratios as nature intended. The synergy of 'whole' oils and combinations is yet to be fully explored. Similarly, routes of administration and time of exposure also need further investigation.

Endocannabinoid system (ECS)

Interest in the modulatory effects of the ECS has extended to include essential oils. A systematic review conducted by Johnson *et al.* (2020) considered 17 pre-clinical studies where the most relevant findings, in terms of pain relief, relate to the sesquiterpene alkene, betacaryophyllene (BCP). The authors report that BCP shares similar analgesic and anti-inflammatory properties to cannabinoids by exerting a selective agonist effect on CB2 receptors. This means it exerts a therapeutic action without the psychoactive consequences associated with CB1 receptor agonists. While Tisserand and Young (2014) consider BCP as generally non-toxic and with a wide safety margin, of striking importance is evidence of non-tolerance with prolonged use. Notably, the anti-inflammatory effect is further enhanced by continued exposure, particularly in neuropathic inflammatory conditions. Further research is required to evaluate the effects of BCP-rich essential oils, including *Copaifera officinalis* (copaiba balsam), *Piper nigrum* (black pepper), *Melissa officinalis* (melissa), *Cananga odorata* (ylang ylang) and *Syzygium aromaticum* (clovebud).

Aromatherapy for the pain of advanced cancer

Evidence-based studies have shown that aromatherapy is consistently effective in the management of nociceptive, acute and chronic non-malignant pain (Buckle 2015), particularly post-operative, obstetric and gynaecological pain (Lakhan, Sheafer and Tepper 2016). There is a paucity of clinical studies specific to the pain of advanced cancer. Primarily, this is attributed to quantitative studies evaluating the pain-relieving effects of aromatherapy in conjunction with other psychological variables of anxiety, depression, insomnia and stress, where pain is not a primary outcome (Boehm, Büssing and Ostermann 2012). However, when pain is evaluated as the primary outcome, it is often examined alongside other cancer-related symptoms, as shown in the revised Cochrane review conducted by Shin *et al.* (2016). Individually, all the studies indicated promising results with aromatherapy massage, including alleviating medium- to long-term pain, anxiety and long-term symptoms in women with breast cancer. However, the clinical significance was compromised by small sample sizes and a consequent lack of statistical power which prevented translation into clinical benefit.

Currently, systematic reviews are unable to offer tangible evidence to support pharmacological interventions (Wiffen *et al.* 2017) or non-pharmacological approaches (Hökkä *et al.* 2014; Candy *et al.* 2020) for adequate pain management in this patient group. This calls for further consideration as to the reasons why the management of advanced cancer-related pain is proving difficult, and the potential of integrating aromatherapy interventions.

The potential of aromatherapy

A striking observation of conventional pain management is the emphasis on pharmacological intervention to address the physical aspects of the patient's pain. Unfortunately, this fails to consider the broader, holistic components contributing to the patient's 'total pain' experience. Ultimately, the success of pain management relies on a comprehensive understanding of the subtle interplay between these holistic aspects.

Assessment from the patient's perspective

Within healthcare, Krishnasamy (2008) lists the principal elements of pain assessment:

- Intensity – how severe is the pain?
- Character – how would you describe your pain?
- Location – where is your pain? Does it go anywhere else?
- Timing – when does your pain occur?
- Associated factors – what makes your pain worse or better?
- Implications of pain – how does this pain affect your daily living?

Pain assessment scales are widely advocated, with the ESMO recommendation of the Visual Analogue Scale (VAS), Verbal Rating Scale (VRS) and Numerical Rating Scale (NRS) (Ripamonti *et al.* 2012). However, personal clinical experience has highlighted the problems many patients encounter when assigning a numerical value to their pain, or even trying to describe their pain experience. This very point was demonstrated by Gibbins *et al.* (2014), who reported that patients found pain-rating scales challenging and identified that the clinical terms 'controlled' or 'non-controlled' levels of pain are generally not part of the patient's vocabulary. From their perspective, 'pain control' is the degree in which pain limits their functional ability.

Functional ability

Accomplishing 'everyday tasks', being able to 'live normally' and maintaining relationships are ways in which patients determine desirable levels of pain management (Gibbins *et al.* 2014; Zelman *et al.* 2004). For patients with severe levels of pain, achieving even modest activity is considered acceptable. Functional ability is central to the patient's self-assessment of pain, as it is to the effectiveness of pain-relieving approaches (Gibbins *et al.* 2014; Hackett, Godfrey and Bennett 2016; Zelman *et al.* 2004).

Critical insights by Gibbins *et al.* (2014) advocate changing the opening question of 'How is your pain today?' to 'When thinking about your pain, what is it allowing you to do today?' Patients will disclose more when asked to describe a pain-free day and what they would want/aim to do with it. Importantly, the patient's functional ability becomes the foundation on which to base future evaluation of pain-relieving interventions.

Beliefs of pain

The fluctuating nature of advanced cancer pain was demonstrated by Hackett et al. (2016), where patients (n=21), interviewed twice in a six-week period, showed notable changes in their pain experience. Significantly, when complex pain disrupted functional ability, patients perceived the escalating pain as an indicator of disease progression, meaning their end of life is approaching. For some patients, the consequent emotional turmoil and increased uncertainty adversely affects them seeking help. Understanding the patient's meaning of pain often overcomes their need to identify its underlying cause and requires the skills and support of a multi-disciplinary team (MDT) approach (Did-waniya *et al.* 2015).

Managing the effects of medication

In order to achieve optimal pain relief without medication side-effects, some patients take sufficient medication just to 'take the edge off' their pain and are often reluctant to take more to completely alleviate it (Gibbins *et al.* 2014; Hackett *et al.* 2016; Zelman *et al.* 2004). Others will exert more stoicism and wait until the pain becomes severe, even unbearable, before taking pain relief. And there are those who manage the effects of the medication and adjust their activities to maximize what is important. For example, a patient may experience drowsiness with opioids and use the sleep it induces to rest prior to spending time with family or going out.

Exploring the patient's pain experience offers greater insight into how pain affects their functionality, mood and existential meaning. Taking into account how they use their prescribed medication, plus any other approaches to alleviate pain, helps to establish a clear picture from which to consider appropriate intervention.

Essential oils as adjuncts

In her chapter on 'Pain and Inflammation' in her 2015 book, Dr Jane Buckle emphasizes the place of essential oils as adjuncts to conventional analgesia. Pain relief can be effected through various combinations, including an essential oil's individual components; the direct and positive influence of aroma on the limbic system and CNS; enhancing the parasympathetic nervous system response through touch; and a placebo effect.

The intimate relationships between the physical, spiritual and psychosocial aspects of pain cannot be separated. Essential oils specific to these areas are outlined in Chapters 5 and 6, in addition to related symptoms of fatigue and insomnia in Chapters 7 and 8 respectively. These dimensions must be considered within the overall formulation and integrated alongside oils where clinical use has identified their pain-relieving properties. In the absence of research-based clinical evidence in this patient group, the essential oils shown in Table 9.3 are drawn from my personal clinical experience and the practice of qualified aromatherapists.

Table 9.3: Examples of essential oils as adjuvants for pain management in patients with advanced cancer

Essential oil Botanical name (common name)	Active constituent(s)	Pain-relieving property	Reference
Anthemis nobilis (roman chamomile)	amyl-angelate plus other esters >70%	Analgesic Antispasmodic Anti-inflammatory	Baudoux *et al.* (2006) Harris (2016)
Artemisia dracunculus (tarragon)	chavicol methyl ether	Antispasmodic	Baudoux *et al.* (2006) Harris (2016)
Cananga odorata (ylang ylang)	benzyl acetate, BCP geranyl acetate methyl benzoate	Analgesic Anti-inflammatory Antispasmodic	Baudoux *et al.* (2006) Holmes (2019)
Citrus aurantium var amara flos (neroli)	neryl acetate	Antispasmodic	Baudoux *et al.* (2006) Holmes (2019)
Citrus aurantium var amara fol. (petitgrain)	l-linalool	Anti-inflammatory	Holmes (2019)
Citrus bergamia (bergamot)	linalool linalyl-acetate	Neuropathic chronic pain	Holmes (2019)
Copaifera officinalis (copaiba balsam)	BCP	Neuropathic Anti-inflammatory	Johnson *et al.* (2020)
Helichrysum italicum (helichrysum)	neryl acetate	Antispasmodic Anti-inflammatory	Baudoux *et al.* (2006) Holmes (2019)
Kunzea ambigua (kunzea)	terpinen-4-ol α-bisabolol	Analgesic Anti-inflammatory	Holmes (2019)
Laurus nobilis (laurel leaf)	1,8-cineole terpenyl acetate α-pinene	Neuropathic Analgesic	Baudoux *et al.* (2006)
Lavandula angustifolia (lavender true)	linalyl acetate	Analgesic	Baudoux *et al.* (2006) Holmes (2019)
Lavandula latifolia (spike lavender)	linalol, 1,8-cineole camphor	Analgesic	Baudoux *et al.* (2006)

cont.

Essential oil *Botanical name* (common name)	Active constituent(s)	Pain-relieving property	Reference
Matricaria recutita CO_2 (german chamomile CO_2)	α-bisabolol chamazulene	Anti-inflammatory	Kerkhof-Knapp Hayes (2015)
Mentha arvensis (cornmint)	menthol	Topical analgesic Antispasmodic Neuropathic	Harris (2016) Holmes (2019)
Mentha citrata (bergamot-mint)	linalyl acetate	Analgesic	Harris (2016)
Mentha x piperita (peppermint)	menthol	Analgesic Topical anaesthetic Antispasmodic Neuropathic	Baudoux *et al.* (2006) Harris (2016) Kerkhof-Knapp Hayes (2015)
Nardostachys jatamansi (spikenard)	patchoulenes β-gurjunene bornyl acetate	Neuropathic Antispasmodic Anti-inflammatory	Holmes (2019) Kerkhof-Knapp Hayes (2015)
Origanum majorana (sweet marjoram)	geranyl acetate terpinen-4-ol	Antispasmodic Anti-inflammatory Neuropathic	Holmes (2019) Kerkhof-Knapp Hayes (2015)
Pelargonium graveolens (geranium)	l-linalool	Neuropathic Anti-inflammatory Antispasmodic	Holmes (2019) Kerkhof-Knapp Hayes (2015)
Pinus sylvestris (scots pine)	α-pinene, BCP terpinolene	Rubefacient Topical analgesic	Baudoux *et al.* (2006) Harris (2016)
Piper nigrum (black pepper)	BCP, eugenol	Analgesic Rubefacient	Harris (2016) Holmes (2019)
Zingiber cassumunar (plai)	sabinene terpinen-4-ol	Anti-inflammatory	Holmes (2019)

Aromatherapy applications
Inhalation
The direct interaction between inhaled essential oils and the neuro-endocrine system, neurotransmitters and neuromodulators within various brain centres has been shown to moderate stress biomarkers

(Schneider 2016) and influence pain dynamics (Schneider 2017). Recommendations are for essential oil concentrations to be high enough to potently stimulate the olfactory system (Schneider, Singer and Singer 2018). Therefore, aromatic inhalation needs to form a significant part of a patient's pain management plan, particularly where emotional and existential distress, and insomnia are foremost in their presentation. A useful option is the aromatherapy inhaler stick.

Educating patients in self-direction of the frequency and duration of essential oil inhalation is equally as important as describing specific situations when inhalation should be used; for example, in episodes of breakthrough pain, where pain intensity can rapidly escalate and conventional 'rescue' medications, via oral or transdermal routes, often take up to 30 minutes to reach maximum effect. While waiting, the simultaneous use of an aromatherapy inhaler stick provides patients with an option to feel emotionally calm with one to three breath cycles, or deeply relaxed with up to eight cycles of breath (depending on the oils used). Involving family and caregivers in these discussions is often helpful.

Massage

Soft tissue massage is an appreciated source of comfort to patients with life-limiting illness. Previous studies have focused on the role of massage for managing symptoms, including cancer-related pain (Calenda 2006; Cassileth and Vickers 2004; Deng and Cassileth 2005; Jane *et al.* 2011; Kutner *et al.* 2008; López-Sendín *et al.* 2012; Post-White *et al.* 2003). Studies incorporating aromatherapy massage for patients with advanced cancer report significant improvement in pain relief (Chang 2008; Shin *et al.* 2016), sleep quality (Soden *et al.* 2004), anxiety (Corner *et al.* 1995a; Imanishi *et al.* 2009; Wilkinson *et al.* 1999; Wilkinson *et al.* 2007) and reductions in stress biomarkers (Hadfield 2001; Stringer *et al.* 2008). Individual RCTs report favourable outcomes in this patient cohort, although a lack of methodological rigour and small samples sizes are frequent reasons precluding several studies from meeting the entry criteria for systematic review (Bardia *et al.* 2006; Candy *et al.* 2020; Hökkä *et al.* 2014).

In contrast, qualitative approaches consider the patient's experience rather than focusing on a single variable, as shown by Cronfalk *et al.* (2009). Patients with life-limiting illness (n=22) were evaluated over a two-week period and received either a hand or foot massage at home. In total, patients received nine massage sessions, each of 25 minutes' duration, using a commercial brand of lightly scented vegetable oil of either citrus or hawthorn. Patients considered massage a caring intervention; they valued the personal attention and trust of a dedicated therapist; they described a sense of respite derived from the experience of 'floating away'; and they reported profound mental and existential peacefulness from the physical connection and feeling of well-being. Of particular significance was the relief in being able to stop for a while; to reach a place of respite from symptoms, to experience a notable decrease in pain, or to just simply experience a sense of being present, as in the here and now. Importantly, this study gives powerful insight into the patients' experience of massage.

Other qualitative studies also report how patients value being able to feel released from their illness for a while, with many identifying such moments as being crucial to a 'desirable day' (Zelman *et al.* 2004). This highlights the complexity of cancer-related pain, where quantitative methodology is simply not identifying the subtle interplay between the emotional, social, spiritual and physical factors involved. Qualitative evaluation is fundamentally important within palliative care if we are to guide clinical practice using evidence-based approaches that truly reflect the patient's pain experience.

Topical application

Topical application for pain management in these patients requires careful consideration of the integrity and condition of the patient's skin, which also influences the choice of base substances. Fixed oils and/or macerates that possess known analgesic, anti-inflammatory or neural properties have the potential to enhance the overall pain-relieving effect. Useful for pain-relief formulations are *Calophyllum inophyllum* (tamanu), *Hypericum perforatum* (St John's wort), *Simmondsia chinensis* (jojoba) and *Arnica montana* (arnica).

Generally, larger surface areas require a concentration range between 3 and 5%, while smaller, highly localized areas require concentrations between 5 and 20%. Dermal pathways for essential oil application are explored in more detail in Chapter 12.

Thermo-related application

Specific to neuropathic pain associated with chemotherapy-induced peripheral neuropathy (CIPN), Harris (2012) advocates utilizing essential oils with known cooling properties, such as menthol-rich *Mentha x piperita* (peppermint) or *Mentha arvensis* (cornmint), alongside oils with known analgesic properties. Dilution of the overall formulation in a base substance, for example a non-oily cream or *Aloe vera* gel, should be between 3 and 5%. Twice daily application is suggested to the peripherally affected areas, namely hands/forearms and feet/knees affected by CIPN, together with the corresponding spinal vertebrae – cervical spine and/or lumbar region.

The cooling effect is largely generated by the monoterpene alcohol, menthol. Pergolizzi *et al.* (2017) describe menthol as a potent agonist of the transient receptor potential melastatin-8 (TRPM8) thermoreceptor. At low concentrations (<1%), menthol will exert a comfortable cooling sensation which is detected by TRPM8. However, increasing menthol concentrations above 1% will simultaneously activate the transient receptor potential ankyrin-1 (TRPA1), which is associated with cold pain. For neuropathic pain, a concentration starting at 1% menthol of the overall formulation is sufficient to be detected by peripheral thermoreceptors, thus moderating the patient's pain to a 'cool' sensation, rather than a painful experience.

Conversely, essential oils with known warming components such as 1,8-cineole, common to *Eucalyptus globulus* (blue gum eucalyptus) and *Eucalyptus radiata* (narrow-leaf eucalyptus), or other essential oils which exert a rubefacient effect such as *Piper nigrum* (black pepper) and *Zingiber officinale* (ginger), can soothe areas of spasm and musculoskeletal tension.

In either situation, where an altered thermo-perception is induced, it is strongly recommended to undertake a patch test first to ensure that the patient is comfortable with the level of cooling or warmth being applied.

Aromatic bathing

Formulating oils to the individual's needs and appropriate to the time of day can further enhance pain relief, such as a warm aromatic bath before bedtime where deep-level relaxation and quality sleep are required. Overall, it provides a balancing effect to the whole person and is an option suited to patients who are more physically able, or those with access to an assisted bath such as an in-patient unit, or for those who treasure the ritual and pleasures of bathing.

Compresses

Localized application of a compress to a painful area can bring immense comfort. Cool compresses are useful where there is heat and inflammation of unbroken skin; where joints are sore and tender; in the event of headaches; where there is pruritus (itch) or restless leg syndrome (RLS); and in some situations to ease the burning sensation associated with neuropathic pain.

Warm compresses deeply penetrate heat to relax and ease muscle tension/spasms, soothe neuralgia, warm cold arthritic joints, and bring immense comfort to those where pain is deeply felt or the cold is penetrating to the bones. For a whole-body approach, where aromatic bathing is not an option, gently compressing warmed, moist aromatic towels along individual limbs, the back and chest can be deeply relaxing. Incorporating hydrosols can also be beneficial (see Chapter 3).

Combining interventions

There is immense value in combining inhaled and dermal applications of essential oils for adjuvant pain management. Depending on the situation, and to avoid overwhelming the patient, an effective option is to start with one aromatherapy intervention, either inhalation or topical application, which relates to the patient's priority of concern. Commonly, this is the inhalation pathway to swiftly address the spiritual and psychosocial manifestations of pain.

Creating such a stepwise approach allows for careful monitoring of the therapeutic effect, how the patient is coping and any adjustments that may be required, and space to determine other appropriate applications. Combinations of inhalation, massage, bathing, compresses and footbaths are useful adjuncts for advanced pain management in the clinical setting and should not be underestimated.

CASE STUDY 9.1: WINNIE'S EXPERIENCE

Referral

With progression of Winnie's disease came an increase in pain intensity of a neuropathic nature, central to the coccyx and accompanied by restless leg syndrome (RLS). Integrative clinical aromatherapy approaches for pain management continued over a 12-month period. The following is a 'clinical snapshot' of her care during the introduction of higher-level, prescribed analgesia.

Aromatherapy sessions

Winnie was lying on her sofa in the mid-afternoon sun. She spoke of her exhaustion, the poor night's sleep and how troubled she felt with an increasing and persistent ache in the coccyx. The RLS was worse when she first got into bed and was often interspersed with episodes of sharp, burning pain, affecting both legs and preventing her getting off to sleep.

The topical aromatherapy pain-relief blend of 3% concentration (due to renal dysfunction) was no longer fully effective and neither was the paracetamol she took as required. She was reluctant to consider further prescribed pain medications, including opioids, and was yet to start the low-dose amitriptyline, recently organized by her doctor for neuropathic pain.

Winnie's family maintained regular contact and she enjoyed their news, especially of her grandchildren. However, her usual social activities and regular lunch with her closest friend had been postponed. Her daily walk to the local shops had reduced and today she decided to remain at home.

We discussed the aromatherapy options. Winnie agreed to a new aromatherapy inhaler stick, formulated from essential oils of her choosing to aid deeper-level psychospiritual relaxation and quality sleep. Additionally, she consented to re-formulation of the pain-relief blend, increasing to a 5% concentration with a change of base substance to a gel. The aim was to enhance a cooling sensation and monitor its effectiveness with the sporadic neuropathic pain accompanying the RLS (see Table 9.4). Unfortunately, cool showers, or footbaths prior to bedtime were not a practical option for Winnie. Details of the session were shared with the MDT.

Table 9.4: Winnie's reformulated aromatherapy regime (1)

Method of application	Botanical products used Botanical name (common name)	Amount used	Directions for use
Topical pain-relief blend 5%	Essential oils Lavandula latifolia (spike lavender) Zingiber cassumunar (plai) Copaifera officinalis (copaiba balsam) Mentha citrata (bergamot-mint) Matricaria recutita (german chamomile) Mentha arvensis (cornmint)	 30% 20% 25% 10% 5% 10%	Patient-assisted Twice daily application to coccyx and legs for two weeks then review
	Base substance Aloe vera gel	100%	
Aromatherapy inhaler stick 'Deep peace and calm'	Cistus ladanifer (cistus) Citrus reticulata (mandarin) Lavandula angustifolia (lavender true) Simmondsia chinensis (jojoba)	1 drop 4 drops 2 drops 1ml	Patient-directed as required at night At each use, 4–8 breath cycles

At the phone call follow-up the next day, Winnie reported a much more settled night. She was able to turn over in bed more easily, with reduced pain in the coccyx. Her RLS was less extreme and eventually eased after releasing the weight of the bedclothes. Winnie connected well with the aromatherapy inhaler stick, choosing to start with three to four breath cycles.

One week later, with an increase in the number of breath cycles of her aromatherapy inhaler stick, Winnie reported feeling calmer in herself and better able to return to sleep during the night. She had been in contact with the MDT about her prescribed pain medication. Her reluctance stemmed from a lifetime of natural approaches and her dislike of the drowsiness she had experienced previously with conventional pharmacology. The MDT remained mindful of their prescribing while minimizing polypharmacy.

Over the course of the next few weeks, at the start of the global pandemic, adjustments were made to the pain-relief gel, changing essential oils with an increase in concentration to 7.5%. Alongside prescribed analgesia, this provided sufficient relief for Winnie while she remained independent within her home. However, the lockdown restrictions of the global pandemic meant Winnie's family were unable to visit. Coupled with the associated fears of Covid-19, the reality of her isolation intensified as lockdown restrictions progressed. This translated into a noticeable increase in Winnie's pain intensity. She described generalized pain, mainly throughout her spine, low back and the upper part of both legs, which was much worse at night. It transpired that Winnie had stopped applying the morning dose of pain-relief gel because 'I have no pain at that time.' We discussed the benefits of regular application of the gel and at the same time, planned a re-formulation of her aromatherapy regime to address the escalating spiritual and emotional distress which was contributing to her pain intensity (see Table 9.5).

The MDT were updated and plans put in place for increased telephone contact by the family support counsellor and clinical nursing team. Winnie's family and friends remained a constant and daily source of strength.

Reformulation of the pain-relief blend took place, with an emphasis on anti-inflammatory/analgesic base substances of rapid absorption, with the inclusion of *Boswellia carterii* (frankincense). This was intentional to assist Winnie's spiritual well-being; it was a familiar aroma which returned her to her beloved Africa and proved to be a deep source of comfort. A minor adjustment was made to the aromatherapy inhaler stick formulation to include *Anthemis nobilis* (roman chamomile), designed to increase the sedatory effect at night.

Table 9.5: Winnie's reformulated aromatherapy regime (2)

Method of application	Botanical products used *Botanical name* (common name)	Amount used	Directions for use
Topical pain-relief blend 10%	Essential oils *Lavandula latifolia* (spike lavender) *Zingiber cassumunar* (plai) *Copaifera officinalis* (copaiba balsam) *Kunzea ambigua* (kunzea) *Boswellia carterii* (frankincense)	 30% 15% 30% 15% 10%	Patient-assisted Twice daily application to coccyx and upper legs for two weeks, then review
	Base substances *Calophyllum inophyllum* (tamanu) *Simmondsia chinensis* (jojoba)	 60% 40%	
Aromatherapy inhaler stick 'Deep peace and calm'	*Cistus ladanifer* (cistus) *Citrus reticulata* (mandarin) *Anthemis nobilis* (roman chamomile) *Simmondsia chinensis* (jojoba)	1 drop 4 drops 1 drop 1ml	Patient-directed as required Daytime 1–3 breath cycles Night-time 4–8 breath cycles

Reflection

We return here to the importance of personal autonomy and the seamless support of a community MDT. Integrating clinical aromatherapy maintained Winnie's lifelong use of natural health approaches and gave her time to process her fear of starting prescribed opioids. Concerns about the complexity of pain and the nature and side-effects of opioids are commonly experienced by patients. Sensitive communication and incorporating other pain-relieving approaches enabled Winnie to continue this regime during the remainder of the pandemic lockdown period with minor adjustment to the formulation and for two subsequent months alongside her prescribed opioid analgesia.

CHAPTER 10

Breathlessness in Patients with Life-Limiting Illness

Cited as a core symptom of four main life-limiting illnesses, breathlessness affects up to 70% of patients with advanced cancer, 95% with chronic obstructive pulmonary disease (COPD), 88% with heart failure (HF) and 85% with motor-neurone disease (MND) (Gysels and Higginson 2011). Additionally, breathlessness affects patients with dementia, advanced age and HIV, and is highly prevalent in patients receiving end-of-life care, particularly in the last three months of life (Kamal *et al.* 2011).

Traditional approaches to breathlessness assessment and management centre on its physiological measurement. However, Bausewein *et al.* (2018) point out that in advanced illness, these objective findings do not fully illustrate the extent of the patient's distress. From my personal clinical experience, far more is revealed about the true nature of the person's experience and the impact of breathlessness on their daily life from their descriptions, such as 'I'm suffocating', 'I can't get enough breath in' and 'There's no air'. Others report breathing as being 'hard work, frightening, painful, or a continuous fight' (BPJ 2012, p.23).

Regardless of the diagnosis, breathlessness (a term often used interchangeably with dyspnoea) is ultimately a patient-centred symptom. This is reflected in the definition from the American Thoracic Society (1999), 'a subjective experience of breathing discomfort that consists of qualitatively distinct sensations that vary in intensity'.

Characteristics of breathlessness within palliative care

Breathlessness in advanced illness is recognized as a complex interplay of physical, psychological, emotional and spiritual factors which should not be separated (Corner, Plant and Warner 1995b). To aid healthcare professionals, Abernethy and Wheeler (2008) describe a biopsychosocial framework, derived from Dame Cicely Saunders' concept of 'total pain', known as 'total dyspnoea'. The authors apply the same physical, psychological, spiritual and social domains to collectively consider the patient's unique experience of breathlessness (see Figure 10.1).

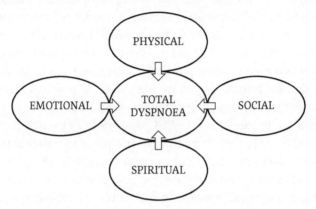

FIGURE 10.1: 'TOTAL DYSPNOEA' MODEL (ABERNETHY AND WHEELER 2008)

Physiological factors

In a review of breathlessness in patients with life-limiting illness, Kamal *et al.* (2011) discuss several causal factors. These are summarized in Table 10.1. It is evident that breathlessness is not solely attributed to the physical disease itself. Often, it can result as a systemic effect of advanced disease processes, for example in situations where cachexia and fatigue are present. Furthermore, in patients with cancer, breathlessness can also be treatment-related, including surgery, radiation pneumonitis/fibrosis, radiation-induced pericardial disease, chemotherapy-induced pulmonary disease and chemotherapy-induced cardiomyopathy (Dudgeon *et al.* 2001).

Table 10.1: Anatomic and underlying disease giving rise to breathlessness (Kamal *et al.* 2011)

Anatomic condition/ symptom	Underlying causal factors
Pulmonary obstruction	COPD, reactive airways, cough/secretions, mass lesions
Pulmonary restriction	Fibrosis or other interstitial disease, effusions, infections, kyphosis, obesity
Perfusion/oxygenation mismatch	Anaemia, pulmonary hypertension, heart failure, pulmonary embolism
Fatigue/weakness	Cancer-related fatigue, multiple sclerosis, amyotrophic lateral sclerosis

Psychological factors

Irrespective of the underlying diagnosis, the association between breathlessness in advanced illness and anxiety, panic attacks, fear and spiritual distress has been well documented (Corner *et al.* 1995b; Gysels and Higginson 2011; Nardi, Freire and Zin 2009; Schroedl *et al.* 2014). An interesting feature of Gysels and Higginson's (2011) qualitative comparison is that patients with cancer, COPD and MND describe the onset and nature of breathlessness in emotional terms, where anxiety, panic and fear feature prominently over physical limitations. In contrast, patients with HF discuss breathlessness in relation to its physical restriction arising from the negative effects of other symptoms.

A small audit conducted at St Christopher's Hospice by Taylor (2007) identified that levels of anxiety and panic in patients referred for breathlessness management are often significantly higher than patients' estimates, or those of their referring clinician. Other emotional manifestations of breathlessness include intense irritability, irrational outbursts, anger, worry and frustration. These may be attributed to depleted oxygen levels (hypoxia), although Taylor (2007, p.26) concludes, 'it can be an understandable emotional response to existential terror'.

Spiritual factors

Many patients experiencing breathlessness report fear of an uncertain future. For those with cancer, Gysels and Higginson (2011) identified that breathlessness, which initially prompted patients to seek medical investigation, became less important when they were given a diagnosis of cancer. Patients then described feelings of 'shock', with an immediate association with death.

In Schroedl *et al.*'s (2014) study of patients with COPD, fear of dying featured prominently, together with fear of losing their independence and of suffering. Consequently, patients report an inability to face the future and cope by taking one day at a time. Living in the present is a strategy Gysels and Higginson (2011, p.7) observed in patients with MND as a means of adjusting to symptoms and the future; for these patients, where there is no known cure, breathlessness reaffirmed the way in which 'the illness affects mechanisms essential to life'.

Social factors

Social isolation is a common and disabling issue for these patients. Psychological and spiritual distress, combined with the physical restriction of breathlessness, inhibits every single movement, limiting daily activities to the extent of rendering patients housebound (Gysels and Higginson 2011; Schroedl *et al.* 2014).

Conventional management of breathlessness

Within the palliative care literature, authors are generally agreed that the goal of breathlessness intervention is to address both the symptom and underlying causes (BPJ 2012; Corner *et al.* 1995b; Kamal *et al.* 2012). However, when causes are no longer reversible, breathlessness, if present, is considered 'refractory' with priority for symptom relief (BPJ 2012). Interventions are categorized into pharmacological and non-pharmacological.

Pharmacological interventions

Kamal *et al.* (2012) highlight opioids, most commonly morphine, as the most extensively researched and first-line pharmacology for the management of breathlessness. Additional effects of opioids lie with treating pain and anxiety, both of which are integral to this complex symptom. Careful dosing and titration have drawn researchers to the same conclusion, that low doses of sustained-release oral opioids exert a significant and continuous therapeutic benefit in breathlessness relief.

Anxiolytics, in the form of benzodiazepines, have been studied both as single agents and in combination with opioids (Kamal *et al.* 2012). However, a Cochrane review identified that this class of pharmacology causes more side-effects, such as drowsiness and somnolence, in the breathless patient and has limited beneficial value (Simon *et al.* 2010). Similarly, intra-nasal midazolam, considered a popular method of application, was also found to have no therapeutic advantage when compared with an intra-nasal placebo (Hardy *et al.* 2016).

Traditionally, supplemental oxygen for breathlessness has been a standard line of management for patients in hospital and palliative care settings when hypoxic. However, its use is complex and its benefit limited (Baldwin and Cox 2016). Abernethy *et al.* (2010) recommend that patients are monitored closely and supplemental oxygen be discontinued if no relief is observed after three days.

Nebulized medications, such as saline solution 0.9% to increase mucous fluidity, or nebulized bronchodilators to relieve airway spasm or constrictions, may be beneficial. Other pharmacology for managing underlying causes of breathlessness is summarized by Balkstra (2010). Treatments are directed at the underlying cause and include diuretics to alleviate excess fluid volume, bronchodilators and corticosteroids for their anti-inflammatory action, particularly in situations of airway obstruction.

Non-pharmacological interventions

Many of the non-pharmacological approaches to breathlessness management are derived from those used by patients with COPD. Through experience, they learn to adapt to the gradual onset of symptoms (Gysels and Higginson 2011). In contrast, patients with cancer generally present with a sudden onset of breathlessness with little time to adjust.

Corner *et al.* (1995b) evaluated the effectiveness of nurse-led strategies for the management of breathlessness in patients with cancer. The success of this seminal study prompted a larger-scale replication (n=119) by Bredin *et al.* (1999). Patients were randomized to receive either nurse-led interventions, as listed below, or best supportive management. Following eight weeks of intervention, improvements in breathlessness, performance status as well as physical and psychological states were demonstrated in patients attending the nurse-led clinics. A striking feature is that nurse-led strategies were tailored to the individual's needs and involved family and caregivers.

- Comprehensive assessment of breathlessness including factors which exacerbated or alleviated symptoms
- Exploration of the meaning of breathlessness, their disease and feelings about the future
- Advice and support for patients and their families on ways of managing breathlessness
- Training in breathing control techniques, progressive muscle relaxation (PMR) and distraction exercises
- Goal-setting to complement breathing and relaxation techniques to help the management of functional and social activities and to support the development and adoption of coping strategies
- Early recognition of problems warranting pharmacological or medical intervention

Within palliative care, Kamal *et al.* (2012) discuss non-pharmacological pulmonary rehabilitation through exercise for patients with COPD. For those with cancer-related breathlessness, increasing air movement by hand-held fans, the use of combination gases such as heliox, acupuncture and nutrition can bring relief. Although several interventions show promise, the authors advocate for further evaluation which is directed to the components of the 'total dyspnoea' model. As such, it is important to examine the clinical evidence and potential of aromatherapy as a plausible non-pharmacological option.

Aromatherapy in breathlessness management: Current clinical evidence

The direct interface between essential oils and the respiratory mucosa offers rapid access and symptom relief, making it an area of intense research interest. Predominantly, the constituent 1,8-cineole, an oxide with bronchodilatory, mucolytic, anti-inflammatory and antitussive properties, is considered the component of choice for respiratory pathologies (Harris 2007). Essential oils rich in 1,8-cineole that are suitable for respiratory pathologies are shown below:

- *Cinnamomum camphora ct cineole* (ravintsara ct cineole)
- *Eucalyptus radiata* (narrow-leaf eucalyptus)
- *Eucalyptus globulus* (blue gum eucalyptus)
- *Laurus nobilis* (laurel leaf)
- *Lavandula latifolia* (spike lavender)
- *Melaleuca cajuputi* (cajeput)
- *Melaleuca quinquenervia* (niaouli)
- *Myrtus communis* (myrtle)
- *Salvia rosmarinus ct cineole* (rosemary ct cineole)

Harris (2007) reports on several studies which have evaluated the benefits of these oxide-rich oils in respiratory illness, including management of COPD. For these patients, improvements were identified in mucociliary clearance, increased ciliary beat, cough relief, lung function, peak flow and dyspnoea, using oral routes of administration.

Alongside 1,8-cineole, Baudoux (2007) advocates other verified essential oil components for respiratory care. These include: the mucolytic effects of ketone-rich oils, such as piperitone in *Eucalyptus dives* (peppermint eucalyptus), camphor and verbenone in *Salvia rosmarinus ct camphor* and *ct verbenone* (rosemary); the antispasmodic, relaxant and anti-inflammatory effects of ester-rich oils such as benzyl benzoate in *Cananga odorata* (ylang ylang), isobutyl angelate in *Anthemis nobilis* (roman chamomile), linalyl acetate in *Citrus aurantium var amara fol.* (petitgrain); the bronchodilatory effects of phenyl methyl ether-rich oils such as anethole in *Foeniculum vulgare* (fennel) and *Pimpinella anisum* (aniseed); the antihistaminic and anti-inflammatory effects of chamazulene in *Matricaria recutita* (german chamomile); and the antitussive effects of various components in *Cupressus sempervirens* (cypress) and *Eucalyptus radiata* (narrow-leaf eucalyptus).

A growing area of interest is the notion of using essential oil components to activate transient receptor potential (TRP) ion channels located within the airways, to increase airflow. Horvath and Acs (2015) detail the physiological mechanisms of TRP channels which are believed to play a key role in respiratory disorders, including COPD and cough. Of particular interest is transient receptor potential melastatin-8 (TRPM8), an ion channel which is thermoreceptive, detects cool temperatures and is activated by the monoterpene alcohol, menthol and, to a lesser extent, the oxide 1,8-cineole. Researchers investigating the inhaled effects of these components in nasal TRPM8 channels report that the cold sensation experienced in the nose is associated with an increased sensation of improved airflow even if airflow remains unchanged (Burrow *et al.* 2009). Such an approach is useful for breathlessness management, an example is given in Case study 10.1.

The potential of aromatherapy

A wealth of evidence-based information exists within the aromatherapy literature which relates to essential oil use in general respiratory care. Although not specific to the management of breathlessness in life-limiting illness, many of the approaches offer potential therapeutic value to these patients.

Assessment from the patient's perspective

The patient's experience of breathlessness, rather than its objective measurement, is paramount. Therefore, assessment must begin with the patient's words and descriptions. Frequent themes arising from qualitative studies highlight the stigma, guilt and self-blame with which patients associate their breathlessness (Gysels and Higginson 2011; Schroedl *et al.* 2014). This is particularly evident in those with COPD, HF and cancer, where causative factors include smoking, environmental influences, poor life choices and lifestyles. To aid our understanding of a patient's experience, Bredin *et al.* (1999) advocate:

- exploration of what breathlessness means to the individual
- how breathlessness impacts their life

- what a patient understands about their illness
- how a patient views their future.

Additional to this holistic approach, factors which exacerbate breathlessness and those which alleviate it are other important considerations. Careful observation of the patient offers valuable insight into the degree of respiratory distress. Sensitive assessment is required which neither exhausts the patient nor provokes their breathlessness. With the patient's consent, family members and caregivers can also be helpful in providing specific details. Characteristic signs of acute breathlessness include:

- Mouth breathing, often 'purse-lipped breathing'
- Lip cyanosis
- Gasping for air
- Excessive use of respiratory accessory muscles which are prominent on inspiration
- Short, hurried sentences
- Evidence of a productive or non-productive cough

It is important to determine what the primary concern is for the patient. This may not necessarily relate to the physical effort of breathing, but more to the management of panic and anxiety associated with not being able to take in sufficient air. Working directly with the patient's priorities is crucial.

Essential oils

Generally, respiratory conditions are most responsive to essential oils with bronchodilatory, mucolytic, anti-inflammatory, antitussive, antihistaminic and relaxing properties (Baudoux 2007; Buckle 2015; Harris 2007). These will be discussed within the context of breathlessness in the patient with advanced respiratory illness.

Anxiety, panic and spiritual distress

Psychological and spiritual distress feature significantly in these patients and includes fear of not being able to take in sufficient breath, of suffocating, suffering and dying. Essential oils with anxiolytic and highly calming properties are obvious choices and do not possess the central nervous system (CNS) side-effects associated with benzodiazepines.

A range of essential oils specific to the management of spiritual and emotional distress are considered in Chapters 5 and 6.

Mucous and expectoration

Clearing mucous secretions can be difficult and exhausting for the breathless patient. For patients who are physically able to cough, the aim of aromatherapy intervention is to reduce inflammation and increase mucous fluidity and expectoration. In a detailed account of mucous management of the bronchi, Hadji-Minaglou and Maeda (2007) recommend essential oils with proven anti-inflammatory, mucolytic and expectorant properties, as shown in Table 10.2.

Table 10.2: Evidence-based essential oils suitable for respiratory mucous management (Hadji-Minaglou and Maeda 2007)

Essential oil *Botanical name* (common name)	Properties
Eucalyptus camadulensis (eucalyptus river red gum) *Eucalyptus radiata* (narrow-leaf eucalyptus) *Myrtus communis* (myrtle) *Laurus nobilis* (laurel leaf)	Anti-inflammatory and expectoration actions on the respiratory tract
Eucalyptus dives ct piperitone (peppermint eucalyptus gum ct piperitone) *Lavandula stoechas* (french lavender) *Carum carvi* (caraway) *Laurus nobilis* (laurel leaf)	Powerful mucolytic actions on the respiratory tract

For maximum effect and to avoid compromising normal function of the mucociliary escalator, Harris (2004) advocates low-dose essential oil intervention. Applications involving steam inhalation aid humidification and consequently mucous fluidity, which may enhance ease of expectoration. However, cautions are indicated which will be subsequently discussed.

Cough

Cough can be problematic for the breathless patient. Designed as a protective mechanism to expel irritants or blockages from the air passages, cough can also result from the disease itself or its pathophysiological consequences. It can be a source of exhaustion and distress for both the patient and their family and needs to be managed carefully.

Cough arising from bronchal spasm may be relieved by essential oils with recognized bronchospasmolytic properties. Harris (2004) and Baudoux (2007) suggest *Carum carvi* (caraway), *Artemis dranunculus* (tarragon), *Cananga odorata* (ylang ylang), *Anthemis nobilis* (roman chamomile), *Citrus aurantium var amara fol.* (petitgrain), *Ammi visnaga* (khella), *Angelica archangelica* (angelica), *Inula graveolens* (sweet inula), *Melissa officinalis* (melissa) and *Ocimum basilicum ct methyl chavicol* (exotic basil ct methyl chavicol).

In some patients, cough suppression may be required. The anti-tussive effects of essential oils such as *Eucalyptus radiata* (narrow-leaf eucalyptus) and *Cupressus sempervirens* (cypress) have proven benefits (Baudoux 2007), in addition to specific oil components of menthol and 1,8-cineole (Morice *et al.* 1994; Plevkova *et al.* 2013).

Cautions and contraindications of essential oil use

In breathlessness related to life-limiting illness, where the effects of aromatherapy have not been fully evaluated, there are specific cautions and contraindications of essential oil use. These are summarized and drawn from the valuable works of Harris (2004) and Tisserand and Young (2014). In patients with heightened odour acuity, hypersensitivity to aromas or airway hyper-reactivity, avoiding essential oils altogether may be more appropriate. For these patients, hydrosols are a plausible alternative. Some cautions and contraindications of essential oils in advanced respiratory care are:

- Increasing mucous fluidity in patients who are physically unable to cough must be avoided
- High concentrations of inhaled essential oils can decrease muco-ciliary function. Employ low-level dosing
- Duration of inhaled essential oils is as important as concentration. Incorporate shorter diffusion or inhalation times
- Oils rich in 1,8-cineole, menthol and camphor possess stimulating aromas which may, for the breathless patient, induce bronchial spasm. Low-level dosing is required
- Other essential oil constituents cited as potential respiratory irritants are the monoterpenes, α-pinene, β-pinene, δ-3-carene and (+)-limonene
- Inhaled menthol or 1,8-cineole therapy should not be applied on or near the face of babies, infants or small children
- Careful monitoring and evaluation of all aromatic approaches is crucial

- In end-of-life care, where decreased mucociliary clearance and ineffective cough reflex result in accumulated secretions in the air passages, avoid essential oils with mucolytic and expectorant properties. In these situations, respiratory congestion is best managed with conventional pharmacology

Supplemental oxygen

The issue of using essential oils or other oil-based botanical products on or near the face/nares (as well as the hair, moustache, upper chest and hands) in patients with supplemental oxygen is an ongoing area of debate. To date, no clear clinical guidelines exist. As oxygen supports combustion, the identified hazard is an increased risk of fire should there be a source of ignition. Given that essential oils and fixed oils are flammable, the argument is that their presence may increase the risk of burns to the patient. Most patient information literature and pharmacist recommendations advocate against using oil, grease or petroleum jelly when handling patients under oxygen therapy (or handling medical equipment associated with the therapy), including products to alleviate oxygen-therapy-induced chapped lips, dry mouth and nares (Bauters, Schandevyl and Laureys 2016). This is an area that requires further evaluation with regard to essential oils, either topically or via airborne diffusion. Aromatherapists working with patients on oxygen therapy should always check the oxygen safety policy related to their place of work.

Hydrosols

Hydrosols can be invaluable for the breathless patient. Generally, patients prefer a cool, well-ventilated environment with circulating air. Combining portable fans with cool hydrosol misting sprays directed at the face can be immensely soothing. Additionally, cold compresses soaked in hydrosol applied to the forehead, nape of the neck or the face can supplement the beneficial effect of fans. Useful options include *Rosa damascena* (rose), *Citrus aurantium var amara flos* (neroli), *Lavandula angustifolia* (lavender true), *Anthemis nobilis* (roman chamomile) or *Cupressus sempervirens* (cypress).

Dry oral mucosa exposed to supplemental oxygen therapy, or through mouth breathing, can be refreshed with oral rinses or ice-chips made with hydrosols. Useful options include *Mentha x piperita* (peppermint), *Origanum majorana* (sweet marjoram), *Satureja montana* (winter savory) or *Abies balsamea* (balsam fir). Refer also to the section on oral health in Chapter 11.

Working alongside patients with breathlessness

A basic understanding of the patient's illness and respiratory function is important. Often, patients have insufficient breath to provide the details. Prior liaison with the multi-disciplinary team (MDT) aids awareness of the underlying pathology, current treatment and medical intervention.

A calm, unhurried and mindful approach brings reassurance and a sense of security to the person with breathlessness. This includes knowing when to reach out with a caring touch, or when to simply sit and be present. It is an opportunity to observe and be alongside the patient, enabling them to invite conversation when they feel able and ready. Aligning yourself to match their slower, considered pace gives them a clear message of not being rushed. Speaking clearly, using shorter sentences and fewer questions, while allowing space for the patient to answer without interruption, provides an opportunity for the person to explore their thoughts and feelings.

Maintaining dignity

Of primary concern to many patients is the increasing loss of independence, and this can manifest not only in social isolation and associated depression, but also in worry about being a burden to others. Combined with the need for symptom relief and alleviation of psychological and spiritual distress are factors underpinning a patient's dignity (Chochinov *et al.* 2002). Practical interventions aimed at preserving dignity are discussed by Taylor (2007) and some examples are listed below. These can be integrated into clinical practice to offer the patient solutions to fulfilling simple activities independently, as well as an opportunity to practise breathing control.

- Dress and undress sitting down; take frequent rests
- Inhale to reach, exhale to bend down
- Put on footwear by crossing the leg at the knee, not bending
- Wear slip-on shoes and front-opening clothes
- Use a stool or chair in the shower
- Avoid very hot water
- Ensure that the bathroom is ventilated
- Wear a towelling robe after a bath or shower to absorb the moisture
- Dry shave in preference to wet shave to reduce prolonged arm movements
- Use an electric toothbrush and avoid strong mint toothpaste

- Remember to pause and pace yourself when eating and drinking as these require advanced breathing control
- Limit time spent speaking on the telephone; there are no visual clues for pacing
- Consider a walking aid, stick or rollator, to provide support and a means of pacing
- Use a self-propelled wheelchair for longer distances

Breathing control

Breathing control is central to breathlessness management. While most patients benefit from sessions with a physiotherapist, there are simple breathing techniques which can be utilized in clinical practice. Taylor (2007) encourages focus on extended exhalation, rather than deep-inhalation techniques which emphasize effort and frustration. By using calm instruction, patients are encouraged to extend their exhalation by simply sighing it out. Reflexively, inhalation will follow, in a less forceful way. Initially, this technique may feel counter-intuitive for patients, but will improve with practice and support, and as Taylor (2007, p.25) states, 'when mastered the effect can be dramatic'.

Readers are also referred to the work of Mackereth, Maycock and Tomlinson (2017) whose chapter 'Easing the Breathing Body' in their book offers exceptional, practical information regarding breathing control. This includes various practices, sniffing/huffing, nostril flaring, box-breathing, straw-breathing and the stretch-breathe-and-yawn technique.

Mindful Moist Mouth

Mouth-breathing is commonplace in these patients, which leads to a dry throat, heat in the body and breathlessness. Mackereth and Tomlinson (2014) developed a simple technique, Mindful Moist Mouth (MMM), where therapists can guide a patient, using mindfulness and imagery techniques, when swallowing water. Mentally tracking where the water touches the mouth and throat then how far the coolness tracks down into the body is a starting point to this extremely effective method. Mindful suspension of the water in the mouth and moving it around the entire mouth before swallowing helps expand their awareness. Finally, returning the patient's attention to how the mouth feels afterwards, and where the coolness has tracked, enhances awareness of the changed physical and relaxed psychological states.

Aromatherapy applications

Any aromatherapy intervention requires careful consideration and needs to be appropriate to the patient's priority of concern and within their physical capability, in addition to allowing for the cautions and contraindications as discussed previously. The most valuable method for breathlessness management is inhalation.

Warm humidified inhalation

The inhalation of warmed, humidified air is known to improve muco-ciliary clearance and decrease air trapping in the bronchus in patients with COPD (Rea *et al.* 2010). Simultaneously, it can also reduce pulse and respiratory rates in these patients when used in the early stages of breathlessness (Kawagoshi *et al.* 2018). A traditional method such as a steam bowl beneath a towel is too hot and claustrophobic for the breathless patient. Suitable alternatives include individual steam-inhalation devices, such as a Clearway®, or using a few drops of undiluted essential oil formulation in a ceramic dish inside the shower cubicle.

Another consideration which utilizes room temperature humidification is to combine essential oils with sodium chloride 0.9%, delivered through a nebulizer system, as described by Kerkhof-Knapp Hayes (2015). Although the question of essential oil dispersion is unclear, it is an interesting area for future evaluation. For patients with high odour acuity, nebulized hydrosols without essential oils are a pleasing alternative.

Aromatherapy inhaler sticks

Air movement is reported as a vital sensation for patients experiencing breathlessness. However, keeping windows and doors open may not be possible during the colder seasons or inner city living with high levels of air pollution. Therefore, an enhanced sensation of airflow can be produced via the cooling effect of menthol-rich essential oil vapours to activate respiratory TRPM8 ion channels, as previously discussed. Low-level essential oil formulation using personalized aromatherapy inhaler sticks offers the patient an intervention which requires minimal exertion, while at the same time optimizing quality of care and comfort. This is exampled in Case study 10.1.

In situations where breathing control is difficult and the patient is unable to co-ordinate nasal inhalation with exhalation via the mouth, a comfortable option is to sit quietly with the aromatherapy inhaler stick close enough to smell the aroma, and breathe for one to two minutes.

Alternately, Bioesse® aromapatches can be useful, or rollerball application of an essential oil blend can be administered to the chest/neck area if continuous low-level aromatherapy is acceptable to the patient and in the absence of supplemental oxygen.

Massage

Massage, using light strokes and shorter treatment times, may bring subjective relief to patients who can tolerate touch and are physically able to sit well supported on a massage chair. Non-oily cream is appropriate to those on supplemental oxygen.

Combinations

Other aromatherapy applications which minimize exertion for these patients include footbaths, compresses, or simple cold-air diffusion of essential oils for short periods.

It is worth remembering that patients with chronic breathlessness have often lived with the symptom for some time. They know their breathing limitations and have mastered what works best for them. Introducing new suggestions often requires a level of diplomacy when inviting the patient to consider other options. Timing is crucial here and experience teaches us to avoid overwhelming the patient with too many suggestions. Or indeed, 'overdoing' the session by trying to address too many issues at once. Less is always more!

CASE STUDY 10.1: ROYDON'S EXPERIENCE

Referral

Roydon, a 76-year-old man, was referred to the specialist palliative care team with chronic COPD. An aromatherapy referral was raised by the clinical nurses for assisted management of breathlessness and associated symptoms of anxiety and insomnia.

Background summary

In his younger life, Roydon enjoyed working in the hospitality industry; it suited his sociable personality, sharp sense of humour and strong family values. However, since diagnosis, he has become increasingly limited in his daily activities due to chronic breathlessness and is mostly confined to his home.

The house is equipped to meet his breathing limitations with the living area adapted to one level, although three steps up to the bathroom remains an insolvable challenge. He receives daily assistance with personal care. For the most part, Roydon spends his time in the lounge with views over the gardens, which he can visit using the rollator walking frame.

Personal goals

Familiar with Rongoā Māori (traditional Māori medicine), Roydon was open to aromatherapy intervention. His priorities of concern were to:

- ease the anxiety when preparing to move
- improve his breathing capacity
- enjoy a relaxed night's sleep.

Aromatherapy session

The first home visit was undertaken jointly with the referring specialist palliative care nurse. Roydon was sitting in his recliner chair trying to capture his breath and gestured for us to sit. His wife told us he had just finished showering and would need a few minutes to settle. While his wife updated the nurse about his medications, I quietly observed Roydon's breathing: the slightly cyanosed and pursed lips, as if sucking each breath through a straw; the short exhalation and rush to take another breath; his fingers gripping the arms of the recliner chair. A window was slightly open, allowing in-flow of the cooler winter air.

When he felt ready, he spoke in staccato-style sentences; the chronic struggle to breathe further evident in his tight neck musculature and barrel-shaped chest. He described how the mere thought of walking to the bathroom distressed him, causing him to worry about whether he would 'have enough puff' to make the few metres across the room plus the three steps. Usually, he would stop at the foot of the steps to catch his breath, although this intensified his anxiety, wondering whether he would regain sufficient breath to reach the bathroom in time.

In answer to my brief questions, Roydon took his time to express a dislike of medicinal smells and strong synthetic aromas, he had no known allergies, his olfactory acuity was good and he was willing to try the oils. At this point, he began speaking in longer sentences and was interested in my suggestions. The oils were selected for their known effects to ease respiratory distress and calm anxiety, fear and panic. Working with one drop of a single essential oil at a time, dried on a strip of tissue, I invited his thoughts on the aroma.

Santalum spicatum (sandalwood) was familiar to him with its woody, musky notes. He enjoyed it equally as much as *Boswellia carterii* (frankincense), describing a sense of peacefulness which he found reassuring. He chose both. *Mentha x piperita* (peppermint) came with a prior caution of drawing the tissue towards him slowly and at a distance when taking in the stronger aroma. Roydon was pleasantly surprised by the sensation it gave him of space within his nostrils, and how it made his breathing feel easier. His curiosity led to a fourth choice, *Agonis fragrans* (fragonia), where he found himself transported to the rugby pitch, describing a rustic mix of grass and mud, which comes from lunging for the ball and driving his body face down to slide across the pitch. When he opened his eyes, he looked alert and alive, smiling at the memory of activity.

His chosen oils were designed to support deep-level relaxation of the CNS, while simultaneously offering the sensation of increased air-flow by activating the TRPM8 receptor. The latter was achieved by combining menthol-rich *Mentha x piperita* (peppermint) and the oxide, 1,8 cineole in *Agonis fragrans* (fragonia). See Table 10.3.

Table 10.3: Roydon's aromatherapy intervention

Method of application	Botanical products used *Botanical name* (common name)	Amount used	Directions for use
Aromatherapy inhaler stick 'Breathe-easy'	*Santalum spicatum* (sandalwood)	2 drops	Patient-directed as required
	Agonis fragrans (fragonia)	3 drops	Hold the device as close as is comfortable and breathe normally for one to two minutes Use before getting up to walk, wait a few minutes for maximum effect
	Boswellia carterii (frankincense)	1 drop	
	Mentha x piperita (peppermint)	3 drops	
	Simmondsia chinensis (jojoba)	1ml	

Roydon quickly grasped the instructions of how to use the aromatherapy inhaler stick, breathing in his usual way for one to two minutes as he took in the aroma. Several minutes later, he excused himself and walked to the bathroom, managing the three steps without needing to stop to catch his breath. On his return, he seemed more agile and with a grin, said, 'I like the minty...more minty!'

Reflection

During Roydon's first session, the emphasis lay with collaboration in oil choices and supporting flexible use of the aromatherapy inhaler stick to suit his needs. In the subsequent follow-up visits, we worked with preventative strategies, such as anticipating the psychological distress of breathlessness prior to mobilizing, and breathing control using the aromatherapy inhaler stick for night-time anxiety. The ensuing sessions allowed for other suggestions to enhance breathing techniques.

CHAPTER 11

Common Gastrointestinal Symptoms in End-of-Life Care

Symptoms of the gastrointestinal tract are commonplace in patients with life-limiting illness and often a source of immense discomfort for the patient, which is distressing to their caregivers. This chapter considers the most prevalent symptoms where integrating aromatherapy approaches can offer considerable comfort:

- Oral health
- Nausea and vomiting in advanced cancer
- Bowel-related symptoms

ORAL HEALTH

Oral health is an important aspect of general well-being and is defined as 'multifaceted and includes the ability to speak, smile, smell, taste, touch, chew, swallow and convey a range of emotions through facial expressions with confidence and without pain, discomfort and disease of the craniofacial complex' (Glick *et al.* 2016, p.322). In the presence of advanced disease, where the patient's health is deteriorating, symptoms of the mouth are increasingly prevalent. Evidence prioritizes these as xerostomia (dry mouth), oral fungal infections and dysphagia, closely followed by mucositis, halitosis, taste alteration, orofacial pain and ulceration (Venkatasalu *et al.* 2020). Individually or in combination, these oral symptoms compromise the patient's quality of life, causing difficulties with eating, talking and being close to loved ones (Fischer *et al.* 2014; Rohr, Adams and Young 2010). Therefore, early diagnosis and treatment of oral health issues in these patients is critical.

Xerostomia

For more than two decades, research has verified xerostomia as the most prevalent and significant oral symptom in patients with advanced cancer (Hanchanale *et al.* 2015; Venkatasalu *et al.* 2020), affecting up to 77% of patients (Jobbins *et al.* 1992). Causes in this patient group are numerous and include the disease itself, age, dehydration, the direct effect of cancer treatments, pre-existing comorbidities such as Sjögren's disease and concurrent pharmacology (Hanchanale *et al.* 2015).

Patients are often prescribed large numbers of different medications, many of which possess anticholinergic properties, including opiates, benzodiazepines, anti-emetics and corticosteroids (Fleming, Craigs and Bennett 2020). Bronchodilators, antihistamines, decongestants and diuretics are also known to cause dry mouth (Agar *et al.* 2009). Sheehan *et al.* (2011) evaluated this 'anticholinergic load' of palliative pharmacology in 199 patients, where 60% received medication with recognized anticholinergic properties in the last 72 hours of life.

Among its key functions, saliva is vital for lubrication of food prior to swallowing and for its antibacterial action. Diminished salivary flow can lead to difficulties with chewing and swallowing as well as taste alteration, resulting in systemic malnutrition and weight loss. As such, xerostomia represents a serious problem for patients in end-of-life care, from general decline, increasing at each stage, through to actively dying (Chen and Kistler 2015). Prompt diagnosis and effective management is paramount.

Conventional management of xerostomia

Unfortunately, research-based treatment options for xerostomia are sparse, with low-quality evidence for artificial saliva, pilocarpine, chewing gum and acupuncture (Hanchanale *et al.* 2015). Standard oral care alleviates dryness in 80% of these patients (Nakajima 2017) and symptomatic relief can be achieved through lubricating the lips and oral mucosa (Kvalheim *et al.* 2016). To reduce an acidic oral environment, Lim (2018) advocates fluoride toothpaste as an essential part of oral care, in addition to topical agents aimed at lubricating the dry mucosa. These can be commercial over-the-counter products or home remedies, such as bicarbonate of soda mouthwash to alkalize and debride the oral cavity, or oral sprays of olive oil or plain water.

Patients tend to self-manage xerostomia by using combination approaches. Fleming *et al.* (2020) identified the most common as sipping drinks, sucking sweets, chewing gum, using toothpaste and mouthwashes alongside pharmacological aids such as salivary sprays and gels. Importantly, over half of the patients in this cross-sectional study (n=135) were also concerned about the mucosal dryness extending to their lips, throat and nasal passages and the impact this had on their ability to swallow, disturbing them throughout the day and waking them at night.

Oral infections

A persistently dry mouth predisposes the patient to dental caries, oral infections and candidiasis (Fleming *et al.* 2020). Oral infections are predominant in 46% of patients with advanced cancer, where the highest reported rates of 67% are in those with oral and maxillofacial disease (Xu *et al.* 2013). Treatments such as chemotherapy, radiotherapy or chemo-radiation for head and neck cancers increases the risk of developing oral infection. Chemotherapy-induced immunosuppression plays an important role in the pathogenesis of oral infection, while radiotherapy treatment can cause mucosal damage, mucositis and xerostomia, which leads to infection (Soysa, Samaranayake and Ellepola 2004).

Conventional management of oral infections

Xu *et al.* (2013) report fungal infections of *Candida albicans* and non-*albicans* species as the most common in this patient group. In their prospective observational study (n=850), candidiasis accounted for more than 52% of patients and is attributed to patients being unable to maintain adequate oral hygiene and nutritional intake. Single-dose fluconazole 150mg orally is reported as being therapeutically effective for most palliative patients with oral candidiasis (55/57 patients), with a significant reduction in the severity of symptoms (p<0.001) and few side-effects (Lagman *et al.* 2017).

Dysphagia

Swallowing difficulties are among the top three oral health problems experienced by these patients (Venkatasalu *et al.* 2020). Oropharyngeal dysphagia is primarily caused by site-specific head and neck cancers; altered anatomy resulting from surgical intervention or radiotherapy for head and neck cancer; chemoradiation-induced mucositis; xerostomia; medication adverse effects; poor oral hygiene and ill-fitting dentures (Langmore *et al.* 2009; Wilkinson, Codipilly and Wilfahrt 2021).

In their detailed account of dysphagia, Wilkinson *et al.* (2021) describe its varying presentations. Patients with oropharyngeal dysphagia often experience coughing, choking, nasal regurgitation, difficulty initiating a swallow, or needing to repeatedly swallow to clear food from the mouth. This may be accompanied by hoarseness of the voice. With oesophageal dysfunction, patients are able to start the swallow reflex but then experience the sensation of food becoming stuck in the oesophagus. Additionally, painful swallowing is indicative of an infective process such as candidiasis or viral oesophagitis.

Conventional management of dysphagia
For patients able to tolerate oral care, Lim (2018) advocates stringent oral hygiene (two to three times a day) involving cleaning of the teeth, tongue and hard palate, using a fluorinated (non-foaming) toothpaste applied with a paediatric toothbrush or gauze-covered finger; flossing or interdental brushes to remove debris between the teeth; alcohol-free oral rinses and a moisturizing ointment for the lips. Early intervention for oral infection is paramount, as is multi-disciplinary collaboration to educate patients and their families in nutrition and dietary modifications appropriate to the individual's situation (Langmore *et al.* 2009; Wilkinson *et al.* 2021).

Evidence-based oral care
Oral health clearly has a profound impact on a patient's overall well-being and is a vital part of holistic care. However, research continues to emphasize common oral symptoms, rather than evaluating the most appropriate ways to manage, improve and standardize oral care procedures. A proactive approach is needed to assess oral health as part of the patient's initial assessment, not only by nurses and clinicians but by other members of the multi-disciplinary team (MDT), including aromatherapists. Making oral health integral to the patient's routine follow-up minimizes the risk of care being missed or even disregarded, and reduces the ambiguity surrounding the point at which the patient is no longer able to manage their own oral care and requires caregiver intervention.

Aromatherapy for oral health in patients with cancer: Current clinical evidence

Clinical evidence for oral aromatherapy interventions in patients with cancer primarily rests with those receiving active treatments.

Aromatherapy for treatment-induced oral mucositis

Chemotherapy approaches and site-specific radiotherapy to the head and neck region can severely damage the delicate mucosal linings of the gastrointestinal tract causing pain, inflammation, ulceration and xerostomia of the buccal cavity, which often extends to the oesophagus. In patients immunocompromised by treatment side-effects, these symptoms can lead to severe oral infections. Researchers continue to evaluate natural sources with protective effects.

Maddocks-Jennings *et al.* (2009) compared an oral mouthwash, one drop each of essential oils of *Leptospermum scoparium* (manuka) and *Kunzea ericoides* (kanuka) in 10–15ml warm water, in patients at risk of radiation-induced oral mucositis, versus a control group receiving standard oral care (n=19). The treatment group were directed to swish the essential oil mouthwash for 15 seconds then spit out, repeat dilution and swallow. This was done 30 minutes before or after meals, smoking or drinking, plus immediately before and after each radiotherapy session. Compared with the control group, the essential oil regime alleviated pain, delayed onset and reduced occurrence of oral mucositis.

In a randomized controlled trial for patients experiencing chemotherapy-induced oral mucositis (n=56), Miranzadeh *et al.* (2015) compared the effects of a routine conventional mouthwash where 1400mg lidocaine, 224mg dexamethasone and 35 000mg/l sucralfate was added to a diphenhydramine solution (control group) versus the same conventional mouthwash in the treatment group with the addition of hydrosol of *Achillea millefolium* (yarrow) at a 50:50 ratio.

After cleaning their teeth, both groups were instructed to perform a three-minute gargle of 15ml of the allocated mouthwash, four times daily for 14 consecutive days. Significant reductions in oral mucositis were reported in the treatment group (p=0.001), with 71% completely healed by day 14.

Aromatherapy for treatment-induced xerostomia

Oral aromatherapy intervention has been evaluated in patients undergoing radioactive iodine therapy for cancer of the thyroid gland, where a common long-term problem is salivary gland dysfunction, rendering patients with xerostomia. In a double-blind RCT, Nakayama, Okizaki and Takahashi (2016) compared aromatherapy inhalation with a control of inhaled distilled water. While hospitalized, the aromatherapy group (n=35) received an essential oil mix of 1ml *Citrus limon* (lemon) combined with 0.5ml *Zingiber officinale* (ginger), with instructions to inhale for ten minutes prior to every meal for two consecutive weeks. The control group (n=36) inhaled distilled water as a placebo. Compared with the control group, increased saliva secretion was reported in patients using the aromatherapy inhalation.

Research interest is also escalating with citrus essential oils. Preliminary results of in-vitro studies conducted by Saiki *et al.* (2018) demonstrated the protective effects of d-limonene, a major constituent found in the epicarp of citrus peel. d-limonene protected the salivary cells of mice exposed to radiotherapy without altering the effectiveness of the treatment on cancer cells. In addition, oral d-limonene was shown to be readily transported into human salivary glands, which indicates positive potential for future clinical studies investigating citrus essential oils in the prevention of salivary gland damage and subsequent xerostomia.

Other resources, such as the dental literature, have an increasing number of publications and reviews related to essential oil use with xerostomia (Saiki *et al.* 2018), halitosis (Dobler, Runkel and Schmidts 2020) and general oral health (Rajesvari and Lakshmi 2013). Pre-clinical studies evaluating essential oils with antimicrobial efficacy related to oral biofilms were reviewed by Dobler *et al.* (2020). The most effective oils include *Cymbopogon citratus* (lemongrass), *Eucalyptus globulus* (blue gum eucalyptus), *Leptospermum scoparium* (manuka), *Melaleuca alternifolia* (tea tree), *Mentha x piperita* (peppermint), *Myrtus communis* (myrtle), *Origanum majorana* (sweet marjoram), *Coriandrum sativum* (coriander), *Satureja hortensis* (summer savory) and *Thymus vulgaris* (thyme). Further clinical studies are required.

The potential of aromatherapy

While the escalating interest in aromatherapy for oral health in patients with cancer is promising, the findings may not be generalizable to those with advanced disease. Deterioration in the patient's health and fragility of the oral mucosa require sensitive intervention with adjustment appropriate to the individual's needs.

Assessment from the patient's perspective

Venkatsalu *et al.'s* (2020) integrative review of 19 studies evaluating palliative oral symptoms highlights the adverse social and functional impact of the patient's experience. Increased feelings of shame, of being a patient rather than a person, of avoiding social contact, of loneliness and feeling less satisfied with life were among the causal factors of psychosocial distress reported by patients with xerostomia. Orofacial pain prevented patients from sharing and enjoying meals. Speech difficulties made it harder to engage in conversation, which limited their participation in social gatherings and reduced the enjoyment of mealtimes. Depression was found to be prevalent in these patients, particularly the elderly, where poor oral hygiene leads to halitosis and causes severe social withdrawal.

Oral care is an intimate aspect of well-being, and patients may not find it easy to disclose the difficulties experienced in maintaining their oral health. Aromatherapists are well placed to facilitate space and time for patients to comfortably share their story, which enables an opportunity to identify the presence of oral symptoms. These may not necessarily be visible, but a vigilant therapist will detect difficulties in talking or swallowing, or observe dry lips, a coated tongue or the presence of halitosis. Skilful communication will help the patient and caregivers to explore these observational findings and work towards a comprehensive oral assessment in conjunction with the patient's MDT.

Essential oils

Spiritual and psychosocial components

In oral palliation, where existential and psychosocial distress can be deeply felt, essential oils can be selected from those discussed in Chapters 5 and 6.

Xerostomia

For xerostomia, if the salivary glands are intact and undamaged, it is possible to enhance salivary function by integrating essential oils which are akin to food flavourings the patient recognizes, such as *Mentha x piperita* (peppermint), *Thymus vulgaris ct linalool* (thyme ct linalool), *Salvia rosmarinus* (rosemary), *Zingiber officinale* (ginger), *Citrus limon* (lemon), *Citrus bergamia* (bergamot), *Citrus aurantiifolia* (lime) and *Citrus sinensis* (sweet orange). See section *Aromatherapy applications* for recommended intervention.

Antimicrobial management

As explored previously, essential oils are a valuable option for oral antimicrobial management. Although clinical evidence in patients with advanced cancer is sparse, an RCT conducted by Kang, Na and Kim (2010) evaluated the effects of an essential oil mouthwash used by hospice in-patients against an oral saline rinse. The intervention group (n=22) used a 0.5% oral solution of essential oils of geranium, lavender, tea tree and peppermint (botanical names unspecified) in 500cc distilled water. The control group (n=21) used 0.9% sodium chloride solution. Both groups were instructed to mouth rinse for seven minutes, twice daily, for one week. The findings suggested an increase in oral comfort and a reduction in oral candidiasis in the intervention group.

Caution: Where undiluted essential oil mouthwashes make direct contact with the buccal mucosa during the rinsing period, caution is required. The mucosal lining of the oral cavity does not possess the same protective keratinized layer as that of the skin, thereby increasing its fragility and permeability. For this reason, Tisserand and Young (2014) advocate against oral ingestion or oral application of undiluted essential oils.

Importantly, essential oils with known irritant properties to the skin and mucosal membranes, such as oils rich in monoterpenic-aldehydes, specifically the constituent citral, should be used cautiously in this patient group and at a low-level concentration. Additionally, the phenolic-based oils are much stronger irritants to the oral mucosa and should not be used with these patients. Examples are shown in Table 11.1.

Safer options with equivalent antimicrobial and antifungal action include *Leptospermum scoparium* (manuka), *Kunzea ericoides* (kanuka), *Thymus vulgaris ct linalool* (thyme ct linalool), *Cymbopogon martinii* (palmarosa), *Commiphora myrrha* (myrrh), *Pelargonium graveolens* (geranium), *Citrus bergamia* (bergamot) and *Citrus limon* (lemon).

Table 11.1: Essential oils with irritant properties
to the skin and mucous membranes

Essential oils with irritant properties related to monoterpenic-aldehydes *Botanical name* (common name)	Essential oils with strong irritant properties related to phenolic components *Botanical name* (common name)
Cautionary use at low-level concentrations in this patient group	Caution: Not to be used for oral care
Cymbopogon citratus (lemongrass)	*Syzygium aromaticum* (clovebud)
Litsea cubeba (may chang)	*Satureja montana* (winter savory)
Melissa officinalis (melissa)	*Satureja hortensis* (summer savory)
Eucalyptus citriodora (lemon eucalyptus)	*Cinnamomum verum* (cinnamon leaf)
Backhousia citriodora (lemon myrtle)	*Origanum vulgare* (oregano)
Leptospermum petersonii (lemon tea tree)	*Thymus vulgaris* ct *carvacrol* and *thymol* (thyme ct carvacrol and thymol)

Base substances and dilution

An appropriate excipient is required to fully disperse essential oils and minimize the risk of mucosal irritation. Low-level essential oil concentration, starting at 0.5% and not exceeding 1%, can be achieved with fixed oils, such as *Simmondsia chinensis* (jojoba) which provides a light film that retains and attracts moisture, *Macadamia ternifolia* (macadamia) or a light *Olea europaea* (olive). The essential oil blend can be gently applied to the buccal mucosa following routine oral care as a spray, or using a finger wrapped in oil-soaked gauze to lubricate the oral spaces. For patients using interdental floss, coating the floss with the oil blend may enhance detailed antimicrobial care. Patients need to be advised not to eat or drink anything for 30 minutes afterwards. Such an approach is particularly effective in situations of oral candidiasis, infection or ulceration.

Alternately, Holmes (2019) recommends 0.5–1% essential oil concentration with a dispersant, for example, Solubol®. This can be further diluted with water, hydrosol or herbal tisane and used as an oral rinse and gargle.

Gel-based substances are another option. Kerkhof-Knapp Hayes (2015) advocates fresh *Aloe vera* gel and the fruit pulp of sea buckthorn which, when combined, forms a useful base substance for essential oils appropriate to the situation. This is particularly useful for dabbing directly onto ulcerated areas and for its additional antimicrobial action and cooling effect on the oral biofilm.

Hydrosols

For palliative oral care, personal clinical experience leads me to these fragrant co-products of essential oil distillation, particularly when undiluted essential oil mouth rinses are too potent for a mucosal lining that is fragile. Patients report less 'stinging' or 'burning' of the oral mucosa, and the immediate hydration of these delicate tissues brings considerable comfort, particularly to those experiencing xerostomia. Diluting hydrosols 50:50 with cooled, boiled water makes for an effective oral rinse or spray. Undiluted hydrosol can be frozen and used as ice-chips as often as required.

In a pilot study, where equal parts of hydrosols of *Satureja montana* (winter savory), *Laurus nobilis* (laurel leaf) and *Salvia officinalis* (sage) were used in palliative patients (n=24), Kovač (2017) reported increased oral hydration, comfort and taste, with reduced halitosis, ulceration, inflammation and candidiasis. The hydrosols were integral to the patients' oral care regime, used as a spray three to five times daily, or applied via sponge sticks to swab the oral cavity twice daily.

Choices are numerous and hydrosols can be used singly or in combination, depending on the individual's situation and their personal taste preference. Popular choices include *Thymus vulgaris ct linalool* (thyme ct linalool), *Mentha x piperita* (peppermint), *Satureja montana* (winter savory), *Salvia rosmarinus* (rosemary) and *Rosa damascena* (rose). In situations of mucosal inflammation, ulceration and oral infection, *Matricaria recutita* (german chamomile) and *Helichrysum italicum* (helichrysum) are unsurpassable (Kerkhof-Knapp Hayes 2015).

Aromatherapy applications

Hydrosol mouthwashes and 'as required' oral sprays can be supported by other essential oil interventions.

Inhalation

Prior to mealtimes, or at any other time of the day, simple aromatherapy inhalation can assist oral salivary flow for those experiencing xerostomia. Collaborative formulation with the patient determines their aroma preference, which can then be prepared as an aromatherapy inhaler stick or, for those with less dexterity, a Bioesse® aromapatch.

Lips and nares

Care of the lips and nares can easily be overlooked. Often in cases of xerostomia and in the active phases of dying, the lips can become sore and cracked, and the nares very dry. Re-moisturization of the lips can be achieved with a simple beeswax balm prepared with either cocoa or shea butter, or vegetable oil. A light application of *Aloe vera* gel, or a simple plain fixed oil, such as *Simmondsia chinensis* (jojoba), to the lips and nares can also restore comfort. However, oil-based substances are contraindicated in patients receiving supplemental oxygen therapy, as discussed in Chapter 10. In these situations, a serum or gel made from a hydrosol, or *Aloe vera* juice, thickened with Amigel® at a concentration of 0.2% (one part Amigel® to nine parts liquid), is a safe and effective option.

Massage
Among its many roles, the parasympathetic nervous system is responsible for rest, digestion and salivation. Where salivary glands are viable and intact, incorporating deep-level relaxation into the patient's care may be beneficial to salivary flow in those experiencing xerostomia. For the patient receiving end-of-life care, massage of the hands or feet is less demanding on their energy consumption.

Gentle, localized massage of the parotid glands, located bilaterally in the cheek area in front of the ears with a 'tail' extending over the lower jaw, may assist with increasing saliva production. Similarly, massaging the submandibular glands located beneath the jaw and tongue, and the sublingual glands located bilaterally beneath the jaw and closer to the chin, can also be effective. Massage of the facial musculature requires a qualified therapist, familiar with muscles of mastication such as the deep masseter muscles, as well as the salivary glands. Short-duration facial massage of between five and ten minutes can be deeply relaxing. Patients and caregivers can also be taught the simple massage techniques for salivary gland stimulation.

Compresses
In the event of massage not being suitable, warm aromatic compresses can be prepared and laid along the jaw line or gently pressed against the cheek to help enhance blood supply to the area, aid muscle relaxation and enhance salivary flow.

NAUSEA AND VOMITING IN ADVANCED CANCER
Cancer is often associated with unpleasant symptoms and distressing treatment side-effects. Among them, nausea and vomiting are commonly encountered by patients with advanced cancer, resulting in

weakness, weight loss and nutritional deficiency which can adversely affect their quality of life (Mannix 2006).

Traditionally, nausea and vomiting are thought to co-exist, although this is not always the case. Nausea may present independently (Singh, Yoon and Kuo 2016) and is often more disabling, long lasting and worse than vomiting (Stern, Koch and Andrews 2011). From my personal clinical experience, the term 'nausea' is unfamiliar to many patients, who tend to use phrases such as 'I feel queasy', 'I can't stomach anything' or 'I'm right off my food.' This may contribute to nausea being easily overlooked and consequently under-treated. Similarly, the term 'vomiting' is referred to by patients as 'being sick' or 'throwing up' and often used interchangeably to describe other problems, including regurgitation and expectoration. Successful management, therefore, begins with clarification of the nature and causal mechanisms involved.

The nature of nausea and vomiting

Nausea is described as an unpleasant feeling of the need to vomit and is often accompanied by autonomic symptoms including sweating, salivation, pallor and fear (Twycross *et al.* 2002). It is entirely subjective in nature and while it may precede emesis, the physical act of vomiting may not always occur. More often, nausea is of greater concern to patients because of its relentless nature.

In contrast, Twycross *et al.* (2002) describe vomiting as generally episodic, highly physical in nature and characterized by the forceful expulsion of gastric contents through the mouth, whereas retching, commonly known as 'heaving', is the repetitive contraction of abdominal musculature in preparation to evacuate stomach contents. For successful symptom management, Glare *et al.* (2011) advise distinguishing nausea and vomiting from other gastrointestinal symptoms, including regurgitation (reflux or oesophageal obstruction), rumination (eating disorder) and dyspepsia (recurrent pain or discomfort in the upper abdomen).

Patients with advanced cancer can experience increasing nausea and vomiting with disease progression and as death approaches (Glare *et al.* 2011). Clinical presentation is often complex with a variety of underlying causes, as shown in Table 11.2. Additionally, modern palliation often includes other concurrent disease-controlling treatments, such as chemotherapy and radiotherapy, and surgical interventions which may also incite nausea and vomiting.

Table 11.2: Chronic causes of nausea and vomiting in patients
with advanced cancer (Harris 2010; Glare *et al.* 2011)

Anatomic area	Underlying causal factors
Biochemical	Medication, e.g. opioids, chemotherapy agents, antibiotics Ischaemic bowel infection Metabolic, e.g. hypercalcaemia, hypernatraemia, uraemia, hyperglycaemia
Delayed gastric emptying	Medication, e.g. opioids, tricyclic anti-depressants Ascites, hepatomegaly, splenomegaly, autonomic dysfunction
Gastrointestinal	Bowel obstruction, radiotherapy-induced colitis, chemotherapy-induced
Cranial	Raised intracranial pressure, e.g. tumour, bleed, meningeal infiltration
Vestibular	Medication, e.g. opioids Vestibular neuritis, labyrinthitis
Cortical	Anxiety, anticipatory nausea, pain, sight, smell, taste

Emetic pathways
Vomiting

Vomiting is understood to arise from a complex reflex arc, co-ordinated in an area of the brainstem traditionally referred to as the 'vomiting centre' (VC). Rather than being a discrete centre, as originally thought, it is now considered a broader, inter-connecting neural network which extends throughout the medulla and is fully within the blood–brain barrier, where it receives afferent input from several other sources (Smith, Smith and Smith 2012; Twycross *et al.* 2002). This is shown in Figure 11.1.

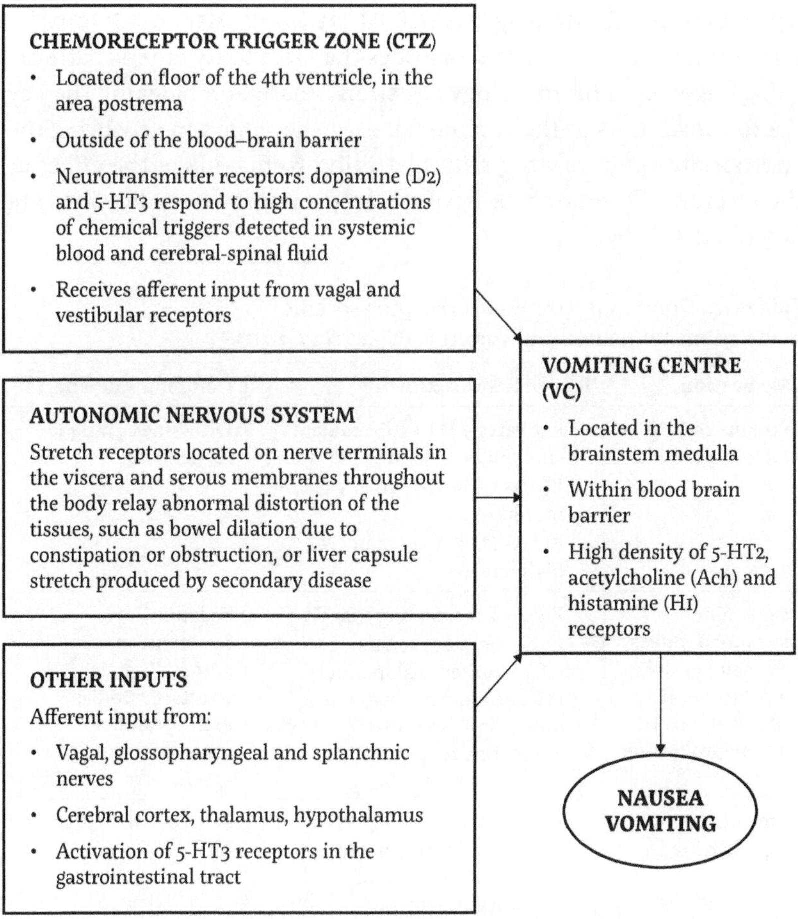

CHEMORECEPTOR TRIGGER ZONE (CTZ)

- Located on floor of the 4th ventricle, in the area postrema
- Outside of the blood–brain barrier
- Neurotransmitter receptors: dopamine (D2) and 5-HT3 respond to high concentrations of chemical triggers detected in systemic blood and cerebral-spinal fluid
- Receives afferent input from vagal and vestibular receptors

AUTONOMIC NERVOUS SYSTEM

Stretch receptors located on nerve terminals in the viscera and serous membranes throughout the body relay abnormal distortion of the tissues, such as bowel dilation due to constipation or obstruction, or liver capsule stretch produced by secondary disease

VOMITING CENTRE (VC)

- Located in the brainstem medulla
- Within blood brain barrier
- High density of 5-HT2, acetylcholine (Ach) and histamine (H1) receptors

OTHER INPUTS

Afferent input from:

- Vagal, glossopharyngeal and splanchnic nerves
- Cerebral cortex, thalamus, hypothalamus
- Activation of 5-HT3 receptors in the gastrointestinal tract

NAUSEA VOMITING

FIGURE 11.1: PHYSIOLOGICAL MECHANISMS OF NAUSEA AND VOMITING (SMITH *ET AL.* 2012; TWYCROSS *ET AL.* 2002)

Nausea

Despite the prevalence and importance of nausea, its causal mechanisms are relatively unknown. A review of studies investigating the pathophysiology of nausea describes a complex interplay between psychological states, the central nervous system (CNS), autonomic nervous system, gastric dysrhythmias and the endocrine system (Singh *et al.* 2016). Currently, it is not known which of these central regions initiate nausea and which are associated with the emotional aspects of the sensation to generate sympathetic nervous system involvement (Sanger and Andrews 2018).

Conventional management of nausea and vomiting

Careful clinical assessment establishes the most likely emetic pathway being triggered. Pharmacology selection is based on blocking the key neurotransmitters at the receptor sites, at the same time ensuring the appropriate route of drug administration to maximize the effect at the receptor. Commonly prescribed receptor-specific medications are described in Table 11.3.

Table 11.3: Commonly prescribed receptor-specific medications for nausea and vomiting (Glare *et al.* 2011)

Medication	Receptor site/action	Common side-effects
Prokinetics, e.g. metoclopramide	• Activates 5-HT4 to stimulate cholinergic system in gut wall • Blocks 5-HT3 to activate gastric motility • Blocks D2 receptors in CTZ in high doses	Drowsiness, fatigue, restlessness
Dopamine receptor agonists, e.g. haloperidol, prochlorperazine, chlorpromazine, levomepromazine	• Blocks D2 receptors in CTZ • Other broad-spectrum effects (except haloperidol) include blocking histaminic, muscarinic, serotonergic, alpha-adrenergic receptors	Sedation, hypotension, anticholinergic effects, dystonias, extrapyramidal symptoms and specifics for each drug
Anti-histamines, e.g. cyclizine	• Block H1 (histamine) receptors in VC, vestibular nucleus and CTZ to reduce mucosal secretory activity	Sedation and specifics for each drug
Selective 5-HT3 antagonist, e.g. ondansetron, granisetron	• Block central and peripheral 5-HT3 receptors on vagus nerve, enterochromaffin cells of peripheral enteric nervous system and in CTZ • Primarily used for chemotherapy-induced emesis • Limited use in palliative care to refractory cases as third-line treatment	Constipation, headache, sedation and specifics for each drug

Other useful adjuncts include corticosteroids, short-acting benzodiazepines (mainly in anticipatory nausea/vomiting), hyoscine, octreotide and cannabinoids (Glare *et al.* 2011).

Non-pharmacological interventions

The focus of research in this area largely surrounds behavioural approaches, acupressure and acupuncture. Techniques of guided imagery (Hosseini *et al.* 2016) and progressive muscle relaxation (PMR) to redirect a patient's focus of attention are effective adjuncts alongside prescribed anti-emetics in patients experiencing chemotherapy-induced emesis (Charalambous *et al.* 2016; Molassiotis *et al.* 2002).

Similarly, a meta-analysis conducted by Ezzo *et al.* (2005) found that acupuncture-point stimulation plus anti-emetic pharmacology significantly reduced acute chemotherapy-induced vomiting, but only marginally decreased acute nausea. Subsequent studies investigating acupuncture of the popular PC6 (Neiguan) and ST36 (Zusanli) acupoints (Hou *et al.* 2021) and acupressure of the PC6 acupoints using motion sickness bands (Lee and Frazier 2011), offer some degree of palliation for chemotherapy-induced symptoms. Further rigorous studies are required to determine dose, frequency and the number of acupoints for effective symptom management.

Massage

A systematic review conducted by Alves, Jardim and Gomes (2017) examined the benefits of massage in patients with cancer and identified four studies where massage exerted a significant immediate reduction in nausea: Ahles *et al.* (1999), Billhut, Bergbom and Stenes-Victorin (2007), Cassileth and Vickers (2004) and Grealish, Lomasney and Whiteman (2000). Additionally, the authors demonstrated evidence of the psychological benefits of massage, concluding that its relaxation effects help with rebalancing the body and a feeling of well-being.

Phytotherapy

Traditionally, *Zingiber officinale* (ginger) has long been the herbal intervention of choice to alleviate digestive symptoms, including nausea and vomiting. Studies investigating its anti-emetic efficacy generally relate to symptoms arising from motion sickness, pregnancy and post-operative situations (Ernst and Pittler 2000; Geiger 2005; Keating and Chez 2002; McParlin *et al.* 2016).

Within the oncology literature, *Zingiber officinale* (ginger) has shown promise as an adjunct in a variety of ways for chemotherapy-induced emesis. This includes: inhaling the essential oil vapours (Lua, Salihah and Mazlan 2015); drinking a fresh infusion made from a 10% decoction of *Zingiber officinale varietas rubrum* (red ginger) diluted in water

(Muthia, Wahyu and Dachriyanus 2013); and ingesting capsules containing a purified extract of ginger root (Ryan *et al.* 2012).

Partial antagonism of 5-HT3 receptors has been demonstrated in animal studies using menthol (Heimes *et al.* 2011), an active constituent of essential oil of *Mentha x piperita* (peppermint) traditionally known for its anti-emetic properties. While herbal infusions made with fresh mint leaves, root ginger or lemon slices are often advocated in situations of mild to moderate nausea, it is the concentrated volatile constituents of plant matter that are of greater research interest.

Aromatherapy in nausea and vomiting: Current clinical evidence

Increasingly, essential oils are being evaluated for their anti-emetic properties, primarily with post-operative nausea and vomiting, and chemotherapy-induced emesis. It is worth considering their use in these situations to determine their clinical effectiveness.

Post-operative nausea and vomiting (PONV)

Despite PONV being a common adverse reaction to all types of anaesthesia, conventional pharmacology is not always completely effective. For over a decade, researchers have examined the potential of essential oils alongside conventional anti-emetics, leading to a Cochrane review in 2012. A revised update, conducted by Hines *et al.* in 2018, set out to evaluate whether the therapeutic effectiveness of aromatherapy justifies its use in PONV.

Sixteen studies met the inclusion criteria, equating to a total of 1036 participants. Inhaled isopropyl alcohol (IPA) was the popular choice of researchers, as a single agent versus standard pharmacology, as well as a comparison with individual essential oils. Others evaluated combinations of essential oils, namely the proprietary blend QueaseEase®, which contains essential oils (botanical names unspecified) of peppermint, spearmint, ginger and lavender (Hodge, McCarthy and Pierce 2014; Kiberd *et al.* 2016), or a mixture of peppermint, spearmint, ginger and cardamom (Hunt *et al.* 2013). In all studies, the aromatics were administered via inhalation and compared with a placebo. Therapeutic effectiveness was reported in terms of nausea intensity and duration, use of rescue anti-emetics and patient satisfaction. Collectively, no differences were found in nausea intensity and severity between the groups.

However, of those who received essential oils, fewer required rescue anti-emetics for PONV.

A striking observation of this latest Cochrane review is that all the studies evaluated the efficacy of essential oils only during the post-operative period. Given that PONV is such a common reaction to anaesthesia and may be influenced by pre-operative anticipatory anxiety, it would seem prudent to engage earlier management strategies. An excellent example is demonstrated by anaesthesiologist Geiger (2005). Over a six-month period, he used a 5% blend of essential oil of *Zingiber officinale* (ginger) in *Vitis vinifera* (grapeseed), delivered nasocutaneously (via a rollerball applicator to the PC6 acupressure points) during the pre-operative period, then concurrently alongside multi-modal pharmacology. Integrating this combined 'anticipatory-approach', he observed that up to 80% of patients he considered at high risk of PONV did not report any symptoms of nausea, or require any additional intravenous pharmacology. Such observations are worthy of further formal evaluation.

Chemotherapy-induced nausea and vomiting (CINV)

Several studies have investigated the potential of essential oil of *Zingiber officinale* (ginger) for CINV, using a variety of applications. Marx *et al.* (2017) systematically reviewed seven RCTs of which five reported positive results with the essential oil of ginger. Unfortunately, small sample sizes, design shortfalls and an inability to determine a suitable dosage for CINV management hindered conclusive therapeutic findings.

When introducing personalized aromatherapy inhaler sticks into a large oncology centre, Stringer and Donald (2011) retrospectively evaluated essential oils of *Mentha x piperita* (peppermint) with *Citrus limon* (lemon) for their general therapeutic efficacy. Inhalation of this essential oil blend settled nausea in 47% of patients (n=123).

The essential oils of *Zingiber officinale* (ginger) and *Mentha x piperita* (peppermint) are promising adjuncts in the management of PONV and CINV. However, few studies have considered their anti-emetic potential in patients with advanced disease.

Aromatherapy for nausea and vomiting in advanced cancer

Gilligan (2005) reported nausea reduction in the majority of hospice in-patients (n=25) using single or combinations of *Pimpinella anisum* (aniseed), *Foeniculum vulgarae* (sweet fennel), *Anthemis nobilis* (roman chamomile) and *Mentha x piperita* (peppermint) essential oils alongside conventional pharmacology. Combinations were considered more effective than single-agent oils and were administered via abdominal compress, massage, personal air spritzer or air diffusion.

In conjunction with standard pharmacology, the inhaled essential oil of *Mentha x piperita* (peppermint) was effective in reducing nausea in 88% (n=8) of hospice in-patients (Seale 2012).

Currently, systematic reviews evaluating end-of-life symptom management are unable to identify any large-scale studies offering evidence-based, non-pharmacological approaches which alleviate nausea and vomiting (Glare *et al.* 2011; Walsh *et al.* 2017). However, this also extends to conventional pharmacology, where a recently updated Multinational Association of Supportive Care in Cancer/European Society for Medical Oncology (MASCC/ESMO) consensus-recommendation concluded that 'the evidence in this field is minimal with largely poor-quality trials or uncontrolled trials and case studies. The level of evidence in most studies is low' (Walsh *et al.* 2017, p.333). This raises the question of why nausea and vomiting management in this patient group is proving difficult and calls for further evaluation of integrative approaches such as aromatherapy.

The potential of aromatherapy

Predominantly, the clinical evidence is derived from studies investigating treatment-induced emesis, which may not always be relevant to the patient receiving palliative care, where the underlying causes of nausea and vomiting are often multi-factorial and relate to disease progression. Comprehensive assessment from the patient's perspective is a crucial starting point.

Assessment from the patient's perspective

Sensitive communication with open-ended questions and using the patient's words encourages exploration of their unique experience to distinguish between nausea, dyspepsia, vomiting, retching, regurgitation or combinations. Gaining insight into their prescribed medications, including what is actually being taken, and when, brings further clarity. This applies to other non-pharmacological approaches or 'home remedies' being used. A perspective of what the symptom experience means to the patient provides a clearer picture as to the frequency, intensity and associated emotional, spiritual and social distress involved. Collectively, this level of detailed information forms a foundation from which appropriate and effective intervention can be considered.

Essential oils

The distinct differences between the CNS pathways for nausea and vomiting directly influence essential oil selection. Vomiting is considered a motor response controlled within the brainstem (Santucci 2020). In contrast, nausea involves a range of sensory, cognitive, emotional and homeostatic dimensions mediated through the limbic system, which affect its severity (Balaban and Yates 2017). Crucially, essential oil selection hinges on a clear assessment of the patient's holistic experience, as exampled in Case studies 5.2 and 11.1.

The selection of essential oils needs to relate to the individual's priority of concern and aroma preference. Two or more oils, aimed at targeting various aspects of the CNS, are generally more effective and will minimize the risk of a negative odour association being created between a single-agent essential oil and nausea or vomiting. Emphasis rests with the patient choosing their own oils. Importantly, essential oils selected from those discussed in chapters relating to spiritual and emotional care (see Chapters 5 and 6) offer calming respite.

Zingiberaceae family

In-vivo studies consistently demonstrate that the pungent principles of *Zingiber officinale* (ginger), 6-, 8- and 10-gingerol, as well as 6-shogaol, possess a direct action on 5-HT3 receptors as well as a prokinetic effect, making it a potent anti-nausea/emetic (Abdel-Aziz *et al.* 2006; Marx *et al.* 2017; Pertz *et al.* 2011). Although the exact mechanisms have not been fully identified, a review of clinical in-vitro and in-vivo studies conducted by Marx *et al.* (2017) concluded that this class of bioactive compounds from the ginger rhizome possess multiple properties. These include: 5-HT3, substance P and Ach receptor antagonism; anti-inflammatory properties; and increased gastrointestinal motility and gastric emptying rates.

For clinical use, Kerkhof (2018) makes an important distinction between extraction processes of the ginger rhizome, where these pungent principles are dominant in carbon dioxide extraction but not in the distilled essential oil. Therefore, *Zingiber officinale* (ginger) CO_2-total extract is an important oil of choice for patients experiencing nausea and vomiting, particularly related to gastroparesis and opioid-induced constipation.

Also within the Zingiberaceae family, *Elettaria cardamomum* (cardamom) has long been valued for its digestive and carminative properties. Comprised largely of 1,8-cineole and α-terpinyl acetate, with small amounts of limonene and α-terpineol, its anti-emetic properties are credited to traces of borneol, known to inhibit acetylcholine pathways (Cabo *et al.* 1986). *Elettaria cardamomum*'s (cardamom) time-revered antispasmodic properties, which are specific to the gastrointestinal tract in reducing pain, flatulence and colonic spasm (Schnaubelt 1998), make it a valuable option.

Citrus oils
Given their fresh, uplifting notes, citrus-derived essential oils are understandably a popular choice and reported by researchers as being effective in the management of cancer-related nausea (Buckle 2015; Price and Price 2012; Stringer and Donald 2011). A review of studies examining the neuro-pharmacological properties of essential oils attributes the anxiolytic and anti-depressant-like activity of *Citrus limon* (lemon), *Citrus sinensis* (sweet orange) and *Citrus aurantium var amara flos* (neroli) to their direct action on 5-HT neurones (Wang and Heinbockel 2018). Considering that the serotenergic system is largely involved in the mechanism of nausea and vomiting, it would seem reasonable to consider citrus essential oils in the overall formulation.

Hydrosols
Sensory innervation of the taste receptors by the cranial nerves (vagus, glossopharyngeal and facial) is in close proximity to the VC and CTZ. As such, taste alteration, xerostomia, oral infections and ulceration resulting from advancing illness and deterioration frequently contribute to symptoms of nausea and/or vomiting in this patient group. A selection of hydrosols (see section *Oral health*), used as an oral rinse/spray or ice-chips, offers hydration and a gentle measure of care. Where altered taste sensation or anticipatory nausea is an issue, frequent changes of hydrosol formulations may be required.

Aromatherapy applications
Inhalation
Aromatherapy inhalation offers direct and rapid access to the CNS via structures of the limbic system, while minimizing gastrointestinal

disturbance. Most effective are aromatherapy inhaler sticks (Dyer *et al.* 2016; Stringer and Donald 2011) and nasocutaneous application via rollerball applicators (Geiger 2005). Other approaches include Bioesse® aromapatches and nasal clips, which have proved useful for managing acute procedural anxiety (Lewis 2018) and offer potential for this patient group with anticipatory symptoms.

Massage
For some patients, incorporating massage, especially foot reflexology or massage of individual body areas, such as the scalp, face, neck and shoulders, or hands, can be deeply relaxing. Calming sympathetic nervous system activity is particularly relevant for patients where anxiety, fear, stress and panic underpin symptoms of nausea and vomiting, as shown in Case study 5.2: Roger's experience.

Compresses
Topical application of cool compresses soaked in hydrosol can soothe the patient experiencing autonomic nervous system responses to nausea. These can be applied to the forehead or nape of the neck.

Combination approaches
Odour-conditioning techniques which combine aromatherapy inhalation with guided imagery or PMR is a personal intervention of choice for these patients. Quiet aromatic inhalation of this nature is particularly useful for patients whose symptoms are persistent, where they feel depleted of energy, exhausted and emotionally fragile, or in situations of intractable and chronic nausea where tender respite is needed. This combination can be undertaken at any time and anywhere, with the added advantage of involving family members, friends or caregivers who are willing to calmly participate.

Further evaluation is needed in these patients to determine the most valuable methods of application and whether the beneficial effects can be extended with essential oils.

CASE STUDY 11.1: JOHNSON'S EXPERIENCE

Referral
Following a 12-month history of advanced prostate cancer, Johnson was referred to the specialist palliative care team with deteriorating health.

Despite a complex medication regime, he continued to experience nausea and vomiting. Referral for aromatherapy intervention was made by the hospice medical director.

Background summary

For 12 months, this gentle Māori elder received hormone therapy as conservative management of his advanced prostate cancer, in addition to a complex drug regime, 're-purposing for cancer prevention'. The 're-purposing regime' amounted to a total of nine separate medications.

Johnson presented with decreasing appetite and weight loss for which the specialist palliative care team had put in place a broad anti-emetic regime, together with prescribed pain relief and supplemental oxygen therapy at home for episodes of breathlessness. Including the 're-purposing regime', the polypharmacy was considerable.

Personal goals

Familiar with Rongoā Māori (traditional Māori medicine), Johnson was open to aromatherapy intervention. His priority of concern was to take his wife to their favourite cafe and share cake and coffee like they used too.

Aromatherapy session

Despite his frailty, Johnson walked proudly into the therapy room at the hospice day centre, holding a beautifully carved walking stick in one hand and accompanied by his lovely wife. Johnson was open to considering other options because his primary concern was to be able to taste and enjoy food again, which invited further exploration.

On gentle enquiry, Johnson spoke of his love of food, particularly how a simple meal or cup of coffee paved the way to unite families, friends and communities. Now though, these social 'get-togethers' had completely changed, because food tasted bland and even the texture was different. Carefully, we broke this down to explore whether this was a particular food, or all food types. He said that most food 'balled' in his mouth. When I asked what this term meant, he described how a piece of food would immediately roll into a dry ball inside his mouth. Initially, this would trigger a cough, sometimes making him breathless, which then made him feel 'queasy'. If he did not manually remove the ball of food in time, in his words, 'I'd throw it back up.'

On inspection, the oral mucosa was dry with no signs of candidiasis, although there was evidence of dental caries. Clearly, he was not producing enough saliva to trigger enzymatic action and activate oral digestion. Consequently, food was rolling into a hard, dry ball which he struggled to expel, exacerbating cough, breathlessness, nausea and vomiting.

We began by discussing several practical measures aimed at adding moisture to his food, including meals with sauces or gravies; yoghurt with his favourite fruits; sucking frozen blueberries or pieces of fresh/tinned pineapple to cleanse and refresh the palate; and avoiding salty, dry foods. Other suggestions included a review of his medication with the hospice medical director to minimize polypharmacy and drugs with anticholinergic effects, which could be contributing to his xerostomia. Johnson also agreed to visit a dental hygienist.

While these were set in motion, we discussed aromatherapy interventions, working together to determine what would be most effective. As outlined in Table 11.4, hydrosols were used to increase oral hydration. An aromatherapy inhaler stick was prepared which utilized the prokinetic and anti-emetic properties of *Zingiber officinale* (ginger) CO_2-total extract; plus, the known anxiolytic and anti-depressant effects of the citrus oils and their direct action on serotonin 5-HT neurones.

Table 11.4: Johnson's aromatherapy interventions

Method of application	Botanical products used *Botanical name (common name)*	Amount used	Directions for use
Oral hydrosol spray and rinse	*Mentha x piperita* (peppermint) *Thymus vulgaris ct linalool* (thyme ct linalool)	Equal parts 1:1 hydrosol Dilution 50% with cool boiled water	Patient-directed *Oral spray:* use prior to mealtimes and as required day or night *Oral rinse:* 10ml three times daily after meals
	Mentha x piperita (peppermint)	Undiluted hydrosol	Prepare ice-chips. Suck as often as required
Aromatherapy inhaler stick	*Zingiber officinale* (ginger) CO_2-total extract *Citrus limon* (lemon) *Citrus bergamia* (bergamot) *Simmondsia chinensis* (jojoba)	4 drops 4 drops 1 drop 1ml	Patient-directed Inhale 4–8 breath cycles at each use, four times daily. Plus, 1–3 breath cycles as required day and/or night

Within 48 hours, Johnson's wife reported that he was connecting well with the aromatherapy products, there had been no further nausea, he had stopped the supplemental oxygen therapy and his pain control had improved. An appointment was organized with the dental hygienist.

Two weeks later, Johnson reported that his taste sensation was recovering, and he was enjoying small meals. He continued to use the oral hydrosol spray and aromatherapy inhaler stick while adjustments were being made to his medications. Most importantly, Johnson announced that he had taken his wife to their favourite cafe, where they had shared cake and coffee. He had been able to taste everything and spoke of how important it was for him to be able fulfil his goal and enjoy the time with his wife.

Reflection

The crucial starting point was to understand the symptoms of nausea and vomiting from Johnson's perspective. Combining active listening skills with reflection of Johnson's terminology and clarification of his words (such as the term 'balling') provided intimate insight into his experience. Listening offered a greater understanding of the challenges he faced while bringing us closer to the underlying causal possibilities.

All too often, patients are disempowered along the illness trajectory, where their normal routines are infiltrated by a clinical focus on disease and pharmacological symptom management. Here, Johnson was able to explore the emotional, social and spiritual importance of food in his life, which led to an achievable goal, a highlight of his everyday living.

The experience of symptoms in a person with life-limiting illness differs considerably to that of a healthy individual. As therapists, it is crucial to understand the physiology of the symptom within its holistic context. Otherwise, we too run the risk of falling into the same trap as the training of our healthcare colleagues, where we will simply reach for an essential oil matched to the symptom. In this case, we would have missed all the other contributory factors of poor dental hygiene, polypharmacy, induced anticholinergic side-effects of prescribed medication, plus the associated emotional, social and spiritual distress this was causing.

BOWEL-RELATED SYMPTOMS

Among the most common gastrointestinal symptoms in patients with life-limiting illness are those related to the bowel. Constipation and diarrhoea affect a large proportion of these patients, arising from primary disease, side-effects of treatment or prescribed medication. Such symptoms are prevalent, often persistent and both adversely affect the patient's quality of life. This section will consider each symptom within the holistic context of patient care and the potential of aromatherapy.

Constipation

Defined as a slow transit of faeces through the large bowel, constipation results in infrequent, difficult or incomplete bowel evacuation, often accompanied by pain and discomfort with the passage of dry, hard and sometimes bulky stools (Candy *et al.* 2011; Larkin *et al.* 2018). Within palliative care, Candy *et al.* (2015) reported the prevalence of constipation ranging between 18 and 90%, which is dependent on whether the primary disease is malignant or non-malignant, and increases substantially in patients receiving prescribed opioids, and the elderly.

Common causes

The underlying causes of constipation in patients with advanced cancer are multiple and typically relate to functional, organic and pharmacological factors (Larkin *et al.* 2018).

Functional factors

- *Dietary:* low-fibre diet, anorexia, reduced food and fluid intake
- *Environmental:* lack of privacy, need for assistance, cultural
- *Other:* inactivity, age, depression, sedation

Organic factors

- *Metabolic:* dehydration, hypercalcaemia, hypokalaemia, uraemia, diabetes mellitus, hypothyroidism
- *Neuromuscular disorders:* myopathy
- *Neurological disorders:* autonomic dysfunction, spinal or cerebral tumours, spinal cord involvement
- *Structural issues:* abdominal or pelvic mass, radiation fibrosis, peritoneal carcinomatosis
- *Pain:* cancer pain, bone pain, anorectal pain

Pharmacological

- *Pharmacological:* opioids, antacids, antitussives, anti-depressants, anti-emetics, neuroleptics, iron, diuretics, anticholinergics and chemotherapeutic agents

The nature of constipation

In a qualitative exploration of the views of patients, caregivers and health-care professionals regarding constipation within palliative care, Hasson *et al.* (2019) identified distinct differences. Healthcare professionals primarily focus on the physical aspects of bowel movements and their pharmacological management, while patients and caregivers describe a complex symptom with physical, emotional and social implications. Patients report physical bloating, abdominal pain, cramps, reduced appetite, rectal bleeding, tearing and haemorrhoids. Emotionally, they describe dread and anxiety at the thought of visiting the toilet and embarrassment caused by frequent trips to the bathroom with no result. Socially, there is a sense of not wanting to leave the house because of the need to be within close proximity of a toilet. Additionally, persistent anxiety and the physical demand of getting to and from the bathroom is fatiguing and of great concern to these patients. Constipation causes considerable suffering, and yet it remains poorly recognized and inadequately treated.

Conventional management of constipation

While disease progression impacts a patient's lifestyle rendering them at risk of developing constipation, researchers agree that in this patient group, constipation is predominantly medication-induced (Aretin 2021; Candy *et al.* 2015; Hasson *et al.* 2019). Generally, first-line approaches are pharmacological, using laxatives.

Oral laxatives

Laxatives are designed to directly soften faecal matter, or increase peristaltic stimulation, or both. In a review of common laxatives used in this patient group, Candy *et al.* (2015) list stimulant preparations such as bisacodyl, sodium picosulphate, and those containing senna or wheat bran, as laxatives which increase propulsive colonic motility. Osmotic laxatives, for example lactulose, increase water content in the colon to soften stools and stimulate peristalsis. Bulk-forming laxatives involve absorption of large amounts of fluids and are deemed unsuitable for patients in palliative care, where achieving sufficient hydration for bowel activity is not always possible.

Peripherally acting mu-opioid receptor antagonists (PAMORAs)

The aim of PAMORAs is to block peripherally located opioid receptors responsible for opioid-induced constipation, while simultaneously sparing the centrally mediated analgesic effects of opioids by not crossing the blood brain barrier. Methylnaltrexone, an injectable PAMORA, is effective in inducing laxation in this patient group where conventional laxatives have failed (Candy *et al.* 2011). Oral forms of PAMORAs have subsequently been developed.

Suppositories and enemas

On digital examination, in the event of a full rectum, suppositories and enemas are a first-line approach. They are designed to soften faecal impaction, and Larkin *et al.* (2018) describes how suppositories also stimulate rectal motility, are quick acting and often effective. Common active ingredients include glycerine, bisacodyl oxyphenisatin and CO_2-releasing compounds, although there are no studies evaluating their effectiveness in patients with advanced cancer. If oral laxatives are ineffective after several days, enemas are often used, although administration carries various contraindications in this patient group, including the risk of perforating the bowel wall (Larkin *et al.* 2018).

Insufficient evidence is available to determine which laxatives are more effective than others in this patient group, or cause fewer adverse effects (Candy *et al.* 2015). These gaps in clinical research were also identified by Muldrew *et al.* (2018), who further highlighted the lack of a standard definition of constipation, an absence of the patient's subjective experience, subjective and objective methods of assessment, as well as non-pharmacological approaches for constipation management in patients receiving specialist palliative care.

Non-pharmacological interventions for constipation

Evidence in support of non-pharmacological approaches in patients with cancer is meagre and largely derived from lifestyle modifications used in healthy general populations.

Lifestyle modifications

Increased dietary fibre, oral fluids and exercise are central to constipation management in healthy individuals. However, in the palliative setting these may not be effective or even possible. In a comprehensive evaluation of constipation management in patients with cancer, Wickham (2017) pragmatically discusses the limited benefit of recommending fibre and oral fluids to the patient with advanced disease. Pre-existing comorbidities, such as anorexia and dehydration, and the severity of constipation in someone taking opioid analgesia, renders increased fibre and fluids counterproductive.

Abdominal massage

Physiologically, abdominal massage has the capacity to increase gastric motility, shorten intestinal transit time, increase rectal loading, relax sphincters and generally enhance abdominal comfort (Wickham 2017). As an adjuvant intervention, it is reported as being effective in a variety of patient groups, including the elderly, those with spinal cord injury, and post-operative ileus and palliative care patients (Sinclair 2011).

Specific to patients with opioid-induced constipation (OIC), Yildirim, Can and Talu (2019) randomized 204 patients with mixed cancer and non-cancer diagnoses into either an experimental group to receive abdominal massage or a control group of best standard practice. Those in the experimental group were instructed in a 15-minute abdominal self-massage and continued this twice daily, after breakfast and dinner, for four weeks. The incidence of constipation was significantly lower in the experimental group ($p<0.001$) and stool consistency, straining, incomplete evacuation and increased number of defaecations were all improved in the experimental group compared with the control group. Across a five-week period, a significant decrease in severity of constipation and straining was reported in the experimental group, together with a decrease in the feeling of fullness in the rectum, severity of gas and pain. Importantly, the authors observed how patients in the experimental group found massage relaxing and were eager to be involved in their own self-care.

Other complementary approaches

Wang and Yin (2015) reviewed various complementary approaches used to manage chronic constipation, including acupuncture, moxibustion, abdominal massage and herbal medicine. While acupuncture and herbal medicine showed promising results for constipation relief, the authors advocated further well-designed studies to determine therapeutic efficacy in all modalities.

ACUPRESSURE

In addition to routine bowel care, Wang *et al.* (2019) conducted a non-randomized study of hospice in-patients with varying cancer diagnoses experiencing constipation (n=30). All participants received an eight-minute acupressure treatment, daily, for three consecutive days utilizing three acupoints: Zhongwan (CV12), Guanyuan (CV4) and Tianshu (ST25). Significant improvements were observed in straining during defaecation (p<0.001), sensation of incomplete evacuation (p<0.001), comfort levels during defaecation (p<0.001) and colonic motility (p<0.001).

ABDOMINAL AQUACARE

Described by Kerkhof-Knapp Hayes (2015, p.289) as 'the number 1 most effective non-pharmacological intervention', abdominal aquacare is a simple method of cool abdominal washing. The aim is to exert an intense effect on the relaxation of the intestines through vasodilation rather than innervation of the intestinal wall. Hand towels or flannel gloves soaked in cool water (22 ° C) are lightly, but confidently, applied to the abdomen using circular 'washing' movements around the umbilicus, in a clockwise direction for 15–20 uninterrupted circles (approximately one minute). This is repeated and the patient left to rest to allow the internal processes of 're-warming' to take place. Kerkhof-Knapp Hayes (2015) assures a good effect in patients experiencing chronic constipation. Clinical evaluation would be invaluable in this patient group.

Aromatherapy for constipation management: Current clinical evidence

Few studies have assessed the effects of incorporating essential oils into abdominal massage for constipation management in this patient cohort. An RCT conducted by Kim *et al.* (2005) investigated aromatherapy abdominal massage versus plain oil massage in a group of elderly patients. Unfortunately, the full publication is not available in English, making it difficult to interpret how effective essential oils of rosemary, lemon and peppermint (botanical names unspecified), excipient and dilution unknown, were as an integrative intervention.

In an RCT conducted by Lai *et al.* (2011), a selection of essential oils of bitter orange, black pepper, rosemary and patchouli (botanical names unspecified) were used in patients with advanced cancer experiencing constipation. Dilution was made in olive oil (percentage unknown). Patients entering the study were randomized to receive either an aromatherapy abdominal massage, plain oil abdominal massage or standard care. The authors reported improvements in physical and support domains of quality of life together with alleviation of constipation in the aromatherapy group.

The potential of aromatherapy

Constipation is often multi-causal in patients with advanced cancer, particularly in patients commencing opioid analgesia where constipation is a major side-effect with little evidence to guide clinical intervention, either pharmacologically or non-pharmacologically. Anticipating the symptom, by starting prophylactic management as early as possible, is crucial. Combination approaches seem the most prudent way forward, although there are several factors to consider in order to achieve successful intervention.

Assessment from the patient's perspective

In a qualitative evaluation conducted by Hasson *et al.* (2019), patients reported that normalizing conversations regarding bowel function were crucial to their understanding of the symptom and what to expect. It also helped to raise discussion about self-management and how to effectively integrate their own strategies with the support of their MDT. Initiating such conversations informed the patient that bowel issues were equally as important as any other symptom and helped reduce the anxiety and fear that many patients experience. Open, honest conversation regarding the patient's experience of constipation, how this affects them emotionally, socially, spiritually and physically, together with what they find effective in their day-to-day management, is a fundamental starting point for any intervention.

PSYCHOLOGICAL

Dhingra *et al.* (2013) identified that in patients with advanced cancer (n=169), depression and increased levels of anxiety are directly associated with constipation. This is to the extent that patients experience internal conflict when weighing up the daily discomfort and distress of constipation against the reason for taking opioids. It was also discovered that patients incorrectly believe that dietary changes are sufficient to manage this form of constipation and that opioid-induced constipation is a sign of rapidly declining health.

The patient's psychological experience of constipation is paramount to any assessment. It may not be achievable in one session and requires the input of the MDT working cohesively. Interventions, both pharmacological and non-pharmacological, must be considered in line with the patient's wishes.

Essential oils

Given the adverse impact of constipation spiritually and psychosocially in this patient group, it is prudent to consider essential oils which support these aspects of well-being (see Chapters 5 and 6). Encouraging the patient to take time for relaxation using aromatherapy interventions can alleviate considerable anxiety and distress which is associated with the pain of constipation and the discomfort of laxative use.

Aromatherapy applications

'When we rest, we digest' is a powerful phrase which, for some patients, reinforces an intimate connection with their digestive function. Educating patients and caregivers in one or two simple aromatherapy interventions can be extremely empowering.

INHALATION

Aromatherapy inhaler sticks are invaluable for these patients, where they can be used at the patient's convenience. Gentle breath cycles, as described in Chapter 3, can be combined with abdominal self-massage, or with simple relaxation after meals, to enhance the therapeutic benefit.

MASSAGE

Abdominal massage can be easily taught, is non-invasive, free from harmful side-effects, cost-effective (McClurg and Lowe-Strong 2011) and, in palliative patients, has a favourable physiological and psychological impact (Preece *et al.* 2002). Guiding patients and their caregivers through a gentle massage routine, using a plain fixed oil, such as *Simmondsia chinensis* (jojoba) or *Prunus amygdalus dulcis* (sweet almond), which could also include an essential oil of the patient's choice, allows the patient time to connect with total-body relaxation. Mackereth and Maycock (2017, p.111) describe a simple 'I Love You' routine for abdominal self-massage by the patient.

Replication of the Yildirim *et al.* (2019) study would be invaluable for these patients at the onset of opioid medication, or early in their transition into palliative care. This would determine the effectiveness of abdominal massage and the length of time it takes for the bowel to become receptive to such regular assistance, and establish whether therapeutic effectiveness is enhanced with the addition of essential oils.

COMPRESSES

Cool abdominal washing has been described earlier. For the patient who prefers warmth as a digestive stimulant, a warm compress passively supplies heat to the deeper abdominal tissues, offering localized comfort and general relaxation to the bowel. The addition of hydrosols brings an olfactory component which can help to further relax the patient.

AROMATIC FOOTBATHS

Creating a soothing space where the patient can enjoy the deep-level relaxation that comes with a warm aromatic footbath can be very restorative. This can be combined with foot reflexology using the reflex points of the colonic tract to aid gastric motility.

Evaluation of all interventions is central to the success of constipation management. To achieve clarity, this must involve follow-up discussions with the patient about their constipation experience and include any self-adjustment of their prescribed pain relief. Inviting the patient to maintain a bowel journal can be extremely useful.

Diarrhoea

Defined as the urgent passage of frequent loose stools (or more frequent than is normal for the patient), diarrhoea in patients with advanced cancer can adversely impact quality of life and social functioning (Aretin 2021). The prevalence of diarrhoea in patients with advanced cancer is not accurately established, although is known to be less common than constipation and is estimated to affect less than 10% of this patient group (Bossi *et al.* 2018).

Common causes

Clinical guidelines produced by ESMO (Bossi *et al.* 2018) identify the common causes of diarrhoea in patients with cancer, including:

- *Cancer-related:* some cancers are associated with the symptom of diarrhoea, including colorectal, carcinoid tumours, lymphoma, medullary carcinoma of the thyroid, pancreatic tumours causing bile malabsorption and pheochromocytoma
- *Chemotherapy-induced:* chemotherapy agents known to induce diarrhoea include 5-fluouracil, irinotecan, capecitabine, taxanes, anthracyclines, platinum salts

- *Site-specific radiotherapy:* widespread pelvic or abdominal radiotherapy
- *Targeted therapy-induced*
- *Immunotherapy-induced*
- *Hormonal therapy-induced*
- *Gastrointestinal infection,* commonly *Clostridium difficile*
- *Other causes,* such as enteral feeding, coeliac plexus block, gastrointestinal surgeries

For the most part, the above causes are related to active forms of cancer treatment. In patients with advanced stage disease who are not receiving oncological therapies, faecal impaction, partial bowel obstruction, malabsorption (e.g. steatorrhea), previous gastrointestinal surgery, fistulae or tumours reducing absorptive surfaces, excessive intake of laxatives and extreme anxiety are also common causes of diarrhoea (Bossi *et al.* 2018).

Conventional management of diarrhoea

Fundamentally, basic management of diarrhoea surrounds a comprehensive assessment of the symptom to determine the underlying cause and administer appropriate treatment based on the results. Infective causes require immediate intervention to minimize cross-infection, where patients are nursed in isolation until a conclusive diagnosis is established.

Rehydration is crucial and the route is dependent on the severity of the diarrhoea, the amount of fluid loss and the well-being of the patient. The ESMO guidelines (Bossi *et al.* 2018) advocate oral hydration for mild forms of diarrhoea, often with the use of oral rehydration solutions. In more severe situations, where dehydration is symptomatic, intravenous fluid and electrolyte replacement is preferable with careful monitoring. Pharmacological intervention in the form of anti-diarrhoeal agents, such as the opioid receptor agonist loperamide, is ultimately the first-line medication, which can extend to other opioids, including tincture of opium, morphine or codeine. In cases where loperamide is insufficient, the addition of octreotide is recommended, although Aretin (2021) cautions as to the anticholinergic side-effects when intensifying therapies, which can lead to a dry mouth that can be discomforting to many palliative patients.

Non-pharmacological approaches

Rehydration and pharmacological intervention are the primary principles of diarrhoea management in this patient group. However, patients
can easily suffer acute electrolyte imbalance, particularly hypokalaemia
and often a transient lactase deficiency with lactose malabsorption.
Cherney (2008) advises avoidance of milk products.

The ESMO guidelines (Bossi *et al.* 2018, p.iv138) advocate that 'mod-
ification of the diet is not recommended for prophylactic purposes but
can be useful when the patient is developing diarrhoea'. Recommendations are for spices such as chilli, and consumption of coffee and alcohol,
to be avoided during acute episodes of diarrhoea, or at least limited.
Nutritional support through a qualified dietitian is also advised.

Probiotics are another approach which has been assessed in the
prevention of radiotherapy-induced diarrhoea. In a review of RCTs
demonstrating the efficacy of probiotics in radiotherapy-induced diarrhoea, Can (2013, p.267) concluded that probiotics improved the patient's
status; however, the safety and efficacy of specific probiotics need to be
evaluated through further research.

The potential of aromatherapy

Diarrhoea in patients with advanced cancer can be extremely debilitating because of the loss of fluid and electrolytes, the repeated effort of
getting to and from the bathroom and the increased anxiety about faecal
incontinence. Consideration must be given to the underlying cause but
generally symptom relief is achieved with conventional management.
However, aromatherapy interventions can be integrated with the aim
of optimizing patient comfort.

Spiritual and psychosocial care

Frequent, urgent and unexpected bowel movements can generate
heightened levels of anxiety, panic, fear and embarrassment in patients
experiencing diarrhoea. Sleep disturbance can also be an issue which
contributes to ongoing fatigue and eventual exhaustion. Creating time
for relaxation and drawing on earlier aromatherapy interventions specific to spiritual, emotional, fatigue and insomnia (Chapters 5, 6, 7 and
8) may assist the patient in experiencing psychospiritual relief of this
distressing symptom.

Skin barrier protection

In patients with advanced cancer, the repeated bowel motions of diarrhoea and its debilitating effects can lead to soiling. Special attention is therefore needed to protect the patient's skin against irritation caused by direct contact with faecal matter, while simultaneously minimizing the risk of developing pressure ulcers/injuries. It must be noted that essential oils should not be applied directly to the delicate tissues of the anus. However, fixed oils such as *Simmondsia chinensis* (jojoba) can be extremely effective. Aromatherapy specific to skin barrier protection and management of pressure ulcers/injuries is discussed in Chapter 12.

Odour management

Managing faecal odour is important to the patient's dignity where diarrhoea inevitably means close proximity to a toilet, or in some situations the need for a commode close to the bed. The option of open windows and circulating fresh air is not always possible and the patient is conscious of being left in a room where the air is saturated with pungent odours. Drawing on the work of Allan and Gray (2017) in managing malodour related to malignant wounds (see Chapter 12), the use of an 'aroma pot' offers the patient control in dealing with the odour as and when their bowel motions occur. The authors recommend 10 drops of an undiluted essential oil mixture placed on a cotton wool ball contained inside a small screw-top jar. The patient can open the lid and allow open air diffusion as required. The cotton wool ball with the essential oils needs to be refreshed daily.

Intermittent cold-air diffusion of essential oils (as per safety guidelines, Chapter 3) can also be an effective method of aromatizing a room. Hydrosol sprays, where the patient can refresh hands and face with a spray mist, are another useful measure of comfort.

From my personal clinical experience, the citrus oils are extremely effective in minimizing room odour, particularly *Citrus aurantiifolia* (lime), *Citrus limon* (lemon) and *Citrus paradisi* (grapefruit). However, inspiration can also be drawn from essential oils used to manage odour from malignant wounds, as discussed in Chapter 12.

Skin-Related Symptoms in Palliative Care

For patients with life-limiting illness, skin-related symptoms can be complex and often notoriously challenging to manage. Coping with chronic deterioration of the skin at the same time as the internal vital organs are failing can render patients socially isolated and suffering psychological distress, which can profoundly impact their quality of life. This chapter considers the most common symptoms and the potential of aromatherapy intervention:

- Pruritus
- Pathological sweating
- Malignant wounds
- Skin failure and pressure ulcers/injuries

Pruritus

Defined as 'an unpleasant cutaneous sensation which provokes the desire to scratch' (Rothman 1941, p.357), pruritus (or itch) can be a source of considerable suffering for some patients. Although regarded as a rare symptom in patients with cancer, it is estimated that between 5 and 24% of patients with advanced stage disease will experience pruritus which adversely affects their sleep, mood, daily activities and consequently their quality of life (Alshammary, Duraisamy and Alsuhail 2017; Kantor *et al.* 2016). Self-consciousness, embarrassment, low self-esteem and low self-confidence are among the most frequently reported concerns by patients, although less commonly reported in research reviews examining pruritus (Kantor *et al.* 2016).

Mechanisms of pruritus

Pruritus can be acute or chronic in nature with complex pathophysiology. For a long time, itch was considered a variant of pain, following the pathway of nociceptive sensory fibres via the spinothalamic tracts of the spinal cord to the somatosensory cortex. However, researchers identified that a proportion of these sensory fibres are unmyelinated C-fibres and myelinated A-delta afferents, dedicated to the transmission of pruritus (Brennan 2016). Of the dedicated C-fibres, Brennan (2016) estimates that 10% are histamine dependent and 90% are independent of histamine. Consequently, antihistamine medications have little therapeutic effect for the majority of pruritus in these patients.

Common causes and conventional management of pruritus

Within palliative care, Alshammary *et al.* (2017) categorize the common causes of pruritus as cholestasis, uraemia, malignancy, opioid-induced, infection and drug reactions.

Cholestasis

This is arguably the most prevalent source of pruritus in this patient group, affecting between 20 and 25% of patients with advanced liver disease and 100% of those with primary biliary cirrhosis. In malignant cholestasis, such as cancer of the pancreas, cholangiocarcinoma or intra-hepatic liver metastases where the biliary duct is compressed or obstructed by tumour, decompression of the common bile duct using stents is the most effective conventional management. However, this may not always be possible and conservative management using pharmacology is proposed. This includes serotonin reuptake inhibitors (SSRIs), paroxetine for severe itch of a non-dermatologic origin, mu-opioid receptor antagonists (Nowak and Yeung 2017) and low-dose anti-depressants (Kouwenhoven, van de Kerkof and Kamsteeg 2017).

Uraemic

This is related to chronic renal disease, and Nowak and Yeung (2017) report that uraemic itch affects both dialysed and non-dialysed patients, increasing in prevalence to as much as 55–80% of patients with end-stage renal disease. Kappa-opioid receptor agonists can directly minimize itch of this nature; SSRIs and the anticonvulsants gabapentin and pregabalin are also beneficial.

Malignancy and paraneoplastic itch

Alshammary *et al.* (2017) describe a range of cancer-related causes for pruritus, including the side-effects of cancer medication or associated complications, such as cholestasis or renal impairment. The symptom of itch may be tumour-specific and localized to the affected area, such as the peri-anal itch of colorectal cancer, vulval itch of cervical cancer and the scrotal itch of prostate cancer.

Malignant haematological diagnoses, including Hodgkin's disease, chronic myeloid leukaemia and polycythaemia vera, are also known to produce paraneoplastic itch arising from direct infiltration of the skin.

Opioid-induced

Generalized itch associated with oral or systemic opioids is reported as less than 1% (Alshammary *et al.* 2017). A paradoxical effect exists, where opioids may simultaneously induce pruritus and analgesia.

Other causes

Alshammary *et al.* (2017) also report concurrent infection and drug reactions as underlying contributors to pruritus.

Non-pharmacological interventions

Regardless of the underlying cause, there are a range of non-pharmacological interventions and general measures known to offer palliation to the intensity of pruritus. These are listed below.

Topical preparations (Elmariah and Lerner 2011)

- Bathing with lukewarm water for less than 20 minutes
- Unscented soaps
- Moisturizers containing glycerol acetate, urea, petroleum, mineral oil and glyceryl stearate. Use regularly, especially after bathing
- Vitamin D analogues
- Menthol 1–2% topically (indicated for localized neuropathic itch)
- Capsaicin (indicated for localized neuropathic itch)
- Lidocaine
- Ultra-violet B therapy (three times weekly) (Yosipovitch and Bernhard 2013)
- Moisturizers with low pH (one to three times daily, especially after showering/bathing)

Oral

- *Oenothera biennis* (evening primrose oil), one to two capsules twice daily (Yoshimoto-Furuie *et al.* 1999)

Other

- Acupuncture (Menanti, Tansinda and Vaglio 2009)
- Transcutaneous electrical nerve stimulation (Yosipovitch, Greaves and Schmelz 2003)
- Imagery and relaxation (Yosipovitch and Samuel 2008)

General measures for patients (Nowak and Yeung 2017; Perdue 2016)

- Ensure a cool environment
- Avoid irritants
- Use behavioural therapy, relaxation, stress reduction
- Encourage gentle rubbing of skin rather than scratching
- Keep fingernails trimmed
- Wear cotton gloves to minimize skin damage
- Apply cold compresses
- Direct air flow onto wet/damp skin
- Wear loose cotton clothing
- Minimize boredom; encourage distraction

Unfortunately, there is no general consensus as to conventional or combined lines of treatment. The latest Cochrane review evaluated 50 studies assessing the effects of 39 treatment approaches for pruritus in patients with advanced disease (Siemens *et al.* 2016, p.57). The authors conclude:

> Especially in palliative care, patients with pruritus may have more than one origin for their pruritus. The fact that itch affects the skin, immune system and the peripheral and central nervous system means that complex and combinatory pathways are likely to be more effective than a single-line approach.

Aromatherapy for pruritus in advanced illness: Current clinical evidence

Clinical evidence for aromatherapy intervention is principally derived from studies investigating itch associated with chronic kidney disease (CKD) in patients receiving haemodialysis. A systematic review conducted by Bouya et al. (2018) identified four studies which have evaluated the specific effect of aromatherapy in this patient group. The results are summarized in Table 12.1.

While it is important to learn from these study interventions, a cautionary observation is that all patients received aromatherapy applications on the same day as their haemodialysis. Rapid excretion of essential oil components may occur via dialysis, which may not accurately reflect the pharmacodynamics and pharmacokinetics of essential oils for other chronic itch states.

Table 12.1: Aromatherapy studies for uraemic pruritus (Bouya et al. 2018)

Reference	Study design number of patients (n=)	Intervention	Results
Abdelghfar et al. (2017)	Quasi-experimental Pre-post testing (n=29)	Essential oil of peppermint blended with sunflower oil* Aromatherapy massage of 15–25 minutes twice daily, three times per week for two weeks	Highly significant positive effect on pruritus (p=0.000)
Curcani and Tan (2014)	Quasi-experimental Pre-post testing (n=80)	Essential oils of lavender and tea tree blended with almond oil and jojoba wax* Aromatherapy massage of 7–15 minutes to region of pruritus, three times per week for six weeks	Significant positive effect on pruritus (p=0.001)
Ro et al. (2002)	Quasi-experimental (n=29)	Essential oils of lavender and tea tree* Aromatherapy massage of seven minutes to entire non-fistulated arm/hand only, three times per week for four weeks	Positive effect on pruritus

| Shahgolian et al. (2010) | Pre-post clinical trial (n=20) | Essential oils of lavender, mint and tea tree at 5% dilution* Aromatherapy massage using 3–5ml blend for seven minutes of non-fistulated hand only, three times per week for two weeks | Significant positive effect on pruritus (p=0.05) |

*Botanical names unspecified

The potential of aromatherapy

Palliation of pruritus in patients with life-limiting illness requires a combination of approaches which are unique to each person, starting with assessment.

Assessment from the patient's perspective

Unfortunately, few studies have evaluated the patient's experience, although Aresi et al. (2019) investigated reasons for under-reporting of uraemic pruritus. The authors identified a lack of awareness of the relationship between itch and CKD, and the available treatment options in patients and healthcare professionals. Patients felt 'itch' was a less important symptom to discuss with their renal team and would wait to be asked unless it had been increasingly problematic.

Personal clinical experience with patients experiencing cancer-related pruritus have described itch as 'worse than the cancer itself' and 'it's like a deep stabbing which moves around and you don't know when you're going to be stabbed next'. The relentless nature of chronic itch readily depletes a patient's energy levels and adversely impacts their resilience. Understanding what the symptom means to the patient and how it affects their quality of life is a crucial starting point to create a management plan which meets their individual needs.

Fixed oils and macerates

Central to the management of pruritus is skin hydration, the aim being to alleviate the intensity of itch by enhancing skin barrier function and decreasing transepidermal water loss (Anh and Son 2016). This is where aromatherapy's long-held traditions of using plant-based fixed oils for skin hydration and protection are invaluable. The moisturizing benefits largely rest with the role of essential fatty acids, particularly linoleic acid, to hydrate and improve skin barrier function. In sufficient quantities, linoleic acid is vital for the maintenance and repair of the skin barrier. Deficiencies lead to dry, scaly hair and skin, and slow-healing wounds. Vegetable oils rich in linoleic acid are shown in Table 12.2.

Table 12.2: Vegetable oils rich in essential fatty acids (Parker 2014; Price and Price 2014)

Vegetable oil *Botanical name* (common name)	% linoleic acid	Comments
Borago officinalis (borage seed oil)	>35%	• 25% gamma linoleic acid (GLA) • Broad range of phytochemicals which additionally provide an anti-inflammatory action in the skin and joints • Careful storage avoiding heat, light and oxygen
Rubus fruticosus (blackberry seed)	>60%	• 15% alpha linoleic acid • Deeply nourishes the skin • Generous phytonutrient content
Oenothera biennis (evening primrose)	>75%	• 10% GLA
Vitis vinifera (grapeseed)	>81%	• Rich in vitamin E
Actinidia chinensis (kiwi fruit seed)	>20%	• 60% alpha linoleic acid • 3:1 ratio of omega-3 to -6 oils beneficial for anti-inflammatory conditions
Passiflora incarnate (passion fruit seed)	>77%	• Contains calcium and phosphorous, minerals to soothe and support nerves • Anti-inflammatory, anti-spasmodic and sedative properties

When applied topically, the fixed oils of Table 12.2 are rapidly and deeply absorbed across the skin layers to nourish and condition the cells (Parker 2014). For these reasons, Anh and Son (2016) suggest that plant-based fixed oils may have a superior effect in alleviating itch, when compared with synthetic skin moisturizers, by mediating symptoms of topical inflammatory conditions to soothe the underlying irritation of itch.

Fixed oils with known anti-inflammatory properties may also offer symptom relief, including *Simmondsia chinensis* (jojoba), *Calendula officinalis* (calendula), *Persea gratissima* (avocado) and *Calophyllum inophyllum* (tamanu) (Bensouilah and Buck 2006). Of note, the strong 'nutty' aroma of *Calophyllum inophyllum* (tamanu) needs introducing to the patient prior to preparation. Thereafter, skilful balancing is required to create an oil blend which is aromatically agreeable. From my personal clinical experience, this is well worth the effort, particularly for pruritus with a painful neuropathic element, to alleviate the lancinating or stabbing sensations.

Fixed oils with moisturizing effects have been widely researched throughout the cosmetic industry and further extend the options for skin rehydration. Examples of fixed oils with known moisturizing properties (Anh and Son 2016; Parker 2014) are:

- *Prunus amygdalus dulcis* (sweet almond)
- *Sesamum indicum* (sesame)
- *Prunus armeniaca* (apricot kernel)
- *Brassica napus* (rapeseed)
- *Helianthus annuus* (sunflower seed)
- *Cocos nucifera* (coconut)
- *Scelrocarya birrea* (marula seed)

Hydrosols

Applying a light mist, or cool compress, of undiluted hydrosols directly to the skin can be deeply soothing for relentless itch. Vasoconstriction is produced by evaporative processes (Bensouilah and Buck 2006), which can be particularly useful when the scalp is a source of itch, or in those hard-to-reach places such as the back, where an able patient has the option to direct a spray. Topical application of hydrosols increases skin hydration and offers additional relief to patients between their regular applications of moisturizing creams or fixed oil blends. The lighter fragrance may be more appealing to the patient with an increased sensitivity to smell.

Gelling agents such as Amigel® can be incorporated with a hydrosol to create a thicker consistency. In its professional reference guide, Essential Therapeutics recommends preparing Amigel® at a concentration of 0.2% (one part Amigel® to nine parts liquid) to make a sprayable or pumpable preparation which can be customized to the patient's preference. The aim is to extend the evaporative process and subsequent vasoconstriction, which in turn alleviates itch for longer periods of time.

Hydrosols of *Matricaria recutita* (german chamomile), *Anthemis nobilis* (roman chamomile), *Lavandula angustifolia* (lavender true), *Helichrysum italicum* (helichrysum) and *Achillea millefolium* (yarrow) are reported within the aromatherapy literature as being anti-inflammatory (Harman 2010; Inouye, Takahashi and Abe 2008; Price and Price 2004). The known anti-inflammatory constituents are shown in Table 12.3.

Table 12.3: Main constituents of hydrosols with known anti-inflammatory properties

Hydrosol Botanical name (common name)	Main constituent(s) with anti-inflammatory properties	Reference
Matricaria recutita (german chamomile)	bisabolol oxide A	Price and Price (2004)
Mentha x piperita (peppermint)	menthol 1,8-cineole	Price and Price (2004) Inouye et al. (2008)
Helichrysum italicum (helichrysum)	α-pinene	Inouye et al. (2008)
Achillea millefolium (yarrow)	1,8-cineole linalool	Price and Price (2004) Inouye et al. (2008)

Essential oils

Wherever possible, essential oils are chosen to address the individual's psychosocial and spiritual aspects of care, as well as their physical symptom of itch.

PSYCHOSOCIAL AND SPIRITUAL DIMENSIONS

In their book *Aromadermatology*, Bensouilah and Buck (2006) dedicate an entire chapter to the relationship between the skin and the psyche. Internal skin homeostasis is maintained through complex, multi-directional communication pathways between the central nervous, endocrine and immune systems and is a commonly known precept within aromatherapy. Utilizing the olfactory pathways with 'sedatory' essential oils, known to depress the function of the CNS, has the potential to reduce the patient's perception and intensity of itch. Popular essential oils in this category include *Anthemis nobilis* (roman chamomile), *Citrus aurantium var amara flos* (neroli), *Citrus bergamia* (bergamot), *Commiphora myrrha* (myrrh), *Lavandula angustifolia* (lavender true), *Santalum spicatum* (sandalwood), *Valerian officinialis* (valerian) and *Vetiveria zizanioides* (vetiver).

Itch intensity often escalates at night, causing serious exhaustion from regularly disturbed sleep and further exacerbating levels of spiritual and psychosocial distress, which is highly relevant to these patients (see Chapters 5, 6 and 8).

PHYSICAL SYMPTOM OF ITCH

From my personal clinical experience, *Anthemis nobilis* (roman chamomile), *Matricaria recutita* (german chamomile), *Helichrysum italicum* (helichrysum) and *Lavandula angustifolia* (lavender true) are beneficial. Kerkhof-Knapp Hayes (2015) further advocates *Styrax benzoin* (benzoin), *Leptospermum scoparium* (manuka) and *Santalum spicatum* (sandalwood). The combination of *Citrus bergamia* (bergamot) and *Cedrus atlantica* (cedar) is also reported as being antipruritic (Price and Price 2012).

ENDOCANNABINOID SYSTEM (ECS)

Dermatology researchers report significant relief of pruritus in differing systemic diseases, including uraemic and cholestatic causes, following use of cannabinoid receptor agonists in pre-clinical and clinical studies (Avila *et al.* 2020). However, the involvement of the ECS and its reputed role with other signalling systems is vastly complex. Readers are referred to the work of Tóth *et al.* (2019) for a detailed analysis of cannabinoid receptors CB1 and CB2 as potent contributors to the sensation of itch.

In view of the similarities that exist between the pathogenesis of itch and pain sensations, it seems reasonable to revisit the range of essential oils discussed in Chapter 9.

Aromatherapy applications

Aromatherapy intervention is directed by the patient's perspective, experience and holistic assessment. Involving family and caregivers in the assessment process is important, particularly where the patient's dexterity is poor, their condition is frail or fatigue is an overwhelming factor.

TOPICAL APPLICATION AND DILUTION

The itch–scratch cycle can perpetuate damage to the skin barrier which further precipitates itch. Topical application, one to three times daily, of moisturizing creams, blends of fixed oils (only), or blends of fixed oils plus essential oils can intensively hydrate the skin and minimize skin barrier dysfunction. Supplementary application of hydrosols, as a spray or cool compress, may further extend symptom relief.

If incorporating essential oils, localized areas of itch require a concentration starting at 5% for topical application and extending to 10%

(Kerkhof-Knapp Hayes 2015). For generalized itch, concentrations of 1% are safe.

MASSAGE

A crucial benefit of relaxation massage, particularly with skin-related issues, lies with its connection through touch. This can make a vast difference to the patient's sense of self-esteem and emotional well-being, while offering immense comfort in the end-stage of life.

Reductions in itch intensity were reported by Bouya *et al.* (2018) in four studies evaluating aromatherapy massage (see Table 12.1), with statistical significance achieved by Abdelghfar *et al.* (2017), Curcani and Tan (2014) and Shahgolian *et al.* (2010). Of importance is the shorter duration of massage, which is highly relevant to these patients (see Chapter 3).

INHALATION

Inhaling 'sedatory' aromas has been shown to reduce the delay in skin-barrier recovery caused by psychological stress (Denda *et al.* 2000). This inter-connectedness between the CNS, skin and the olfactory element of aromatherapy in managing the itch–scratch cycle makes essential oil inhalation a valuable route of intervention.

SAMPLE FORMULATIONS

Table 12.4 highlights sample formulations drawn from my personal clinical experience with patients suffering chronic pruritus. Generally, an aromatherapy intervention would include:

- hydrosol formulation
- fixed oil/macerate blend
- aromatherapy inhaler stick of the patient's choosing or intermittent cold-air diffusion
- if permissible, an oral administration of *Oenothera biennis* (evening primrose oil), one to two capsules daily.

Table 12.4: Sample formulations for the management of chronic pruritus

Application	Sample formulation	Amount used	Direction for use
Topical hydrosol spray or cool compress	**Undiluted hydrosols of:** Formulation 1 *Anthemis nobilis* (roman chamomile) *Matricaria recutita* (german chamomile) *Lavandula angustifolia* (lavender true)	30ml 30ml 40ml	• Patient-directed as required • Liberal spray to areas of itch as required, particularly after bathing/showering and between skin moisturization • Alternatively, a cool compress applied to areas of high intensity itch. Allow the compress to absorb the body heat
	Formulation 2 *Helichrysum italicum* (helichrysum) *Matricaria recutita* (german chamomile)	60ml 40ml	
	Formulation 3 *Lavandula angustifolia* (lavender true) *Matricaria recutita* (german chamomile)	60ml 40ml	
Fixed oils and macerated oil blends	**Fixed oils and macerates of:** Formulation 1* *Vitis vinifera* (grapeseed oil) *Calendula officinalis* (calendula) *Simmondsia chinensis* (jojoba)	25ml 15ml 10ml	• Patient-directed • After light hydrosol spray, apply 5–10ml oil blend, one to three times daily, especially after showering • Alternatively, fixed oil blends can be dabbed on areas of localized itch as required • Caution: check for nut allergies prior to using nut-derived fixed oils
	Formulation 2* *Prunus armeniaca* (apricot kernel) *Prunus amygdalus dulcis* (sweet almond) *Borago officinalis* (borage seed oil)	25ml 15ml 10ml	
	Formulation 3* *Calendula officinalis* (calendula) *Simmondsia chinensis* (jojoba) *Calophyllum inophyllum* (tamanu)	25ml 15ml 10ml	
	*Essential oils can be added to these fixed oil blends as per dilution criteria in *Topical application* section		

cont.

Application	Sample formulation	Amount used	Direction for use
Aromatherapy inhaler stick	Essential oils with sedatory properties as per section *Psychosocial and Spiritual Dimensions* Other essential oil suggestions: *Rosa damascena* (rose) *Agonis fragrans* (fragonia) *Santalum spicatum* (sandalwood) *Cananga odorata* (ylang ylang) *Canarium luzonicum* (elemi)	4–8 drops essential oil in total	• Patient-directed • Inhale 4–8 breath cycles as required, to reduce itch intensity
Alternatively intermittent cold-air room diffusion		2–3 drops essential oil	• Intermittent diffusion, as per Chapter 3
Oral route	*Oenothera biennis* (evening primrose oil)	1–2 capsules orally	• Once daily (with permission of medical team)

Pathological sweating

Excessive sweating can be extremely debilitating to the patient with advanced cancer, severely impairing sleep, causing excessive daytime somnolence and fatigue, leading to mood disturbance and an increase in carer burden (Oxberry and Edwards 2005). Although excessive sweating is considered a significant problem in these patients (Mercadante *et al.* 2013), surprisingly the research-based evidence to guide clinical practice is sparse.

Mechanisms of sweating

The everyday mechanism of sweating relies on the thermoregulatory system. Oxberry and Edwards (2005) describe how receptors located within the skin, spinal cord and brainstem relay information directly to the pre-optic and anterior hypothalamus. Central signalling continues in higher cortical areas plus other regions of the brain, including the hippocampus, amygdala and mid-brain reticular formation, which also contributes information to the thermoregulatory centre. Thermoregulatory responses are initiated via sympathetic efferent pathways to innervate eccrine sweat glands and blood vessels within the skin. Eccrine glands are concentrated in the palms of the hands, soles of the feet, axillae and face.

Excessive sweating associated with cancer

Most patients experiencing troublesome sweating will report an abnormal increase, commonly known as hyperhidrosis (excessive sweating). Sweating that is specific to night-times is known as nocturnal diaphoresis. In relation to advanced disease, hyperhidrosis is usually secondary to pathological processes which can be of a localized or generalized nature. Underlying causes are shown in Table 12.5.

Table 12.5: Common causes of pathological sweating in patients with cancer (North Haven Hospice 2020; Oxberry and Edwards 2005)

Underlying cause	Comments
Infection	• A common cause of sweating which can be resolved by treating the source of the infection
Malignancy	• Non-Hodgkin's lymphoma, Hodgkin's lymphoma, carcinoid tumours, mesothelioma, neuroendocrine tumours, hepatic metastases, and breast, prostate and bone cancers • Advanced malignancy of any origin can also cause profuse sweating, particularly in the end-stage of life
Endocrine	• Hormone levels can change as a result of the tumour itself or cancer treatments, e.g. chemotherapy, radiotherapy, surgery, hormone therapy • Oestrogen deficiency such as that induced by oestrogen-depriving medications, e.g. tamoxifen in women with breast cancer
Medications	• Opioids, tricyclic anti-depressants, oestrogen-depriving medications, withdrawal from certain medications, alcohol
Emotions	• Stress, fear and anxiety are common causes of profuse sweating, as is intense pain

Conventional management of pathological sweating

In the absence of evidence-based management strategies, clinicians rely on skilful diagnosis to determine the underlying cause of excessive sweating, and clinical guidelines specific to their palliative care unit for appropriate intervention. Table 12.6 sets out the recommendations of the *Primary Palliative Care Guidelines* for Hospice New Zealand (North Haven Hospice 2020). This utilizes pharmacological and non-pharmacological interventions to palliate presenting symptoms.

Table 12.6: Primary palliative care guidelines for
pathological sweating (North Haven Hospice 2020)

Non-pharmacological interventions	Pharmacological interventions
• Manage body temperature. Keep as consistent as possible • Ensure hygiene practices are adhered to • Ensure light clothes are worn when necessary • Ensure towels/cloths are available to 'mop up sweat' • Use of fans as needed • Minimize alcohol intake (if a precipitating factor) NB: Be aware of this common symptom especially for those with hepatic metastases and lymphoma	• NSAIs, e.g. diclofenac • cimetidine 400–800mg nocte • steroids, e.g. dexamethasone • paracetamol 1g four times daily

Additional to these guidelines, other evidence-based approaches to minimize excessive sweating include case studies utilizing acupuncture (Hallam and Whale 2003; Ramasamy and Taylor 2017) and oral cannabinoids (Carr *et al.* 2019), which offer promising results.

Aromatherapy for pathological sweating: Current clinical evidence

Generally, the skin is porous to essential oils. However, when excessive sweating is present, skin-permeability may be significantly reduced, which may be a contributory factor to the absence of clinical studies evaluating aromatherapy in this patient group. For the most part, research-based evidence is derived from studies investigating hot flushes in healthy menopausal women. Significant effects were reported in reducing vasomotor flushing, melancholia, arthralgia and myalgia ($p<0.05$) with aromatherapy massage using essential oils of lavender, rose-geranium, rose and jasmine (botanical names unspecified) in a 4:2:1:1 ratio, diluted in almond (90%) and evening primrose (10%) oils, to a concentration of 3% (Hur, Yang and Lee 2006). Kazemzadeh *et al.* (2016) reported significant reductions in hot flushes in women receiving inhaled lavender ($p<0.001$) for 20 minutes, twice daily for 12 weeks, in comparison with the placebo of inhaling vapours of diluted milk.

The potential of aromatherapy

Although the clinical evidence is sparse in these patients, the potential of aromatherapy in managing excessive sweating rests with activating central mechanisms within the limbic system, to minimize stress and calm vasomotor function.

Assessment from the patient's perspective

Personal clinical experience has highlighted the intense psychosocial distress patients endure when living with the constant uncertainty of breaking into a profuse sweat at any given moment. The spontaneity of social outings, meeting with friends and family, is lost to the anxiety it creates. Close relationships and intimacy are negatively impacted, rendering a person fearful of the reactions of their loved ones and embarrassed by the loss of control over the way their body is functioning.

The qualitative work of Kamudoni *et al.* (2017) offers profound insight into the patient's experience, the lengths taken to disguise or conceal sweating, and the significant time required each day for repeated showers, changes of clothing and bedlinen. Patients describe the discomfort of 'being in wet clothes day in day out', 'having wet feet' and 'sweat dripping into their eyes'. Excessive sweating is also attributed to other common problems, including skin soreness, cracked skin, fungal foot infections and eczema. Although the study group were healthy patients with primary hyperhidrosis of a non-malignant nature, their experience offers a very real perspective of living with excessive sweating.

Skilful and sensitive communication is critical, together with inclusive decision-making to determine botanical products and applications appropriate to the individual's situation.

Essential oils

Cupressus sempervirens (cypress) is well known for its antiseptic and astringent properties, particularly for overhydrated skin and to calm excessive sweating of the feet (Battaglia 2018; Price and Price 2012). The astringent, antimicrobial and anti-fungal effects of *Citrus limon* (lemon) are useful for circulatory and skin-related issues (Kerkhof-Knapp Hayes 2015). Additionally, *Salvia sclarea* (clary sage) is recommended for excessive sweating (Battaglia 2018) and has the additional benefit of being an important oil of choice for the CNS (Holmes 2016).

INFECTION

Specific to fungal infections, essential oils of *Melaleuca alternifolia* (tea tree), *Leptospermum scoparium* (manuka) and *Pelargonium graveolens* (geranium) are among several well-researched oils demonstrating anti-fungal activity (Chen *et al.* 2016; Nazzaro *et al.* 2017; Tisserand 2015).

Where skin infections are present, see the section *Malignant wounds* for essential oils with known antimicrobial activity.

MENTHOL

Topically applied essential oil of *Mentha x piperita* (peppermint) has traditionally been renowned for its refreshing and cooling effects on the skin, particularly the feet. The potent agonist-action between menthol and the skin's thermoreceptors, where it can readily exert a cooling effect, has been described in Chapter 9. Additionally, menthol acts as a vasodilator, although the mechanism of action is unknown. Therefore, caution must be exercised when using menthol-rich essential oils in patients with excessive sweating to ensure menthol concentrations are less than 1% of the overall formulation.

Aromatherapy applications

INHALATION

Excessive sweating interferes with normal pathways for dermal absorption of essential oil blends. Therefore, inhalation, ideally via aromatherapy inhaler sticks, is a valuable starting point, particularly where psychospiritual distress, fatigue and insomnia feature prominently (see Chapters 5, 6, 7 and 8).

TOPICAL

Shower products, prepared with liquid Castile soap and the addition of essential oils with known astringent, deodorizing, antimicrobial and anti-fungal properties, may be beneficial in controlling bacterial colonization of the skin and minimizing odour (see section *Essential oils*). Similarly, lukewarm aromatic footbaths can alleviate the discomfort of lower-limb sweating. It is also a practical measure where fungal foot infections are present.

COMPRESSES

Hydrosols diluted at a 1:5 ratio with water and applied as a cool or warm compress can be comforting to the patient who is unable to shower/bathe independently. These can be applied to localized or generalized areas of sweating as required. The beneficial effects of hydrosols for pathological sweating are further discussed in Chapter 8, under the section *Difficulty with temperature regulation*.

Malignant wounds

'Do you have an essential oil for malodour?' is one of the most commonly asked questions I receive from palliative care professionals, particularly those working within in-patient units, where the noxious odour of a malignant wound can rapidly infuse rooms and corridors, and even infiltrate personal clothing and uniforms. Odour-elimination becomes a central focus for staff who, among their armoury, turn to air fresheners, synthetic fragrances and essential oil diffusion. Visits to numerous hospices have led me to the conclusion that continuous essential oil diffusion in patients' rooms and public areas is commonplace. Complex combinations of oils are used, often of high pungency and concentrations which exceed essential oil safety criteria.

While essential oil diffusion can be effective, particularly in minimizing airborne odour molecules, it is a 'band-aid' which unfortunately does not address the underlying cause of malodour. Odour control is only one aspect of malignant wound management. A greater understanding is needed of malignant wounds, particularly from the patient's perspective, which can offer powerful insight into their experience, the causative factors and appropriate patient-centred intervention.

What is a malignant wound?

Cancer-related wounds predominantly arise from primary skin cancers, but also include recurrent or metastatic spread from a primary cancer elsewhere in the body, or erosion of the skin surface from an underlying advanced pathology (Maida *et al.* 2009). Researchers estimate between 5 and 10% of patients with advanced forms of cancer are likely to develop malignant wounds (Maida *et al.* 2016). Unless the tumour is responsive to adjuvant cancer treatments, uncontrolled cell proliferation will continue. This leads to extensive destruction of local tissue, loss of vascularity, tissue necrosis and ulceration (Probst, Arber and Faithfull 2013b). Further complications include infiltration of adjacent blood and lymphatic vessels (Maida *et al.* 2016; Probst *et al.* 2013b), as well as fistula development in gastrointestinal, genito-urinary and gynaecological organs (Grocott 2000). Such chronic conditions create ideal environments for aerobic and anaerobic bacterial colonization, resulting in malodour, profuse exudate and impaired healing (Edwards-Jones 2018). Sadly, malignant wounds are an indication of advanced and progressive disease with relatively few treatment options.

Presenting symptoms

Commonly, patients will present with more than one wound and clusters of unpredictable symptoms. Maida *et al.* (2009) identified the symptoms most reported by patients with malignant wounds (n=67), as shown in Table 12.7.

Table 12.7: Patients' reported symptoms of malignant wounds (Maida *et al.* 2009)

Commonly reported symptoms	% of all wounds with symptoms
Pain	31.20%
Mass effects (of wound)	24%
Aesthetic distress	19%
Exudate	14.60%
Malodour	10.40%
Pruritus	5.20%
Bleeding	4.20%
Crusting	1.50%

These pose a challenge to clinical management, primarily because malignant wounds extend beyond the physical boundaries of a progressive disease, to a complex situation of how symptoms impact an individual's spiritual, psychological and social well-being.

Wound-related pain

From my personal clinical experience, patients commonly describe the pain as 'like someone's stabbing my breast', 'really terrible pain' and 'relentless night and day'. Pain can arise from pressure of the tumour against adjacent structures/organs and increased localized swelling manifesting from impaired capillary or lymphatic drainage (Probst 2010). Additionally, nerve damage or exposure of nerve endings through the skin, tissue ischaemia, inflammation, infection (Maida *et al.* 2016) and mismanaged dressing changes (Woo and Sibbald 2010) are other causal factors. Malignant wound pain is inextricably linked with spiritual and psychosocial elements, often resulting in a complex pain situation.

Mass effects and aesthetic distress

A key observation of Maida *et al.*'s (2009) study was the high percentage of patients (24%) reporting difficulties with the 'mass effect' of a malignant wound. Physical impairment, through reduced mobility of the limbs and spine, turns simple, everyday activities, such as getting showered and dressed, into major challenges. Anatomically speaking, medical dressings may not conform to the changing wound contours, resulting in a bulky appearance and an altered body image. Eventually, patients are forced to relinquish their regular wardrobe for loose-fitting clothes of fabrics that can sustain repeated laundering. This represents additional losses of body-image, self-confidence and sexual identity to a progressive wound of an unpredictable nature (Reynolds and Gethin 2015).

Exudate

Exudate originates from biochemical processes generated by bacterial colonization of the wound. These trigger the breakdown of necrotic tissue by proteases which liquefy to produce exudate of varying amounts and frequency (Grocott 2000). This enzymatic action of wound exudate is caustic and can severely damage the surrounding skin, particularly when the amount exceeds the capacity of a dressing (Woo, Santos and Alam 2018).

Multiple dressing changes are needed, day and night, to contain the copious quantities of exudate these wounds can produce. Each dressing change can be demanding on time, energy and resources, often involving complete changes of clothes, a great deal of dressing supplies, as well as the increased burden of laundry and distress (Probst, Arber and Faithfull 2013a). This leads to social withdrawal and consequent feelings of isolation.

Odour

Complex bacterial colonization underpins malignant wound odour. Edwards-Jones (2018) explains how the interplay of anaerobic bacterial colonization, common wound pathogens, together with other offensive odours, such as putrescine and cadaverine released from the breakdown of amino acids in necrotic tissue, creates a malodour which causes deep anguish to patients, their families and the healthcare professionals involved (Alexander 2010; Taylor 2011; Probst et al. 2013b).

Patient descriptors include 'putrid, fishy' and like 'spoiled meat' (Maida et al. 2009) which adversely affects their quality of life as 'a smell that never goes away' (Piggin and Jones 2007).

Patients spend a great deal of time attempting to hide the odour through frequent washing of the wound and careful packing with self-made dressings to minimize leakage of exudate and permeation of odour (Probst et al. 2013a; Probst et al. 2013b). Consequently, this renders them housebound and socially isolated, even marginalized within their own home (Reynolds and Gethin 2015).

Bleeding

Less than 4.2% (n=67) of patients experience wound bleeding (Maida *et al.* 2009), which mostly stems from the tumour eroding small capillaries and venules; fragility of the wound tissue; altered clotting and fibroblast activity, and can be exacerbated through dressing changes (European Oncology Nursing Society (EONS) 2015). Depending on the anatomical site, arterial erosion is possible which can result in haemorrhage. In their study, Maida *et al.* (2009) report that every patient who experienced bleeding expressed a fear of potentially 'bleeding to death'.

Other reported symptoms

Although less commonly reported, pruritus and crusting are other symptoms which can cause intense pain, felt inside the wound as well as the surrounding peri-wound (Maida *et al.* 2009; Probst *et al.* 2013b).

Conventional management of malignant wounds

Palliative treatment options for malignant wounds are limited. Conventional approaches of radiotherapy and/or systemic chemotherapy are possibilities for some patients where tumour reduction may alleviate advancing wound symptoms (Young 2017). However, these established treatments are often accompanied by unwanted side-effects, and so require careful consideration between the clinician and the patient as to risk versus the potential benefit.

Conventional wound management is a central aspect of nursing care, where the aim is to keep wound beds moist and, over time, granulation processes lead to a reduction in size and circumference of the original lesion (Naylor 2005). However, for patients with malignant wounds, these approaches are unsuitable because the humidity of the wound is already excessive and the invasive spread of the tumour often extends beyond containment of conventional dressings (Agra *et al.* 2017).

Evidence-based conventional strategies to manage the symptoms of these complex wounds are summarized in Table 12.8.

Table 12.8: Evidence-based conventional management for malignant wounds

Conventional approach	Current evidence
Odour control *Wound cleansing* Gentle irrigation with normal saline (0.9%), clean tap water or careful showering as often as required	• Helps remove necrotic tissue and reduces bacterial load (EONS 2015)
Antibiotics Metronidazole	• Renowned for treating bacterial and protozoal infections. Cochrane review concluded insufficient evidence to use oral route for odour management in malignant wounds (Ramasubbu *et al.* 2017) • Attributed to poor blood supply of the wound hindering therapeutic antibiotic levels, plus systemic side-effects of nausea and neuropathy (EONS 2015) • Topical forms of metronidazole, either solution (0.8%), powder or gel (0.75%) applications, identified as therapeutically effective (Winardi and Irwan 2019). Long-term efficacy in controlling rapid colonization of multiple bacterial strains in malignant wounds is questionable (Stringer 2017)
Dressings Primary dressings of activated charcoal; hypertonic solutions of sodium chloride; antimicrobial (silver) and ionized hydrogel. Secondary dressing of hydrocellular foam	• Containment of volatile substances underpinning odour is crucial. Most effective are any of the primary dressings combined with secondary dressing of hydrocellular foam (Agra *et al.* 2017; da Costa Santos, Pimenta and Nobre 2010)
Pruritus *Dressings* Hydrogel sheets	• Enhances moisture content of wound bed to ease itch (EONS 2015)
Transcutaneous nerve stimulator (TENS)	• Overrides and prevents painful nerve messages to CNS (EONS 2015)
Natural fabrics in clothing and bedlinen	• Aims to minimize other counterirritants (EONS 2015)

cont.

Conventional approach	Current evidence
Exudate	
Dressings	
As per odour management utilizing highly absorbent dressings	• High absorbency dressings are crucial which conceal wound. Menstrual pads are often chosen but this requires sensitive discussion prior to use to ensure patient's approval (EONS 2015)
Bleeding	
Dressings	
Non-adhesive	• Minimizes disturbing fragile tissue at wound bed which can trigger bleeding (EONS 2015)
Topical haemostatic preparations	
Natural preparations, e.g. calcium alginate, collagen or oxidized cellulose	• A range of topical haemostatic interventions to suit the patient's individual situation (EONS 2015)
Sclerosing agents, e.g. silver nitrate	
Fibrinolytic antagonists, e.g. tranexamic acid	• If haemorrhage is anticipated, preparing the patient and family is essential, together with actioning a medication plan and emergency measures to help minimize the patient's distress (EONS 2015)
Astringents, e.g. alum solution, sucralfate	
Vasoconstrictors, e.g. adrenaline	
Pain	
Pain assessment	
Adjuvant pharmacology	• Vital to understand the patient's pain experience. Determine the most appropriate intervention aligning with WHO (1996) analgesia ladder. Adjuvant pharmacology may be required to manage chronic neuropathic wound pain (EONS 2015)
Pain at dressing changes	
Prescribed opiates	• Administer pre-procedural doses of the patient's prescribed opiates (EONS 2015)
Use low adherence dressings	• Minimizes dressing adherence and protects exposure of nerve endings
Maintain a moist wound bed	
Irrigate rather than swab wounds using warm saline	• Reduces stimulation of exposed nerve endings (EONS 2015)
Topical administration of low-dose opioids	• Morphine 6.25–15mg combined in 8g hydrogel offers continued pain relief while minimizing systemic absorption (Graham *et al.* 2013 cited in EONS 2015)

Non-pharmacological approaches

Most malignant wounds are associated with bacterial colonization and/ or infection which underpin symptoms of odour and exudate. Characteristically, such colonization leads to the formation of biofilms, where structured communities of bacterial species are encased in a protective exo-polysaccharide substance which adheres to the wound's surface (Clinton and Carter 2015). Biofilms act as a barrier to many antibiotic treatments and the patient's innate immune system, adversely affecting healing processes. This increased resistance has led researchers to evaluate other antimicrobial agents, derived from selected natural resources.

Honey

The deodorizing and wound debridement properties of medicinal honey in malignant wounds have been reported (Lund-Nielsen *et al.* 2011; Praptiwi 2017). Among several mechanisms of action, Yaghoobi, Kazerouni and Kazerouni (2013) detail the hygroscopic nature of honey, which dehydrates bacteria with the aid of honey's high sugar content. Its increased osmolarity rapidly debrides and deodorizes a wound, while its acidic nature (pH 3.2–4.5) suppresses bacterial colonization to reduce infection. Honey also triggers complex physiological sequences to enhance anti-inflammatory activity within a wound. As such, oedema and exudates are reduced, which in turn alleviates compression on nerve endings. The authors conclude that further research is required, particularly in determining specific properties of different kinds of honey to ensure its most appropriate use for specific wound management.

Phytotherapy

Systematic reviews of the literature report potential therapeutic benefits with green tea teabags applied as a secondary dressing to minimize malodour (da Costa Santos *et al.* 2010; Gethin, McIntosh and Probst 2016), which is further enhanced when combined with topical metronidazole powder (Winardi and Irwan 2019).

Curcumin ointment, which utilizes the active phytochemical compound of *Curcuma longa* (turmeric), known for its anti-inflammatory properties and potential anti-neoplastic activity, has been cited. When curcumin ointment was applied directly to the wound, three times daily for four consecutive weeks, 90% of patients (n=62) reported a reduction in wound odour (Kuttan, Sudheeran and Joseph 1987).

Aromatherapy in malignant wound management: Current clinical evidence

The antimicrobial activity of essential oils has a well-established history and remains an area of significant research interest. Primarily, this relates to the individual components of an essential oil, particularly terpenes and phenolic compounds, known to exert antibacterial activity with little to no development of antimicrobial resistance and the benefit of minimal side-effects (Negut, Grumezescu and Grumezescu 2018; Schelz, Hohmann and Molnar 2010). The precise mechanism of action is central to most studies, with recent reviews summarizing the pharmacodynamics of essential oil components (Negut *et al.* 2018; Schelz *et al.* 2010).

In-vitro studies

Table 12.9 shows essential oils known to exert antimicrobial activity. The information is derived from reviews of in-vitro studies which have examined single essential oils or their individual components. Further reference to the antimicrobial activity of essential oil components can be obtained via online scientific databases, such as Dropsmart.

Table 12.9: Commonly researched essential oils which exert antimicrobial activity

Essential oil *Botanical name* (common name)	Component(s) contributing to antimicrobial activity	Reference
Thymus vulgaris (thyme)	thymol, carvacrol y-terpinene	Maver *et al.* (2018); Schelz *et al.* (2010)
Melaleuca alternifolia (tea tree)	terpinen-4-ol 1,8-cineole	Maver *et al.* (2018); Negut *et al.* (2018); Schelz *et al.* (2010)
Origanum vulgare (oregano)	thymol carvacrol	Maver *et al.* (2018); Negut *et al.* (2018); Schelz *et al.* (2010)
Lavandula angustifolia (lavender true)	linalool linalyl acetate	Cavanagh and Wilkinson (2002); Maver *et al.* (2018)
Matricaria recutita (german chamomile)	α-bisabolol chamazulene	Maver *et al.* (2018)
Ocimum basilicum (basil)	linalool	Maver *et al.* (2018)
Cinnamomum verum (cinnamon bark)	linalool α-terpineol	Maver *et al.* (2018)

Clinical setting

Utilizing 'whole' essential oils and combinations rather than single isolates for malignant wound management offers a wider sphere of synergistic or antagonistic interaction against microbes, particularly where biofilms are complex and often polymicrobial (Stringer *et al.* 2014). This is evidenced in the clinical setting where two studies in the complementary and alternative medicine literature met the eligibility criteria for critical review by Gethin *et al.* (2016). Both studies evaluated essential oils as topical agents in this patient group.

First, there was Mercier and Knevitt (2005), who developed an aromatherapy protocol for the palliative care setting incorporating a topical essential oil cream. Equal proportions of *Melaleuca alternifolia* (tea tree) and an essential oil of the patient's choice were prepared in an aqueous cream at 2.5–5% concentration. Patients with malignant wounds (n=13) received topical aromatherapy intervention to good effect during their end-of-life care. Although the anecdotal nature of this study details four cases, the basic clinical recommendations are a useful starting point for malignant wound care (see Table 12.10).

Table 12.10: Basic recommendations for clinical use of essential oils (Mercier and Knevitt 2005)

Clinical presentation of malignant wound	Essential oil application
Malodour apparent only at dressing changes	Essential oil diffusion of the room during the dressing change
Low-level malodour is noticeable	1–2 drops of essential oil applied directly to the outer dressing
Continuous and distressing level of malodour	Essential oils prepared in an aqueous cream at 2.5–5% concentration for direct application to the wound surface

Second was an observational study conducted by Warnke *et al.* (2006), which evaluated an antibacterial essential oil mix known as KM-PT70, Klonemax® (see Table 12.11), to rinse malignant wound ulcers in patients with advanced head and neck cancers (n=30). Additional to a five-day, standard course of oral clindamycin (600mg twice daily), the authors report that twice daily rinses of the ulcers using 5ml Klonemax® resulted in complete resolution of malodour in all patients within three to four days of treatment. Furthermore, in some patients, re-epithelialization of ulcers was noted, which the authors attribute to the anti-inflammatory action of the oil rinse.

Table 12.11: Components of KM-PT 70, Klonemax® (Warnke *et al.* 2006)

Essential oils pre-prepared in 40% ethanol base	Dose per gram
Eucalyptus*	70mg
Tea tree*	5mg
Lemongrass*	45mg
Lemon*	45mg
Clove-leaf oil*	7mg
Thyme*	3mg

*Botanical names and chemotypes unspecified

Interestingly, an earlier study conducted by Warnke *et al.* (2004) reported complete amelioration of malodour in a similar cohort of patients (n=25), using twice daily rinses with 5ml of Megabac®, an essential oil mix of tea tree, grapefruit and eucalyptus (botanical names unspecified). The authors stated that when this was integrated alongside conventional therapies of clindamycin and chlorophyll, an average of 23 days' treatment was required to eradicate the malodour.

Given the relatively small numbers of patients with malignant wounds, clinical teams tend to share their experiences through detailed case studies. Ames (2006) describes a 52-year-old lady who presented with a fungating breast tumour and personal goals to decrease the intense odour and minimize the discomfort of dressing changes which often caused profuse bleeding. Patient-selected essential oils included 10 drops of *Boswellia carterii* (frankincense) and 5 drops of *Thymus vulgaris ct linalool* (thyme ct linalool), prepared in olive oil infused with calendula. Gauze squares impregnated with the aromatic blend were packed into the wound daily. Bleeding at dressing changes was managed with a direct application of 1 drop of undiluted *Pelargonium graveolens* (geranium) to the fragile area, with a 30-second haemostatic effect reported. The odour was minimized sufficiently for this lady to enjoy a planned retirement celebration during her end-of-life care.

Allan and Gray (2017) reviewed a combination approach using topical and diffusion of essential oils to manage the severe odour of a large malignant breast wound (15cm x 15cm) and its impact on the quality of life of an 86-year-old patient. The treatment regime is outlined in Table 12.12.

Table 12.12: Aromatherapy interventions for malignant
wound odour management (Allan and Gray 2017)

Essential oils *Botanical name* (common name)	Amount used	Method of application
Melaleuca alternifolia (tea tree) *Lavandula angustifolia* (lavender true) *Citrus limon* (lemon) Aqueous cream	75 drops 100 drops 75 drops 500ml	Daily wound dressings Liberal application direct to wound bed and peri-wound (to replace metronidazole gel)
Eucalyptus radiata (narrow-leaf eucalyptus) *Citrus limon* (lemon) *Thymus vulgaris ct linalool* (thyme linalool ct linalool)	Equal quantities of each	10 drops added to an 'aroma pot' created using a small screw-top jar containing a cotton wool ball impregnated with the essential oil drops Patient-directed as required, for room fragrance prior to visitors

Comparative photographs showed visible reductions in peri-wound erythema and notable changes to the wound itself after eight weeks' use of the essential oil cream. The wound was drier and more compact, with intact tissue and no evidence of localized bleeding. The patient found the cream 'very comforting'. Within one week of this combination approach, the community nurses reported a noticeable reduction in odour. Although the patient herself had no sense of smell, her quality of life was improved by feeling more comfortable and receiving visitors again to her home.

A qualitative service evaluation, conducted by Stringer *et al.* (2014), considered patients with malignant wounds (n=24) who received a topical essential oil cream applied beneath a secondary dressing. A subjective improvement in the patient and family's quality of life was reported. Although the essential oils were not listed, a subsequent case study presented by Stringer (2017) utilized the principles of clinical aromatherapy by pairing the aims of intervention with specific essential oil components for a young man with a complex malignant wound. Combined with prescribed metronidazole gel, an essential oil cream was used effectively as a supplementary support to manage symptoms of odour, exudate and peri-wound skin excoriation.

The potential of aromatherapy

Malignant wounds are complex and rare. Clustering of symptoms is common and complicates the situation to the extent that the patient's daily life is replaced by their attempts to control a progressive wound. This is an insurmountable feat, which ultimately leads to the loss of the life they once knew, to the loss of a functioning body they once trusted, and the loss of personal dignity (Probst *et al.* 2013b; Reynolds and Gethin 2015). The visible advancement of a malignant wound, combined with deteriorating health, generates intense suffering as succinctly summarized by Probst *et al.* (2013b, p.44): 'Psychologically they (the patients) experienced deep suffering due to the consequences of living a marginal life in an unbounded body and the feeling that no one could help them.'

Assessment from the patient's perspective

Integrative clinical and holistic aromatherapy approaches have the potential to ease the intense suffering of these patients. It begins with a comprehensive assessment to sensitively explore the patient's experience of living with a malignant wound and identify their priorities of concern. Customary goals of wound care, in terms of healing, are prevented by the complexity of a progressive wound, concurrent disease and limited lifespan (Naylor 2005). Therefore, precedence rests with incorporating aromatherapy applications to palliate the patient and family's spiritual and emotional distress (see Chapters 5 and 6) and resilience (see Chapters 4 and 13), particularly during the end-of-life transitions (see Chapter 14).

Aromatherapy applications

ESSENTIAL OILS

Managing wound-related symptoms is achieved through integration of botanical products drawn from the clinical evidence of the previous section, earlier relevant chapters and Case study 12.1. Where possible, involving the patient in essential oil choices is an important factor which imparts a sense of control and personal involvement in the decision-making process. This is reflected in the works of Mercier and Knevitt (2005) and Ames (2006).

OTHER BOTANICALS

Topical application of essential oils requires an appropriate excipient which is readily absorbed to minimize exudate and enable wound dressings to remain in place. Among a list approved by the Committee on Herbal Medicinal Products for wound management, Maver *et al.* (2018) explore the various anti-inflammatory, analgesic, astringent and antibacterial properties of *Hypericum perforatum* (St John's wort); the antimicrobial, anti-inflammatory and antiviral activity of *Calendula officinalis* (calendula); and the anti-inflammatory and wound-healing properties of *Aloe vera*. Where pruritus or neuropathic pain elements are present, *Calophyllum inophyllum* (tamanu) and *Hypericum perforatum* (St John's wort) are unsurpassable. Collectively, this range offers promising potential as adjuncts to malignant wound management.

HYDROSOLS
The value of hydrosols in wound care has not been fully evaluated. And yet, there is a place for well-stored hydrosols to tenderly cleanse and soothe the malignant wound bed and minimize exudate and odour. For patients with breast or genitalia wounds who identify as female, rinsing with hydrosols of *Lavandula angustifolia* (lavender true), *Citrus aurantium var amara flos* (neroli) or *Rosa damascena* (rose) can create a sense of femininity.

End-of-life care

During end-of-life care, repeated dressing changes may no longer be a viable option for the patient entering the active dying phase. The emphasis on supportive aromatherapy continues through these end-of-life transitions and is discussed more fully in Chapter 14.

CASE STUDY 12.1: DARYLYN'S EXPERIENCE

Referral

At the age of 43, Darylyn was referred to the specialist palliative care team for symptom management associated with an advanced cancer of the ethmoid bone. She was unable to smell the intense oronasal malodour being produced by the tumour; an odour which caused her immediate family and friends immense distress. Referral for aromatherapy intervention was initiated by the specialist palliative care nurses.

Background summary

This lady's family had expressed concern to the clinical team regarding the offensiveness of Darylyn's oronasal malodour. The nasal rinse prescribed by the ear, nose and throat (ENT) team was no longer effective and the cloying nature of the malodour was causing her children, family and friends to distance themselves and spend less time with her.

At the first session, Darylyn quickly settled into the therapy room, delighting in the hand-stitched quilt covering the massage table, and the cheerful colours. She made no mention of the fragrance of the roses in the vase on the table. We began by exploring what she wanted to gain from the session. She paused momentarily, then started from the point when she first knew that 'something was wrong'.

Seven years earlier, the joy of being pregnant was suddenly shattered by the experience of excruciating facial and eye pain. Initial diagnosis surrounded hormonal changes associated with her pregnancy which further precluded appropriate pain-relief options. Physical relief was achieved by pressing the side of her face hard against a cold pane of glass.

A few months after the birth of her baby, the pain returned. The route to diagnosis was complex because her presentation was considered 'unusual in someone so young'. Radiotherapy and chemotherapy followed and brought significant challenges to her as a young mother.

It was several years before the cancer returned, this time more invasive, with symptoms that were adversely affecting her quality of life. Unable to smell or taste anything, Darylyn relied on her family to remind her to use the nasal rinse prescribed by the ENT team for the malodour. This consisted of rock-salt, Listerine® mouthwash, baby shampoo and water, which she administered between two and eight times daily, to 'clear the debris'. Recently, this had started to cause heavy bleeding, forcing her to stop the rinses and resort to strong peppermints to mask the malodour.

Personal goals

It was deeply humbling to listen to the detail of Darylyn's cancer journey, where for years she had lived 'feeling shadowed by death' and all the while her single goal was to share quality time with her children.

Aromatherapy intervention

Despite the disease-induced anosmia and absence of taste, Darylyn was open to receiving aromatherapy. We discussed ways to minimize the malodour and nasal exudate. Essential oils were selected for their antimicrobial and anti-fungal properties, with the deliberate inclusion of oils indigenous to New Zealand. Despite not being able to smell them, Darylyn felt a sense of connection with plants familiar to her upbringing.

Given the limited range of movement of her jaw, her inability to gargle and the increasing levels of fatigue, the most practical methods of application were explored. Darylyn settled on a nasal rinse, an oral rinse and aromatic steam inhalations (see Table 12.13).

Table 12.13: Darylyn's aromatherapy interventions (part 1)

Application	Botanical products used Botanical name (common name)	Amount used	Direction for use
Nasal rinse	**Hydrosols of:** *Thymus vulgaris ct linalool* (thyme ct linalool) *Helichrysum italicum* (helichrysum)	Equal parts of hydrosol Dilute with cooled boiled water	Patient-assisted Nasal rinse twice daily *At each rinse:* 10ml hydrosol combination 100ml cool boiled water ¼ teaspoon salt
Oral rinse	**Hydrosol of:** *Mentha x piperita* (peppermint) Boiled water Honey **Mixed with essential oils of:** *Leptospermum scoparium* (manuka) *Kunzea ericoides* (kanuka) *Cymbopogon martinii* (palmarosa)	100ml 100ml 5ml 2 drops 2 drops 2 drops	Patient-assisted Oral rinse four times daily Rinse in mouth for one minute, spit out Do not swallow
Steam inhalation	**Essential oils** *Melaleuca alternifolia* (tea tree) *Lavandula angustifolia* (lavender true) *Helichrysum italicum* (helichrysum) *Cymbopogon martinii* (palmarosa) *Eucalyptus radiata* (narrow-leaf eucalyptus)	30% 30% 5% 20% 15%	Patient-assisted One drop essential oil mixture (undiluted) via a Clearway® Steam inhalation, four times daily for one week, then review

The multi-disciplinary team (MDT) were fully informed of the clinical aromatherapy plan. Darylyn and her sister were educated in how to administer each application. A referral was made to the family support counsellor to optimize Darylyn's time with her children.

On day two, with her sister's help, Darylyn was finding the aromatherapy regime 'straightforward'. Her sore throat had reduced from 8/10 to 1/10 on a visual analogue scale and the family reported a significant reduction in odour intensity.

By day four, the oronasal odour had completely diminished and Darylyn's children were going freely in and out of her room.

On day six, at a doctor's appointment, Darylyn was advised by the clinician to discontinue the aromatherapy interventions because 'aromatherapy doesn't work' and instead prescribed oral metronidazole for odour and exudate management.

Five months later, Darylyn made contact again. The side-effects of long-term metronidazole had caused persistent candidiasis and the drug was discontinued. Tumour progression resulted in a high level of malodorous exudate discharging from the ear, with associated halitosis. The nasal exudate was now less problematic. Darylyn's family expressed how effective the aromatherapy intervention had previously been and wished to restart the regime.

Due to the heat of the summer months, the aromatic steam inhalation was not a comfortable option. The application was changed to deliver the essential oil mixture via cold-air room diffusion. Additional interventions were formulated, as per Table 12.14.

Table 12.14: Darylyn's aromatherapy interventions (part 2)

Application	Botanical products used **Botanical name** (common name)	Amount used	Direction for use
Nasal rinse	Discontinued		
Oral rinse	As Table 12.3		Patient-assisted Oral rinse four times daily
Cold-air diffusion	Essential oil mixture of Table 12.3 (steam inhalation)	1–2 drops	Patient-assisted Cold-air diffusion of room for 20 minutes, three times daily, prior to children entering room
Ear cleanse	**Hydrosols of:** *Thymus vulgaris ct linalool* (thyme ct linalool) *Lavandula angustifolia* (lavender true)	80ml 20ml	Patient-assisted 10ml hydrosol mix, twice daily to cleanse the ear pinnae, surrounding skin and hairline. Dry area thoroughly

Ear gel 3%	**Essential oils of:**		Patient-assisted
	Melaleuca alternifolia (tea tree)	30%	Following ear cleanse, twice daily application of
	Lavandula angustifolia (lavender true)	30%	pea-size amount of gel blend
	Cymbopogon martinii (palmarosa)	25%	
	Leptospermum scoparium (manuka)	15%	
	Aloe vera	20g	

Reflection

Throughout her end-of-life care, Darylyn's priority of concern was being with her children. This was achieved in the first instance by managing the exudate and malodour of her malignant wound, which enabled her to feel less isolated. Central to these interventions was a high level of mindfulness and compassion. Seamless communication between the MDT enabled further support through family counselling and holistic management of other symptoms related to her end-of-life care. In those remaining weeks, Darylyn was able to share time with her children and died peacefully at home in the tender care of her family.

Situations with malignant wounds are rare and as a therapist, it was sad to discover that an effective clinical aromatherapy regime was discontinued by a health professional without prior consultation. However, the experience highlighted the lack of knowledge which exists within healthcare and the need for education in the advances of clinical aromatherapy. If we are to integrate clinical aromatherapy successfully, working collaboratively with our healthcare colleagues becomes a critical part of our role. It takes courage, plus a tonne of patience and resilience, to bridge the gaps which exist.

Darylyn's situation was the catalyst which inspired me to develop education programmes for healthcare and allied-health professionals, to assist their understanding of the fundamentals of clinical aromatherapy within palliative care. Conference presentations, team discussions and active involvement as a member of the MDT followed. Gradually, the medical referrals came forward and advancement of integrative approaches began to take place.

Rest peacefully, dear Darylyn. You brought about significant changes which have contributed to the advancement of clinical aromatherapy within palliative care; this is deeply appreciated.

Skin failure and pressure ulcer/injuries

Despite being the largest organ of the body, the skin is often overlooked as an organ susceptible to failure as the patient's health deteriorates. As end-of-life approaches, the complex nature of advancing cancer and its associated comorbidities results in gradual failure of the internal organs which ultimately cannot support the function of the skin and its underlying structures. The body starts diverting blood from the skin to the vital organs as a means of maintaining internal organ system function. Over time, this hypoperfusion of the skin leads to eventual skin failure, which often manifests as visible areas of deterioration and loss of skin integrity (Langemo and Brown 2006).

Pressure ulcer/injuries

Within palliative care, skin failure, deteriorating health, compromised mobility and physical inactivity are primary factors associated with the development of pressure ulcer/injuries (formerly known as pressure ulcers, decubitus ulcers or pressure sores) (Ferris, Price and Harding 2019; Langemo 2005). Despite the best precautionary measures and care, pressure injuries are not always preventable, with an overall prevalence of 12.4% in patients receiving palliative care in a variety of settings (Ferris *et al.* 2019). Older patients are more at risk, where skin hydration, elasticity and perfusion are already depleted and the changes associated with the ageing process, such as diminishing epithelial and fat layers, loss of collagen and elastin, poor vascularity and decreases in gaseous exchange, result in slow tissue regeneration (Langemo 2005). Collectively, or in combination, this makes the skin more susceptible to damage from pressure, trauma, friction, moisture and malnutrition.

In the presence of advancing disease and organ failure, normal skin-healing processes are severely impaired, leading to pressure injury development. Generally, these occur over bony prominences susceptible to high levels of pressure. Common locations include the sacrum, buttocks, hips and heels, more often identified in stages 1 and 2 (Ferris *et al.* 2019), as shown in Table 12.15. For these patients, skin deterioration can be rapid and extensive and is often a visible indicator of the extent of failure occurring within the internal organs.

Table 12.15: Definitions of pressure injury staging (compiled from the European Pressure Ulcer Advisory Panel *et al.* 2019)

Stage	Definition
I	Intact skin, non-blanchable redness usually localized over bony prominences Area may be painful, firm, warmer or cooler than surrounding tissue Difficult to detect in people with dark skin tones
2	Partial thickness skin loss presenting as a shallow open-wound bed May present as an intact or open serum-filled blister No bruising. If noted, bruising indicative of deeper pressure injury
3	Full thickness skin loss, which may show exposed subcutaneous fat Bone, tendon or muscle is not visible Slough may be present but does not obscure visibility of wound depth
4	Full thickness tissue loss with exposed bone, tendon or muscle Slough present on some parts of wound bed
Unstageable	Full thickness tissue loss in which the base of the ulcer is covered by slough or eschar, so depth unknown
Suspected deep injury	Purple or maroon localized discolouration of intact skin or blood-filled blister due to damage of underlying soft tissue

Conventional management of pressure injuries

The unpleasant nature of pressure injuries and skin deterioration can be aesthetically distressing, painful and malodorous, requiring precise and skilful intervention which is pivotal to nursing care. Management strategies include a comprehensive assessment of risk, with prevention being a priority. However, for patients entering the active phase of dying, Ferris *et al.* (2019) highlight a myriad of factors which impair skin healing, resulting in pressure injuries being neither preventable nor treatable and where wound healing is no longer a viable option, such as:

- Impaired immune function
- Biochemical abnormalities
- Physiological stress
- Systemic and localized hypoxia
- Prescribed medications, e.g. steroids
- Palliative treatments, e.g. chemotherapy
- Poor localized blood supply
- Hypotension

- Dehydration
- Excess moisture, including continence issues, fistulae
- Malnutrition

At this stage, the patient's comfort becomes a priority over intensive wound management strategies. For example, modifying repositioning in line with the patient's comfort; minimizing painful dressing changes; and maintaining skin and continence care with the least disruption to the patient (Ferris *et al.* 2019). This requires sensitive, honest communication with the patient and their family to determine the most appropriate way forward.

For specific conventional wound management prevention and treatment strategies, readers are referred to the exceptional guidelines compiled by the European Pressure Ulcer Advisory Panel *et al.* (2019).

Aromatherapy in pressure ulcer management: Current clinical evidence

Several of the aromatherapy management strategies discussed in the previous section, *Malignant wounds*, are transferrable to pressure injury care, particularly management of wound pain, exudate, bleeding and the associated spiritual and psychosocial distress of coping with visible deterioration of the physical body.

The potential of aromatherapy

As death approaches, no one can take away the burden of disease and all that it entails, but aromatherapy can offer a richness of care and comfort that is quite different from any other form of support.

Spiritual and psychosocial care

Integrating aromatherapy interventions for pressure injury management relies solely on the decisions and wishes of the patient. Sensitive and compassionate communication aligns with the gravity of what the patient is facing. Conversations may not necessarily relate directly to the wound itself. More often patients will want to quietly explore what a pressure injury represents: the gradual deterioration of health; the decline of their physical body; the reality that their end of life is approaching and what this means to them; and a reflection on their life (see Chapters 5 and 6).

Prevention

In the early stages of pressure injury development, general preventative measures can be enhanced with aromatherapy preparations.

DEHYDRATED SKIN

For the patient with dry skin, optimizing hydration and skin integrity can be achieved by using blends of fixed oils with high essential fatty acid content, as per Table 12.2, and moisturizing properties, as in the list in section *Fixed oils and macerates*. Although the therapeutic benefits of massage will not prevent pressure injury development, fixed oils minimize further friction when lightly applied to the skin.

An additional benefit of an oil blend is that it lends itself to the relaxing strokes of effleurage to the limbs. The therapeutic comfort achieved by touch of this nature is undeniable and has the potential to connect the patient with deeper levels of relaxation while simultaneously hydrating the skin.

MOIST SKIN

Skin integrity is further at risk in the presence of excess moisture, for example urine, faeces, leakage from a wound or fistulae. In these situations, preventative barrier oils and creams which protect the natural pH of the skin can minimize the caustic damage caused by excess moisture. Moisture damage of this nature can be rapid and painful and readily expose the patient to infections of open pressure-related wounds.

With a molecular structure that is similar to sebum, *Simmondsia chinensis* (jojoba) is highly compatible with the skin. Its exceptional ability to lay a light film over the skin's surface to maintain moisture, while at the same time allowing the skin to breathe (Parker 2014), makes it a first choice for skin barrier prevention. Also, it can be an effective alternative to soap and water, where its use as a skin cleanser, for wound leakage or faecal matter for example, prevents the skin from overworking to replenish losses of natural lipids removed by soap and water.

When formulating a protective base oil, the anti-inflammatory, analgesic, anti-bacterial and cicatrisant effects of *Calophyllum inophyllum* (tamanu) cannot be overlooked (Raharivelomanana *et al.* 2018). The same applies to *Hypericum perforatum* (St John's wort) with its known healing capacity for damaged nervous tissue (Price and Price 2014), making it particularly useful where there is neuropathic pain from nerve damage of an eroding pressure ulcer.

The anti-inflammatory effects of *Calendula officinalis* (calendula) are well known within palliative care settings for soothing radiation dermatitis (Cruceriu, Balacescu and Rakosy 2018) and it offers a beneficial component to a protective skin oil blend. A sample formulation for a protective fixed oil base is listed in Table 12.16. Essential oils, as outlined in earlier sections of this chapter, can be incorporated dependent on the individual's situation.

Table 12.16: Protective fixed oil blend for those
at risk of developing pressure injuries

Fixed oil/macerate *Botanical name* (common name)	Percentage used in fixed oil blend
Simmondsia chinensis (jojoba)	45%
Calendula officinalis (calendula)	25%
Calophyllum inophyllum (tamanu)	20%
Hypericum perforatum (St John's wort)	10%

The anti-inflammatory effects can be further enhanced with the addition of the essential oil *Calendula officinalis* (marigold) CO_2-total extract. Kerkhof (2018) advocates a percentage of between 0.1 and 2.5% (dependant on the situation) of the total formulation and emphasizes the importance of warming the required amount of fixed oil in a bain-marie prior to adding the total extract, to avoid it solidifying on contact.

End of life

As the end of life approaches, the emphasis of pressure injury prevention changes to meet the wishes of the patient and family. Patients may no longer be able to endure regular re-positioning to alleviate direct pressure, or voice to a busy nurse or caregiver that changes of wound dressings are causing pain and discomfort. Aromatherapists are well placed to utilize their skilful communication and observational skills to advocate other tender and therapeutically effective approaches which optimize the patient's quality of life across these end-of-life transitions (see Chapter 14).

CHAPTER 13

Fostering Resilience in Caregivers

Home-based palliative care is globally advocated because it is associated with improved symptom control and quality of life for the patient, as well as reducing the use of healthcare resources (Rabow *et al.* 2013). Living with relatives and having extended family support are also strong determinants for patients to choose end-of-life care at home (Gomes and Higginson 2006). However, family caregivers may not necessarily be included when these decisions are made, leaving some feeling under-prepared, under-supported, or even ambivalent about their ascribed role as caregiver.

Assuming the role of caregiver requires individuals to integrate the responsibilities of caring into their daily life. In reality, this is often concurrent with rearing a family and continuing paid employment. Or in the case of the elderly caregiver, simultaneous to managing their own health problems and other impairments. Moreover, the unpredictable nature of the patient's progressive illness and symptoms, combined with an unknown duration, can take a tremendous toll on the well-being of the caregiver, leaving them increasingly overburdened (Benson *et al.* 2019).

Resilience in caregivers of patients with life-limiting illness

Until recently, little has been known about the specific problems family caregivers encounter and what is most likely to be of support. Predominantly, researchers have evaluated anxiety, depression and psychological distress and conclusively agree that an escalation occurs in caregivers of patients with life-limiting illness (Harding, Higginson and Donaldson 2003; Oechsle *et al.* 2013; Williams, Wang and Kitchen 2014), with the psychological burden often exceeding the patients as death approaches (Oechsle 2019). Among the myriad of difficulties caregivers face are coping with anticipatory grief, adjusting to the patient's progressive deterioration and symptom complexity, managing emotions, struggling with acceptance, adapting to different environments of care, as well as coping with how care influences relationships within the family dynamic (Limardi *et al.* 2015; Oechsle 2019).

Despite the multi-dimensional burden, caregivers with a greater range of coping resources tend to be more adaptable and able to source help as it is needed. Hwang *et al.* (2018) demonstrated associations between high levels of caregiver resilience and perception of good health, absence of depression and positive social support. Coping strategies such as acceptance, planning and positive reinterpretation influenced moderate to high levels of resilience in 77% of caregivers (n=57) of patients with metastatic brain cancer (Saria *et al.* 2017). While both studies highlight resilience as a protection against caregiver burden, further evaluation is needed to determine the factors underpinning resilience.

Factors influencing resilience in caregivers

By the time the patient is referred for specialist palliative care, many caregivers have already provided supportive care for many months, even years, along the patient's illness trajectory. Throughout, caregivers intimately share the critical stages of the patient's journey and the numerous challenges faced. And yet, little is known of their experiences and the factors influencing their capacity to handle such adversity.

Psychosocial and circumstantial resources

Despite the absence of definitive data, Payne (2009) identifies caregivers as predominantly female, the spouse of the patient and in the later years of their life, and categorizes the factors influencing resilience as: socio-demographic; personal and family resources; material and social resources; and circumstances of care. Several of these elements align with those identified by Seiler and Jenewein (2019), who examined resilience and post-traumatic growth in patients across the cancer trajectory (see Chapter 4). However, generalizability of their findings cannot be assumed in caregivers of patients with cancer, or other life-limiting illness. The needs and capacities of caregivers and those of the patient can differ tremendously throughout the illness trajectory. As such, it is important to consider the caregiver's perspective independently.

Caregivers' perspective

Traditionally, qualitative studies have provided valuable insight into the experience of caregiving within palliative care (Bremault-Phillips *et al.* 2016; Harding *et al.* 2003; Oechsle *et al.* 2013). However, only two studies, conducted by Roen *et al.* (2018) and Skorpen-Tarberg *et al.* (2019), have specifically evaluated caregiver resilience with the aim of enhancing home-based care and appropriate healthcare intervention.

Through semi-structured interviews with caregivers of patients with advanced cancer (n=14), Roen *et al.* (2018) identified four consistent themes:

- Being seen and known
- Available palliative care
- Information and communication about illness, prognosis and death
- Facilitating a good carer-patient relationship

The findings of Roen *et al.* (2018) dovetail with those of Skorpen-Tarberg *et al.* (2019), whose qualitative study evaluated the involvement of family caregivers (n=11) across the patient's illness trajectory. Interviewed within 12 months of bereavement, caregivers gave rich and invaluable insight into their caring role throughout the different phases of palliative care. These were categorized into four themes, with the main experiences and needs of caregivers summarized in Table 13.1.

Table 13.1: Summary of family caregiver's experiences and needs (Skorpen-Tarberg *et al.* 2019)

Phase of palliative care	Caregiver's experiences and needs
Early phase Point of transition into palliative care	• Healthcare professionals (HCPs) focus on palliative nature of the patient's disease • Decisions for home-based palliative care mainly defined between HCPs and patient. Caregivers experienced limited involvement in planning palliative care • Felt unable to converse with HCPs in front of the patient to address their specific preparatory needs for end-of-life care • Informational needs of the patient and caregiver often differed • Wanted more information on the process of dying, the disease trajectory, what to expect in their role as caregiver and how this would affect the family

cont.

Phase of palliative care	Caregiver's experiences and needs
Middle phase Emphasis on patient-centred care	• Felt the patient's wishes were taken seriously by HCPs. However, caregivers only felt listened to in discussions specific to the patient's illness and needs • Needs often incongruent with the patient's, e.g. wanting additional home support but the patient refuses • Often a feeling of too much responsibility • Services accessed too late because caregiver was under-prepared
Dying phase Lack of preparation	• Felt a lack of involvement in planning for the patient's end-of-life care • Wished palliative care services had been involved earlier • Wanted more information about the process of dying and what to expect • Often felt isolated in end-of-life care at home. Felt left to handle tasks alone • Perceived day and night continuous caring at home as challenging and frightening • Valued the importance of being able to contact the palliative care team as needed
Bereavement Lack of systematic follow-up	• Expressed a need for a systematic follow-up after the patient's death • Felt that an opportunity to speak with the nurse present in the last days/hours of life was supportive. Further questions about the dying process could be asked. This adversely impacted their mourning if left unanswered • Receiving contact from an HCP served as a support to process their sorrow and move on with their life

For caregivers, practical information about the process of dying, the abilities required of a caregiver, combined with an understanding of available support and resources are considered crucial in the early stages of the patient's illness. Feeling prepared and knowledgeable about the disease and its related symptoms is known to reduce emotional distress, enhance the capacity to cope and positively contribute to the caregiver's quality of life (Bremault-Phillips *et al.* 2016; Ferrell and Kravitz 2017; Payne 2009).

The holistic nature of resilience

As discussed in Chapter 4, the complex interplay of resilience in patients with life-limiting illness aligns with the holistic care model, where an individual is an integrated whole, comprising physical, psychological, social and spiritual dimensions. This also applies to the caregiver who, like the patient, needs to be considered as an individual in addition to being an integral part of their family unit.

In reality, the caregiver's needs, particularly anticipatory guidance, practical information and provision of support in their distress, may easily be overshadowed by healthcare professionals prioritizing patient-centred care. Involving the caregiver in key decision-making conversations throughout the process of end-of-life care is essential. In fact, Payne (2009) calls for a major shift from *'patient-focused care'* to *'relationship-focused care'*, where healthcare professionals take a pro-active stance to give equal priority to the needs of the caregiver and consider how the palliative experience and services would work if they were structured around the wishes of all family members.

Barriers to resilience in caregivers

Resilience is complex, multi-faceted and characterized by how an individual adjusts to the circumstances of adversity (Seiler and Jenewein 2019). For caregivers of patients with life-limiting illness, where the demands fluctuate and resources vary, maintaining positivity, equilibrium and a sense of control of the situation can be challenging. Bremault-Phillips *et al.* (2016) identified several barriers to resilience which are associated with:

- the demands on a caregiver's time and resources
- changing roles and responsibilities within the family dynamic
- the caregiver's personal emotional responses to the situation
- the challenge of learning about medical conditions
- being involved with medical interventions
- exhaustion and sleep deprivation
- financial constraints
- personal health issues.

Caring involves increased vigilance over the patient, advocating for their needs, such as symptom relief, while being mindful of the patient's autonomy. A deep level of emotional support is crucial, particularly where anxiety and depression on the patient's part places additional strain on relationships and communication within the family. Added to which, caregivers are often central to organizing medical appointments, transport, finances and assisting with the patient's personal affairs, such as advance directives, power of attorney, and renewing wills, all the while keeping the extended family and friends informed and maintaining routines of daily life. Unsurprisingly, exhaustion is commonplace in caregivers who are struggling to maintain a level of 'normalcy' within the household. Often it takes someone outside their situation to tenderly suggest accepting help and taking time for self-care.

Autonomy

Autonomy, in varying dimensions, was central to Benson *et al.*'s (2019) qualitative analysis of caregiver resilience when caring for patients with life-limiting illness at home (n=25). Tensions surfaced when the patient attempted to maintain or regain autonomy, raising the question of who had control, which was a common source of conflict for caregivers. Conversely, if the patient was unwilling to participate in making their own decisions, or advocating their needs, this presented caregivers with a different set of frustrations. Autonomy as the primary caregiver was also frequently challenged by extended family, who created a sense of mistrust in the way the patient's care was being delivered, or seemingly accused the caregiver of withholding information about the patient's state of health.

Within the family unit, feelings of resentment can arise where personal autonomy is lacking and other family members are not recognizing or offering support that is needed. Caregiver narratives uphold the immense frustration experienced when family members passively avoid involvement in the care required, or do not appreciate the severity of the patient's deteriorating health, or the demands of caregiving (Benson *et al.* 2019).

Being vigilant to family conflict is important and may not always present itself overtly to the healthcare professionals involved. Benson *et al.* (2019) identified caregivers' expressions which are suggestive of family conflict as:

- resentment
- sadness
- a longing to return to life as it was prior to the caring role.

Early recognition, combined with timely and sensitive psychosocial support by the multi-disciplinary team (MDT), can minimize distress, defuse conflict situations and improve communication, and is considered an essential part of fostering resilience.

The potential of aromatherapy

With hindsight, many caregivers report how they would have approached the role differently, particularly in accepting support at an earlier stage to restore balance (Bremault-Phillips *et al.* 2016; Roen *et al.* 2018; Skorpen-Tarberg *et al.* 2019). This calls for vigilance on the part of the MDT to identify caregiver distress and offer appropriate intervention. Aromatherapy is a potential source of comfort to many over-burdened caregivers.

Spiritual and psychosocial support

Payne (2009) advocates for 'relationship-focused care'. This includes the hopes and aspirations of all family members involved in the patient's end-of-life care, which aligns with the World Health Organization's (2020) definition of palliative care to also support the needs of the family. Employing positive working partnerships with the patient and the important relationships within each family facilitates a greater understanding of the factors influencing resilience within the family unit, particularly in caregivers.

From my personal clinical experience, an aromatherapy session offers a safe and supportive space for caregivers to be heard and acknowledged. The notion of addressing a tired back, or increased muscle tension, or simply having time to themselves, can feel less confrontational for caregivers than facing the emotional and spiritual distress yet to surface. Often, the profound level of relaxation achieved by tailoring interventions to their individual needs and experiences can bring the caregiver closer to recognizing the gravity of their distress and acceptance of help.

Essential oils

As discussed throughout this book, the same principles apply in terms of inviting the caregiver to choose from a selection of essential oils suited to their priorities of concern. Incorporating oils which address their spiritual and emotional capacities is particularly beneficial, as outlined in Chapters 5 and 6.

Aromatherapy applications
Massage
Aromatherapy massage is often a popular treatment choice. However, caregivers frequently experience high levels of stress which may preclude their ability to determine the depth of pressure, or to sustain long periods of massage. Exercising caution is necessary to ensure that the

emphasis is maintained with slow-stroke relaxation massage, of short duration, to a specific area of the body, for example back/neck/shoulders, or hands, feet or face. Incorporating a longer rest period afterwards is often deeply appreciated.

Inhalation

Simple aromatherapy inhalation can be a practical and highly effective solution to the caregiver who may not wish to receive massage. Utilizing the breath cycles, as described in Chapter 3, offers the caregiver the option of an immediate emotional uplift with one to three breath cycles, or four to eight breaths for a deeper physiological effect. Aromatherapy inhaler sticks using 4 to 8 drops of essential oil or rollerball applicators (3%) are appropriate choices.

Aromatic anchoring

Combining aromatherapy inhalation with the aim of anchoring the caregiver to the relaxation session can deeply soothe an overburdened sympathetic nervous system. As described in Chapter 3, three consecutive sessions can firmly embed the profound level of relaxation experienced. Other useful interventions include combining aromatherapy inhalation with guided imagery, hypnosis, meditation and progressive muscle relaxation.

Aromatic footbath

Often caregivers are living within time constraints. In these situations, a warm aromatic footbath can be extremely relaxing and something which can be suggested as a self-care option at home.

Self-care

A simple technique which is invaluable to my personal clinical practice, especially with caregivers with insufficient time for self-care, is acupressure of the facial stress-relief points. In her book *The Blossoming Heart*, Robbie Zeck (2014, p.147) describes how this three-minute technique instils stability and calm, while simultaneously regulating circulatory supply to the cerebral cortex to restore a resourceful state of mind. Adapted for the palliative care setting, the details of this technique are outlined below. Preparing the blend in a rollerball applicator enables the caregiver to continue using this powerful relaxation technique at home.

- Ensure that the caregiver is seated or lying comfortably

- With their eyes closed, begin with a few minutes of gentle breath cycles (as in Chapter 3), emphasizing exhalation through the mouth
- When they are relaxed, ask the caregiver to bring the emotion or difficult situation into their thoughts
- Using a single drop of a diluted essential oil, or oil blend (1%), invite the caregiver to rub the oil drop between the tips of their middle fingers
- Place the tips of the middle fingers lightly on the frontal eminences of the forehead (approximately 3cm above the centre of each brow), slightly stretching the skin outwards
- Hold and resume gentle breath cycles for a minimum of three minutes
- Tiny pulses synchronizing beneath the fingertips signal completion of the process

CASE STUDY 13.1: KAREN'S EXPERIENCE

Referral

Karen's partner had recently been diagnosed with an advanced brain tumour and was under the care of the specialist palliative care team. Aromatherapy was integral to supporting the couple.

Background summary

Invested as a caregiver, Karen maintained a high level of attention to detail in the care of her partner, who had been receiving aromatherapy intervention for some time. Advancement of her partner's disease was evident in the changing pattern of symptoms and increasing dependence and they both knew that the prognosis was limited to a few months. Suddenly, their normal, carefree life had been overturned and Karen was coming to terms with her new role as caregiver and the intense, continuous process of grieving.

At each home visit, we made time to talk, generally over a cup of tea. It was evident that lack of sleep and Karen's constant vigilance were taking their toll. She declined offers of an aromatherapy session, massage, or any other form of relaxation therapy, as these were not part of her usual self-care routines.

During one of these visits, when it was time to replenish her partner's aromatherapy inhaler stick, Karen spoke of how she loved its aroma.

She would assist her partner, unscrewing the device and ensuring the nozzle was positioned the right way up. She described the gentle way in which her partner would then inhale and exhale, savouring the essential oil aromas. Tenderly, I offered to make one for Karen, where she could use it side-by-side with her partner. Although she agreed, Karen did not want to choose her oils, preferring 'something similar' to her partner's (see Table 13.2).

Table 13.2: Karen's aromatherapy intervention

Method of application	Botanical products used *Botanical name* (common name)	Amount used	Directions for use
Aromatherapy inhaler stick (purple) 'Deep peace'	*Cupressus sempervirens* (cypress) *Elettaria cardamomum* (cardamom) *Canarium luzonicum* (elemi) *Citrus limon* (lemon) *Simmondsia chinensis* (jojoba)	2 drops 1 drop 2 drops 3 drops 1ml	Self-directed as required At each use, inhale 4–8 breath cycles, day/night

The MDT were updated with the clinical aromatherapy interventions and follow-up. Karen quickly reported how much she was enjoying the process. Sitting alongside her partner, who had taken to teaching her how to inhale and savour the aroma, and not to rush the sanctity of the ritual, filled Karen with joy. These became tender moments of mutual love and affection as partners, where the role of caregiver momentarily stepped aside.

Reflection
Adaptability was central to this 'impromptu' session, where a blend was created purely on the basis of observation, rather than a shared, inclusive approach as would normally happen. Soothing an over-burdened sympathetic nervous system underpinned the essential oil selection for Karen, while maintaining an overall similarity to her partner's blend.

Central to the blend was *Cupressus sempervirens* (cypress), chosen for its structure, strength and protective nature when change is imminent (Zeck 2014). This monoterpene and sesquiterpenol-rich essential oil is recommended for its ability to restore calm to an over-burdened central nervous system (Fischer-Rizzi 1990). Holmes (2019) advocates how, via inhalation, it evokes existential contemplation during major life transitions. In doing so, a safe refuge is created which supports inner stability and resilience.

It was moving to observe the tranquillity experienced by Karen using this blend and the special moments where her partner shared wise counsel, despite the advancing disease, to help Karen as a caregiver to take rest and time throughout the day for stillness of the mind. Such cherished moments are known to enhance resilience (Bremault-Phillips *et al.* 2016).

CHAPTER 14

Aromatherapy for End-of-Life Transitions

For the patient with progressive cancer and their family, cessation of active treatment is an event which brings reality to an advancing disease and finality to the possibility of a cure. Where active treatment is not an option at initial diagnosis, these patients are suddenly confronted with an incurable illness and the unbearable realization that their life will soon come to an end. Such transitional processes require sensitive end-of-life discussion with the patient and their family, where priorities and choices are made on how to live out the precious remaining time.

End-of-life discussion

Crossing the threshold from active cancer treatment, where cure or prolongation of life is the central goal, to palliative care, where the emphasis lies with quality of life, can be a challenging process. The question of how to implement these tender conversations with the patient and their family remains a fundamental concern for clinicians tasked with this responsibility. Even with a high level of experience and communication skills, oncologists face complex questions of the practicalities involved, estimated time-frames, and existential concerns, all of which are foremost for the patient and family. This presents a broad spectrum of discussion to the oncologist's time and expertise. Kitta *et al.* (2021) identified that patients sense these clinical time pressures and consequently feel unable to explore details of their future. Primarily, this is because they are unable to process what has been said or have not had the opportunity to express their initial thoughts and feelings. Oncologists tend to use this hiatus to discuss manageable specifics, such as additional investigations or treatment options of a palliative nature. Patients viewed this approach as avoidance of clear communication of their subjective experience. Inevitably, many patients cross this critical threshold without having come to terms with the fact that their illness is life-limiting.

Palliative care

Referral to the palliative care team may have been suggested, but for many patients this is a feared option. Zimmermann et al. (2016) conducted semi-structured interviews to determine the perceptions of palliative care among patients and their families (patient n=48; caregiver n=23). Prior to referral, a prevailing theme among patients is that palliative care is synonymous with death and the last weeks of life. The authors conclude that this negative stigma associated with the active stage of dying originates from healthcare professionals and the way patients receive information about palliative care services. Similar findings were identified by Kitta et al. (2021), where oncologists used euphemisms with the intention of alleviating misconceptions, but instead explanations about the concept and purpose of palliative care services were avoided. Patients were left to make their own assumptions. However, once contact was made, patients reported that palliative care teams instilled confidence and contributed to their quality of life (Zimmermann et al. 2016).

Professional collaboration

Clinical experience has taught me that these sensitive end-of-life conversations cannot be accomplished in a single session. It is a process, requiring protected time and appropriate professional support. Clinicians initiating these conversations need to repeat the sessions to ensure the patient and their family are adjusting to their new reality, and interweave these clinical encounters with their palliative care colleagues. Simultaneous collaboration of this nature is crucial, particularly when it is widely known that early integration of palliative care has proven benefit for the patient's quality of life and for support of the family (Detering et al. 2010; Pringle, Johnson and Buchanan 2015; Teno et al. 2007; Zimmermann et al. 2014).

Unfortunately, a seamless transition is not always straightforward. Medical advances have blurred the lines between curative and palliative treatment options (Kitta et al. 2021). Clear and concise information is paramount when treatment options of a palliative nature are being offered. Integral to these end-of-life discussions, Mannix (2017, p.135) advocates for clinicians to 'ensure that the right people are present to hear it, to reflect upon it and support each other in dealing with it. This allows families to share their sadness or worry and avoids locking anyone away in the Cage of Lonely Secrets.' This is where the expertise and diverse experience of the palliative care team is invaluable, to support end-of-life discussions which are timely to the patient's individual needs and with information they feel ready to receive.

Advanced care plan (ACP)

For the most part, patients want to remain in control of their life and make their own decisions. Focusing on their wishes, hopes and fears, as well as their treatment preferences, is important. This includes determining acceptable medical interventions, as well as those which the patient considers would be futile in the event of a sudden deterioration in their health. Preference for their place of death, particular rituals and practices they wish to be honoured during their end-stage care and in the event of their death need to be recorded. Open discussion of this nature has the potential to reduce the fear about what lies ahead, for all involved, by offering a sense of preparedness.

An ACP provides a useful opportunity to approach end-of-life conversations with the patient and their family. Making these details known clearly communicates their specific wishes. This is particularly relevant should the patient lose the capacity to communicate their preferences regarding their end-of-life care.

While an ACP gently guides the patient, it is an intimate and deeply personal experience which raises a myriad of feelings, thoughts and emotions. As their illness progresses, symptoms increase and their general health deteriorates, the patient may find their wishes also simultaneously change. Appropriate plans need to be in place to enable regular, open review of the ACP and make revisions accordingly.

The potential of aromatherapy

Aromatherapy has the potential to bridge the gap by easing the passage of transition into palliative care; to reconnect patients with what matters in their life; to empower them with approaches where they have a sense of control; and to support their loved ones across the entire illness trajectory and through the inconceivable loss that comes with the finality of death. While much has been discussed throughout this book, particularly in relation to the spiritual and emotional aspects of integrative aromatherapy, there are several areas of relevance to consider.

Transitions within palliative care

Fringer, Hechinger and Schnepp (2018, p.2) characterize transitions as events where patients experience 'a change due to deterioration or improvements of their health status'. This can include a change in place of care, for example hospital to home, or home to hospice, a change in levels of care and goals of care, or combinations. However, less is written about the various and continued transitions patients and their families will experience throughout their end-of-life journey. To be precise, the time between their realization that life is limited by a progressive disease, to the patient's actual death. This interim space is usually accompanied by an unspecified time-frame and marks the point at which 'normal life' is upended and in its wake, potential disruption and turmoil ensues.

Supportive aromatherapy intervention

Throughout this period, where the patient and family are 'living with dying', support is crucial to minimize distress and facilitate seamless transitions. The holistic nature of aromatherapy practice offers a person-centred and relationship-centred perspective. It creates space for the patient and their family to process the news of their changing situation, while remaining flexible and compassionate to their needs, and comes as welcome reassurance.

Supportive aromatherapy intervention by a skilled and compassionate therapist, which addresses the complexity of working with both the patient and the family, has been discussed throughout this book. Specifically, there are chapters which tightly interweave with these transitions of end-of-life care, including Chapter 5 that explores the existential aspects of facing one's own mortality, alongside the physical manifestations of distress, where relationships and skilled communication are central. Chapter 6 rests with the emotional impact of a cancer diagnosis, where anxiety can take a strong foothold and over prolonged periods of time, depression can develop. Chapters 4 and 13 look at ways to strengthen the patient's and caregiver's resilience, where the individual's innate capacity to cope and quality of life become the predominant factors. And they consider the role of caring: what is involved and the challenges of maintaining a level of 'normalcy' in a situation of constant flux.

By gently exploring the patient and family's priorities of concern, and by guiding them to opportunities with the multi-disciplinary team (MDT), we can help optimize symptom management, life review, self-directed life closure and communication within the family. Collectively, this inter-disciplinary approach contributes to the overall goal of supportive care, aimed at enriching their quality of life.

Loss and grief

Integral to these end-of-life transitions is the insurmountable loss. Working alongside patients and their families has brought me face-to-face with the patient's loss of health; the loss of employment and consequent financial toll; and the subsequent change in family dynamics as others step in to fulfil household roles. Deteriorating health often requires physical alterations within the home, for example bringing the patient's living space downstairs and installing hospital equipment. This comes with the loss of privacy and an increased number of visitors, including healthcare professionals.

There is the loss of self-esteem, when roles are relinquished, when changes to the patient's body-image become apparent, where treatment interventions have left scars, prosthetics, a stoma bag, or a urinary catheter. Uncontrollable body functions, or odours being produced by a deteriorating body and advancing disease, can lead to the loss of dignity. This can be accompanied by the loss of sexual intimacy.

Coping with a future that is forever changed, the loss of celebratory milestones, hopes and dreams of a life unfolding, can be deeply felt by all involved, often to the extent that it raises fearfulness about dying, and internal questions of how it will happen and when. And what will happen to their loved ones?

Managing symptoms

Patients value support with specific symptoms and describe how reassuring it feels to experience a 'still functioning body', which is considered a vital proof of life (Fringer *et al.* 2018). Frequently, patients report symptoms being worse than the disease itself and often more distressing at night. Nocturnal thought processes can quickly escalate, exposing the patient to disturbing feelings connected with death, which can quite easily become all-consuming. Throughout this book, the role of aromatherapy has been explored in terms of bringing additional comfort to numerous symptoms commonly encountered by these patients.

Accompanying the dying patient

In the last weeks of life, the patient begins to withdraw socially. Gradually, their world becomes smaller, their focus progressively turns inward and there are noticeable signs of physical deterioration (Carlile 2016).

This is known as the 'active dying' phase and is a time when the patient deepens their self-reflection to draw meaning from a life that is fading. They may seek to reconcile differences with others or make peace with their own life circumstances or establish their legacies to ensure future provision for their loved ones.

For those who follow a religious path, this is a time when spiritual counsel is sought; when the priest, minister, rabbi, imam or another spiritual adviser is called. It is a time of contemplation, forgiveness, redemption and consolement. In her professional reflections, Mannix (2017, p.317) describes this as the point where the patient 'adjusts their hope from avoiding death to embracing each day as death approaches'.

A renewed sense of perspective is carried in the knowledge that everything the patient holds close is coming to an end. With it comes a broader vision which extends beyond self, to the focus of everyone and everything. Sand, Olsson and Strang (2009) describe this as 'togetherness', an important coping strategy for patients, where there is a newfound discovery of the ordinary, the significance of being present and taking time to appreciate their surroundings and all life forms. Gratitude and appreciation are prominent and more easily expressed for a kindness received, or in being able to overlook the shortcomings of others and see only their warm, positive qualities. Fulfilment is experienced through being present in every living moment, as exampled in 'A final encounter with winter'.

A FINAL ENCOUNTER WITH WINTER

Early in my nursing career, a patient in the hospice asked if I would take her outside. It was a bitterly cold day, where an overnight snowfall had blanketed the gardens and the air was crisp and carried the breath in billowing clouds. With help, I transferred her from her bed into a wheelchair, then swaddled her in warm blankets. Downstairs, in the foyer of this converted English manor house, a log fire had just been stoked; the crackle and smell of fresh pine touched our senses. I drew alongside the bay window, which framed the gardens like a scene from a Christmas card, then leant over to set the brakes of the wheelchair.

'Not here,' she said. 'Outside...please.'

'But it's freezing out there.'

'I know,' she said, her sunken eyes fixed on the view beyond the windows. Even now, I recall my hesitancy, where every fibre of my being was fearful of taking this dying lady out into the winter cold. She remained steadfast, and anxiously, I followed her wishes.

Outside, she tilted her chin slightly, greeting the icy wind as if it were an old friend, smiling as it pricked at her face. On the other hand, I felt its sub-zero temperature already penetrating my skin and suggested we return indoors.

She shook her head, 'A few more minutes.'

For several moments, her gaze took in the gardens and came to rest on a nearby tree. At its base, the ground was pinpricked with snowdrops.

'Have you seen a snowdrop?,' she asked.

My eyes darted to them quickly, 'Yes, aren't they lovely?,' but my attention was caught up with the increasing cold and being fearful of her demise.

'Carol, have you *really* seen a snowdrop?' Her insistent tone diverted my attention back to the flowers. 'Pick one, I'll show you.'

I followed her instruction and knelt by her side. Together, we marvelled at the little flower-bud hanging like a tiny drop of milk from its green stem. Encased within perfectly shaped petals was a miniature trumpet of white, tipped with tiny splashes of green.

She smiled as she caught my expression of wonder and said, 'Now… you've *really* seen a snowdrop.'

Those few minutes had a profound effect on my perspective and future nursing care. My initial reaction had been to talk this lady out of going outside, and instead, take in the view from the foyer. But her wish was to experience the vibrancy of winter; delight in creating frozen clouds with her breath and feel the wind pricking her face like shards of ice. It revitalized her senses to experience a greater connection with 'being alive'. Insightfully, she had drawn me into her 'presence', teaching me to temper my haste and experience the moment. It was only later that I came to realize this was about taking time to treasure the ordinary. And the only way to fully experience this is by totally immersing oneself in it. These sacred moments would never have been the same had we stayed indoors where this lady would have been denied her final encounter with winter.

The process of dying

For aromatherapists who may be new to palliative care or have not experienced death as intimately as this, it is helpful to understand the process of dying to be able to empathize with the patient and family's experiences and offer appropriate and timely support. While this is a summary, readers can be further guided by the sensitive works of Carlile (2016) and Warner (2013).

As death approaches, there is an ongoing slowing and failing of the systems and functions of the body. Blood is redirected from the skin and peripheral areas to the central core to help maintain a beating heart and breathing lungs to circulate oxygenated blood to the vital organs. Gradually, as the level of oxygenated blood wanes, the process of closing other organs begins to take place.

The patient's interest in food tapers off as the entire digestive tract slows, and absorption of food and water diminishes. The swallowing reflex becomes less pronounced, making tablets difficult to take, and eventually the absorption of liquid medications becomes less effective. Changes in medication and their routes of administration start to take place as the patient's deterioration extends. This is where we see sub-cutaneous routes of administration via the continuous infusion of a syringe driver or bolus injections of medication through in-situ butterfly needles.

As kidney function declines, the patient becomes less interested in fluids, although they may continue to experience a dry mouth. The urine becomes concentrated and dark in colour and there is less output. Excess fluid is redirected into the subcutaneous tissues as kidney failure extends, causing swelling of the lower limbs and abdomen.

Skin failure becomes increasingly evident, with reduced peripheral perfusion and cold extremities (see Chapter 12). Numbness and tingling indicate that the central nervous system is also slowing down and there may be associated restlessness initially in the legs and arms which can extend to a generalized inability to sustain one position for any length of time.

Lucidity waxes and wanes as levels of oxygenated blood decline. In moments where the patient is aware of their surroundings and those in vigil, their focus rests with important matters of what needs to be said or done. These are crucial moments in the final closure of the life lived and need to be honoured and respected as far as possible.

Eventually, death becomes imminent, where levels of unconscious-ness deepen and the rate and pattern of breathing changes. Congestion of fluid within the lungs, and saliva collecting in the throat, can become audible as the patient breathes and the swallow reflex diminishes. Med-ications are often administered to alleviate further fluid congestion and patients can be gently turned onto one side to drain accumulation within the mouth. These final stages of death can sometimes take a few days, particularly if the patient is 'waiting for someone' to arrive or requires permission from their loved ones to make the final transition.

Aromatherapy applications

Even though the patient is no longer conscious, there remains a level of awareness which must be respected. Talking to the patient as interventions take place, holding their hand or simply sitting in silent contemplation, honours these closing moments of life. Compassionate aromatherapy intervention can be immensely helpful during this final phase of dying. Draw on the practices discussed within this book, particularly the oral care of Chapter 11, managing restless legs in Chapter 8, skincare in Chapter 12, as well as the defining Chapters 5 and 6 for spiritual and emotional aromatherapy intervention. This extends to the family involved.

It is during this period of social withdrawal and the accompanying physical deterioration where patients may turn to rituals and healing to support the transition from their physical being towards their spiritual path. Several religions incorporate oils sacred to this final transcendence (see Chapter 5). These traditional ceremonies or other end-of-life rituals can help the patient in their preparation for death by relinquishing anxiety and emotional unrest, as well as facilitating forgiveness (Warner 2013).

Anointing

Anointing is the devotional act of applying sacred oil to specific parts of the body. This ancient ritual forms part of many religious ceremonies and is a practice which has become commonplace in non-religious spiritual celebrations, blessings and healings. Traditionally, anointing is performed by one person to another, such as a priest offering sacramental graces to the sick. However, this act of benevolence has extended to other areas, including self-anointing, where the giver also becomes the receiver. This can take place in any number of settings and situations and is common within aromatherapy practice.

In the active dying phase, patients may request a blend of oils for their personal anointing rituals. Conversations will guide decisions on oil preferences and appropriate methods of application. Patients may have their own specific blend or wish to use personalized blends which have brought them comfort during transitional times along their cancer journey. In practical terms, preparing a rollerball applicator is useful for self-anointing rituals. Alternately, creating a mist spray using hydrosols can be equally consoling.

Self-anointing

Self-anointing is a ritual I use in my clinical work for holistic preparation. Setting an intention with a sacred oil blend, or a mix of hydrosols,
prior to the session sharpens the focus and brings clarity. It is a moment
of stillness, of meditation in reverence of those about to come into my
care. The physical touch of the oil, or hydrosol, to the forehead, heart
space and to the palm of each hand is a symbolic gesture of intent. And
in closure at the end of the working day, after showering, a single drop
of the oil blend warmed in the palms of my hands comes to rest on my
heart space in gratitude of the work that has been shared.

Essential oils and dilution

Essential oils which seamlessly harmonize with this final transition
include *Agonis fragrans* (fragonia), *Angelica archangelica* (angelica),
Canarium luzonicum (elemi), *Commiphora myrrha* (myrrh), *Myrtus communis* (myrtle) and *Rosa damascena* (rose).

Throughout the active dying phase, the concentrated vapours of
a single essential oil can be over-powering. Reducing the level of concentration is necessary, even as low as 0.2% which equates to one or
two drops of essential oil in 100ml fixed oil, such as *Simmondsia chinensis* (jojoba), *Prunus armeniaca* (apricot kernel) or *Calendula officinalis*
(calendula).

Another useful staple among my aromatherapy treasures are tears of
Boswellia carterii (frankincense) resin. Place two or three tears (depending on their size, approximately 25g) in a 100ml jar, immerse in a fixed
oil, for example *Simmondsia chinensis* (jojoba) and leave in a cool dark
place to infuse for three to six months (expiry is the date of the fixed oil).
Gently invert the bottle each month to enable infusion of the delicate
fragrance. This can be used for all sacred interventions during end-of-
life care.

Hydrosols

The delicate fragrance of hydrosols can be used for anointing rituals,
mist sprays, added to the patient's bathing water during personal care
and via warm compresses applied to the entire body (see Chapter 3). In
final cleansing rituals of the patient's body after death, hydrosols can
create a positive lasting memory for those in grief, as highlighted in
Case study 14.1.

Inhalation

Essential oil inhalation may be familiar to the patient throughout the transitions within palliative care. However, as death approaches and the patient becomes more frail and less lucid, managing an aromatherapy inhaler stick requires assistance from caregivers. Alternatively, a single drop of an essential oil synergy on a tissue or small pillow placed near to the patient, or using a Bioesse® aromapatch, or a rollerball applicator, ensuring low-level concentration as appropriate to the individual, are other useful methods of application.

To avoid overwhelming a fragile patient with intense and sustained aromatic diffusion, judicious use is advised. If needed at all, one or two drops of essential oil diffused for short periods of time (five minutes once or twice per day), and at a distance from the patient, is ample. Subtlety is paramount in this preparatory time of sacred transition and can be equally achieved by bringing small quantities of fresh foliage or aromatic herbs from the garden into the room, or occasional sprays of quality hydrosol, in preference to the concentrated aroma of essential oils.

Massage

Touch is such a vital component of human connection and its marriage with essential oils has the capacity to enhance deep level peace and relaxation. However, during the active phase of dying, massage or even light touch may cause the patient disturbance or unrest and may no longer be needed. For those who work esoterically, this is a time to warm a small amount of essential oil (0.2%) in both hands and without physically touching the patient's body, tenderly connect with their energy field to allow the oil's life force to harmonize with theirs.

For family and caregivers, where sleep has been disturbed and long periods of the day are spent seated in close watch of the patient, gentle massage of the hands or feet, back and shoulders, or even a light head massage, can bring welcome sustenance.

Endings matter

As death approaches, close family and friends often gather in support to accompany the patient in their final days and hours of life. For those who sit in vigil, the experience is uniquely shared with the others involved. Carlile (2016) describes this as a time of mutual benefit, where the patient is surrounded by familiar voices, comforting handholding, favourite music, fragrances, or rituals customary to their life. Affirming the patient's worth is common, where family and friends share stories and cherished memories, conveying meaningful insight into the ways in which the patient has touched and enriched their lives. At the same time, it brings conscious reality to those in vigil of the patient's impending death.

Unfortunately, not every death is a smooth transition, moving from phase to phase with orderly progress. Sometimes death can be prolonged, where moments of significant deterioration are followed by periods of seeming strength as the patient rallies, although this is rarely to the level they were before. The emotional peaks and troughs that accompany such episodes can place enormous strain on everyone involved. And if overly prolonged, they can cause loved ones to have thoughts of just wishing for a peaceful ending and it all to be over – thoughts which may later return to trigger guilt.

Most vigils are peaceful. However, where families are estranged or blended, in terms of marriage and children, relationships of those in vigil may be strained by the presence of others. Similarly, relationships may have deteriorated and opportunities to reconcile differences have not happened. There may be distress for both parties where forgiveness has not been sought or been given. Emotions are heightened throughout this period, and it takes a sensitive team to facilitate diplomacy in the presence of the dying patient. In these situations, working alongside those in vigil by incorporating meditation, mindfulness, prayer or contemplation may ease the burden. This can be enhanced by inviting each person to warm a single drop of essential oil, diluted to 0.2%, between their palms in peaceful reverence of their loved one.

While this final phase of life is a preparatory time for those in vigil, the moment of death is profound and still comes as a shock. Suddenly, the senses are filled by the reality of not being able to share a conversation again, or to hear their voice or their laughter, or be able to hold them close and absorb their warmth or savour their familiar smell. In that moment, life is forever changed.

Endings matter because what we experience when someone close dies is taken into our conscious thought to circulate and consider our own mortality. It raises questions about whether this is how we would wish to die. Who would we want to accompany us on our transitional journey? Whether the experience has made us less or more fearful of death. Endings matter because they shape the way we approach the future.

Approaching the future

Death is a profound event and with it comes the onset of grief. For the caregiver, the experience of grief may have started long before the patient's death. 'Anticipatory' or 'preparatory' grief as it is also known, can start as early as the original diagnosis, where there is a heightened awareness of mortality and an inability to plan for a future. Bearing witness to the continual deterioration of the patient and their gradual retreat from the life once shared encompasses many progressive losses, past and future. Consequently, caregivers can experience separation anxiety, anticipation of death and future absence of the patient, denial, and relational losses (Coelho, de Brito and Barbosa 2018).

The grieving process

Inevitably, grief engages more fully from the moment the patient dies. Carlile (2016, p.232) succinctly explains that loss is 'the event and grief is how we respond to the event'. When someone close dies, grief is the reaction and is unique to each person, expressed individually, and is subjective in nature. No two people will experience grief in the same way and while there may be more than one significant loss in a person's life, the experience of grief for each bereavement will also differ.

In her seminal work, Kübler-Ross (1969) described five stages of grief where denial, anger, bargaining, depression, and acceptance are commonly observed reactions to grief. Although most bereaved may experience all five stages at some point, grief itself does not follow a linear pathway. Grief is unpredictable. There is no 'right' or 'wrong' way to grieve; no secret antidote to resolve grief; no rules or set time period. Grief is inescapably felt physically, emotionally, socially and spiritually. It changes with each person, altering throughout their lifetime without ever completely disappearing (Rosenblatt 2017).

The immediate weeks following the patient's death are accompanied by a maelstrom of emotions and feelings for the newly bereaved, including intense sadness, shock, anger, anxiety, regret, denial, pain, restlessness, hope and shame, which can last anything from a few moments to many hours (Carlile 2016). During this period, there are often visitors, including friends dropping by with meals and messages of condolence. However, for those grieving, it can feel impossible to engage with anyone because of the sheer force and nature of emotions that accompany the death of a loved one (Worden 2009). At first, all that is possible is to be alone, in silence, or in the space of their inconsolable crying. Sleep disturbance and consequent exhaustion are common, as are forgetfulness, and the loss of appetite and interest in what is happening around them (Hone 2017).

Among the full brunt of these emotions, where the reality of the patient's death is being realized, comfort comes in segments of remembrance. Memories can act like a salve, soothing the intense emotional pain, little by little, while adjustment to the new reality of their loved one no longer being there begins to emerge. This is where our senses unlock a deeper connection to our memories, through smell, touch, sight and sound.

Stroebe and Schut (1999) observed how, over time, the attention of the bereaved oscillates between being confronted by their loss and being distracted or seeking respite by concentrating on something else. This ebb and flow of grief is a strategy the authors advocate as being necessary for mental and physical health adjustment. Such flexibility brings space for recovery and strengthens resilience before re-engaging with the grief process.

In her profound and deeply insightful account of bereavement after her daughter's sudden death, Dr Lucy Hone (2017, p.104) advocates distraction 'because grieving is an exhausting business. Do whatever occupies your thoughts and consumes your attention. Don't be hard on yourself: if that means watching an entire TV series, or getting lost in movies, or listening to talking books.' Distraction of this nature is a positive means of enabling the bereaved to gently test the water of the real world.

Aromatherapy intervention for the bereaved

Predominantly, the literature which explores grief in cancer care is derived from evaluation of commonly encountered emotional reactions, where *time* inevitably is the healer. Less is reported on what would be helpful for the bereaved to be able to get through one day at a time. Having listened to Dr Lucy Hone present her personal account of grief, I felt both humbled and inspired by her 'practical strategies for resilient grieving'. At its core, the relationships we establish and nurture throughout life underpin resilience (see Chapters 4 and 13) and represent a fundamental part of our capacity to cope in the most adverse of circumstances, as in the death of a loved one.

In my clinical experience with those in bereavement, aromatherapy has been widely embraced as one such practical intervention to be used throughout the grieving process. In the words of one client, Donna Penney:

> when dealing with grief, time is not linear. I have huge blanks of memory; however, I can definitely remember that the aromatherapy treatments you provided to my husband and I, during the late stages of his illness, were outstanding. So healing, gentle and nurturing. We valued them greatly. I miss Keith every single day but I'm also ok. I am grateful for the gift of the home he built and the beautiful nature I have around me. I am grateful to have experienced such a great love.

Working alongside the bereaved

Every bereavement is different and as aromatherapists, it is crucial to remain mindful of this when working alongside those who are grieving. Active listening is central to the session, where the person feels safe and comfortable with their personal experience being acknowledged and accepted without judgement. Grief needs to be shared to ease some of the intense sadness and bring the person closer to accepting the death of their loved one. This is a fundamental part of healthy grieving (Hone 2017; Carlile 2016).

The experience of the patient's death, where it happened, who was there, what the funeral was like and who attended, are details the bereaved often recount several times over. Others may prefer to discuss the tasks which were once shared and now have become additional responsibilities to shoulder. And some may simply need the space to experience a time of stillness, away from what has become a life of constant flux. Interspersed in these conversations are moments of reminiscing, a valuable part of grieving.

It also needs to be acknowledged that family caregivers have to deal not only with the death of their loved one, but also with the impact of the caregiving experience itself. Therefore, many will begin their bereavement emotionally and physically depleted. Aromatherapists are well placed to observe and explore the individual's grief and monitor and report any signs of concern regarding adverse health issues to the MDT.

Essential oils

The death of a loved one is associated with significant increases in mental and physical health problems in the bereaved, although the precise mechanisms are not fully understood (Seiler, von Känel and Slavich 2020). Arguably, the field of psychoneuroimmunology has identified the closest research-based links between life stressors and their effects on the autonomic nervous system, and neuroendocrine and immune processes, which are highly relevant to bereavement (Glaser and Kei-colt-Glaser 2005; Hansel *et al.* 2010; Seiler *et al.* 2020). The broad range of essential oil pharmacology, combined with the holistic approach to oil selection, makes it a valuable option for modulating the stress response and palliating an over-stimulated hypothalamic adrenocortical axis (HPA).

Incorporating essential oils as discussed in Chapters 5, 6, 8 and 13, which consider spiritual and emotional care as well as insomnia and fostering resilience in this time of grieving, is invaluable. Additionally, a few essential oils I keep close at hand for psychospiritual bereavement work include *Agonis fragrans* (fragonia), *Canarium luzonicum* (elemi), *Cistus ladanifer* (cistus), *Citrus aurantium var amara flos* (neroli), *Citrus aurantium var amara fol.* (petitgrain), *Citrus bergamia* (bergamot), *Citrus limon* (lemon), *Citrus sinensis* (sweet orange), *Cupressus sempervirens* (cypress), *Lavandula angustifolia* (lavender true), *Nardostachys jatamansi* (spikenard), *Origanum majorana* (sweet marjoram) and *Pelargonium graveolens* (geranium).

For those inconsolable in their grief, struggling with anxiety, or in the event of the death of a young person, Warner (2018) advocates *Viola odorata* (violet leaf). The moments preceding and immediately after the death of a loved one can bring feelings of catastrophic loss to some which requires the deeply calming comfort of *Cistus ladanifer* (cistus). Zeck (2014, p.77) advocates, 'Gently rub Cistus over your heart centre to bring serenity to your soul in the midst of crisis.' For those experiencing uncontrollable anxiety and panic attacks, *Cananga odorata* (ylang ylang) can be highly relaxing (Kerkhof-Knapp Hayes 2015).

Grieving involves high levels of prolonged stress, which adversely impacts immune system function, rendering the bereaved susceptible to opportunist infections and other stress-related health issues. Useful oils for this purpose include *Abies alba* (silver fir), *Cinnamomum camphora* (ravintsara), *Citrus limon* (lemon), *Commiphora myrrha* (myrrh), *Eucalyptus radiata* (narrow-leaf eucalyptus), *Kunzea ericoides* (kanuka), *Lavandula angustifolia* (lavender true), *Leptospermum scoparium* (manuka), *Picea mariana* (spruce black), *Pinus sylvestris* (scots pine) and *Zingiber officinale* (ginger) CO_2-total extract.

Selecting essential oils for psychosocial and spiritual care alongside oils known to support immune system function offers a rounded approach which is central to holistic intervention.

Aromatherapy application
Inhalation

Gentle essential oil inhalation is primarily the route of choice to man-age the emotional and spiritual experiences of grief. Clinical practice has taught me the value of aromatic anchoring (see Chapter 3), often deeply connecting the bereaved with aromatherapy inhaler sticks in combination with visualization drawn from their personal stories, or with massage or a warm aromatic footbath and foot reflexology.

Working with gentle breath cycles (see Chapter 3) creates physical movement of the chest, where even a small expansion brings a sense of space to ease the central burden of emotional grief. Such a routine can be useful in times where grief catches the bereaved person unaware, and where a few moments of conscious aromatic breathing can help pave the way to be able to move forward. Additionally, incorporating oils from the conifer family, such as *Abies alba* (silver fir), *Picea mariana* (spruce black) and *Pinus sylvestris* (scots pine), all of which have a natural affinity with the respiratory system, is beneficial. This is particularly relevant to those whose pastimes include forest walks, and is enhanced by the addition of *Citrus limon* (lemon) (Benavides 2021).

Massage

The absence of touch, particularly for those who are bereaved of a partner and living alone, can be deeply felt. Incorporating relaxation massage can achieve immense physical, emotional and spiritual comfort from tender human reconnection. The emphasis here rests with 'relax-ation', using slow-stroke massage, rather than remedial or deep tissue work. Relaxation massage is recommended even when musculoskeletal tension arising from prolonged stress and the physical demand of car-egiving is evident. And it is particularly relevant in the newly bereaved, where the senses are in disarray and the experience of numbness and shock may obscure the person's reality of the depth of pressure being applied. Release of muscle tension can be quite easily achieved by apply-ing moist, warm heat to the skin (using towels), prior to introducing essential oils. This facilitates fascial release as well as rapid absorption of the oil blend being used. Tender, gentle care is important to enable rest and to rebalance the central nervous system and HPA.

An additional benefit of massage with the bereaved client rests with vigilance of the general condition of their skin. Simple observation of whether the skin is hydrated and nourished, or dry and scaly with signs of superficial infection, and whether there is weight loss or weight gain (over time), can indicate how the bereaved client is caring for themselves and whether intervention from the MDT is required.

CASE STUDY 14.1: FAREWELL TO GAIL

Gail took her last breath quietly and alone in the interim space between the nurse's tending her comfort and her partner and close friends taking a break from their vigil. It was only a few minutes, but enough for Gail to know she had been surrounded by those who loved her and use the space of those solitary moments to make her final transition.

Sometime later and with permission from Gail's partner, one of her close friends and myself undertook the final preparations. Each person in the vigil had brought a gift for her transition, a vase of wildflowers, a spray of orchids, a scented candle, photographs of loved ones, a pair of silk trousers, her favourite top and a gift of hydrosols, a rose quartz heart and music sacred for the occasion.

The lights were dimmed, a window opened and space cleared so that we could work either side of our friend. We lit the candle and drew the table of flowers closer. Her partner joined us in the room as we talked Gail through our acts of devotion, cleansing her body in the delicately fragranced waters of *Agonis fragrans* (fragonia) and *Rosa damascena* (rose), the music quietly accompanying us. We dressed her in the silk trousers and top, laid a fresh blanket over her and invited her partner to tend to her hair because neither of us was able to get it right. With a deft flick of the fingers, her partner fleetingly lifted Gail's hair and let it fall loosely into the tousled look that was familiar. It brought a momentary smile, a tender appreciation of their love and closeness. A final mist of hydrosol of *Citrus aurantium var amara flos* (neroli) was created over Gail's body. Her partner placed the orchid sprays and remarked how peaceful she looked, as if she were sleeping, and how beautiful she looked. A lasting memory captured.

CASE STUDY 14.2: HAZEL'S EXPERIENCE

As a young woman dying from advanced ovarian cancer, Hazel was looking for something to bring comfort. Not just the physical relief from her pain medication, it was more than that, she wanted to feel weightless. Her petite frame was heavily burdened with abdominal ascites and her only relief came from immersion in a warm bath, where she felt a sense of buoyancy. However, her diminishing strength and increasing frailty meant bathing was no longer a practical option.

Hazel felt too weak to receive massage, but in the stillness of the therapy room, she was content to lie on the massage table, her bony prominences supported with an array of soft bolsters and pillows. She rested beneath a patchwork quilt, hand-stitched by one of the hospice volunteers, as the warmth from the heated table began to penetrate. It reminded her of hot New Zealand summers and lazy afternoons. I asked her to describe what that meant to her. After she finished, we worked together with the oils to create something light and fresh, a reminder of her summers in our citrus-growing region (see Table 14.1).

Table 14.1: Hazel's aromatherapy intervention

Method of application	Essential oils used	Amount used	Directions for use
Aromatherapy inhaler stick 'Summer'	*Citrus limon* (lemon) *Citrus paradisi* (grapefruit) *Cupressus sempervirens* (cypress) *Simmondsia chinensis* (jojoba)	3 drops 2 drops 1 drop 1ml	Patient-directed as required At each use, inhale 4–8 breath cycles

That evening, I received a text from Hazel: 'Thank you for being wonderful this morning. This afternoon's gift from you was, the sense of a summer afternoon, where a friend shares happily the first lemons from his garden, which he has crafted into fluffy clouds of curd. The curd has high points of tart lemon, and a gentle soft lemon, full of love.'

Reflection
Actively listening for the important cues in conversation and expressing an interest in the person beyond their illness is crucial. Human life is made meaningful by the stories which shape it, and these become central when determining what has been significant in the patient's life. Reconnecting with these memories, of favourite pastimes, places they have visited or wished to visit, can be achieved through the aromas of essential oils, or with the fragrance of other non-botanicals. Reconnection of this nature can bring considerable comfort and reassurance.

For Hazel, in these last days of her life, when it was no longer feasible to take a bath for the physical buoyancy, it was possible to achieve a sense of weightlessness in body, mind and spirit. Creating an oil blend which reconnected her to a favourite moment in time and combining it with visualization enabled her to take rest, as often as needed, in a compassionate space of memory.

CHAPTER 15

The Way Forward

Throughout this book, the central issues relevant to patients with life-limiting cancer have been explored within the context of common symptoms, their conventional medical management, non-pharmacological approaches and aromatherapy intervention. Gaps exist and central themes are evident. This chapter will therefore consider the way forward to aid practitioners, healthcare professionals, allied professionals, clinical researchers, students and those with an interest in optimizing the quality of life of patients with life-limiting illness and their families.

Gaps in healthcare

In *Complementary Therapies in Cancer Care*, Kohn (1999) highlighted how patients seek out such therapies as adjuncts to their conventional medical interventions because it offers them touch, time and the opportunity to talk. Similar findings have since been reported by patients with life-limiting illness (Armstrong *et al.* 2019a; Armstrong *et al.* 2019b; Candy *et al.* 2020). However, clinical gaps exist, many of which are evidenced throughout this book.

Holistic approach

Within healthcare, it is apparent that the emphasis of the biomedical model primarily rests with the physical aspects of disease, symptoms and their pharmacological management. A clinical imbalance exists where the patient's emotional, social and spiritual capacities, combined with a comprehensive understanding of their unique ability to cope, are areas requiring attention. It is therefore crucial that these holistic capacities of the patient are not separated and remain a fundamental part of patient-centred and relationship-centred care.

Environment

No one wants to embark on the cancer trajectory, an arduous and unpredictable journey filled with critical stages unique to the individual. High levels of existential and psychological distress accompany the patient and their caregivers from diagnosis onwards and yet, clinical environments are not always conducive to private conversation or the opportunity for open communication. How is it possible to be forthcoming when the healthcare professional is hurried and working within overburdened time constraints? Consequently, issues of importance to the patient are easily overlooked. Space and time are of paramount importance for the patient and their family to be able to take stock of what is happening, consider the options and review these within the context of their life situation. This is a view upheld by Armstrong *et al.* (2019b).

Early referral

As part of the multi-disciplinary team (MDT) approach, complementary therapies offered early in the cancer pathway provide patients with the option of interventions which can help them to manage their situation more easily. Early referral offers the patient and caregivers sessions dedicated to their relaxation and well-being. Within a safe and trusted space they can choose to explore their priorities of concern, where spiritual and psychosocial care are central and symptom management is considered within a broader holistic context. Collectively, this has the potential to strengthen their capacity to cope with the challenges being faced (see Chapters 4, 5, 6 and 13).

Integrating complementary therapies into specialist palliative care enhances regular symptom management, increases comfort and is a valuable addition to the MDT (Berger *et al.* 2013). More often, the clinical reality is that referral occurs when all other conventional avenues of symptom management have been exhausted. Establishing clear lines of communication is therefore essential. This can be achieved by attending MDT meetings where active participation in discussions facilitates sharing of ideas and insights and enhances collaborative decision-making. It allows for another viewpoint, incorporating aromatherapy and other complementary approaches for symptom management, while also reinforcing the holistic dimensions of care. Many healthcare professionals are unaware of the diversity of clinical aromatherapy, making the MDT meeting a valuable forum to educate healthcare colleagues and raise awareness of aromatherapy services while simultaneously advocating earlier referral.

A pragmatic approach, when starting a new service, is to begin with one symptom. A good example is insomnia, where evaluation of aromatherapy intervention with the MDT can unravel a host of intimate existential and psychosocial issues, as well as any physical causal factors which may not necessarily be responding to conventional pharmacology. It is a simple starting point that provides the team with a realistic insight into holistic and clinical aromatherapy intervention.

From my personal clinical experience, working as part of an MDT is a deeply rewarding experience. The wealth of expertise and the diverse skill set creates an inspiring environment, where all professional disciplines collaborate to support the choices and wishes of the patient and family.

Communication

Terminology is a consistent feature throughout this book, where the words and phrases used by healthcare professionals may not always align with those of the patient. Medical terminology needs to be translated into a form the patient will understand. Vigilance is required when listening to the patient's narrative, where a considerable amount can be learned from their descriptors. This brings depth and gravity to what they are experiencing and requires active listening, the appropriate use of silence and reflective summary which incorporates their exact words.

Assessment and evaluation

Assessment involves a clear understanding of the patient's situation and issues which are foremost in their concerns. Background information regarding their diagnosis and medications, together with an overview of their medical and social history can be obtained from the MDT in advance of seeing the patient. More often, patients will present with a diverse range of problems that are complex and multi-factorial.

The holistic approach is integral to any assessment of symptoms the patient may be experiencing, where its dimensions remain interconnected and the patient's perspective is central. Guidance to assist symptom exploration with the patient and aid clinical assessment involves exploring the following:

- What does the symptom mean to the patient?
- How does the symptom affect their everyday life?
- What is the patient's understanding of their illness?
- How does the patient view their future?

The SYMPTOM model for reviewing the role of aromatherapy in symptom management, as described by Mackereth and Maycock (2017, p.107), is a useful acronym for practitioners to follow, as summarised in Table 15.1.

Table 15.1: The SYMPTOM acronym for reviewing aromatherapy interventions (Mackereth and Maycock 2017, p.107)

S	Symptom definition and causation
Y	Your patient's experience of the symptom
M	Medical management
P	Purpose of you providing aromatherapy
T	Technique/treatment delivery/route
O	Options/advice
M	Monitoring/maintaining symptom control

Working cohesively with the MDT enables continuous assessment which minimizes overburdening the patient and family. Not everything can be achieved in a single session, and input from individual professionals helps to create a broader picture. Assessment forms an essential baseline for all therapeutic interventions and must include meticulous evaluation.

Evaluation

Evaluation is commonplace in palliative care, where effectiveness of pharmacology and conventional intervention is monitored with thoroughness. Clinical aromatherapy interventions require equal attention to monitor changes, determine therapeutic effectiveness and monitor patient compliance. Discussion with the MDT is necessary to include ongoing monitoring of prescribed interventions as part of the patient review processes.

On a broader scale, the use of patient-directed audit tools, such as Measure Yourself Concerns and Wellbeing (MYCaW) and Measure Yourself Medical Outcome Profile (MYMOP) (Ishaque, Johnson and Vohra 2019), provide tangible evidence of individual clinical interventions while also determining overall service provision.

Clinical research in palliative care

Evidence-based practice is fast becoming an integral part of an aromatherapist's requirement to practise within healthcare settings, particularly palliative care. However, accurately capturing the patient's experience of aromatherapy interventions, the supportive role of the therapist, the increased feeling of well-being and the respite this brings to their process of dying is impossible to achieve within the rigid framework of quantitative studies. This is evident throughout the chapters of this book, where a striking observation is the shortage of high-quality clinical research within palliative care, including clinical aromatherapy. Few aromatherapy studies meet the eligibility criteria of systematic review and meta-analysis. Of those that do, many individual studies indicate promising results, but the clinical significance is often compromised by small sample size, poor methodological rigour and lack of statistical power which prevents translation into clinical benefit. As such, this requires consideration of appropriate research methods, including the differences between efficacy and effectiveness studies.

Efficacy studies

To minimize bias, the efficacy of an intervention (or its performance) is evaluated under strict criteria. This is to demonstrate the intervention as being the only possibility responsible for the effect, which often involves a considerable deviation from the 'real world' into placebo-controlled, double-blind, randomized controlled trials. Generally, this requires strict entry criteria of a defined homogenous group of single morbidity, where participants have the same or a similar diagnosis, illness or condition. Highly standardized interventions ensure that every participant receives the same dose, timing and method of application. Concurrent medications are also often restricted. In most situations, a team of qualified researchers with access to high-level resources to maximize patient compliance and data collection undertake the overall management of RCTs.

Clinical reality

Within palliative care, the clinical reality is patients with a diverse range of life-limiting illness, often of an older age group and commonly with multiple co-morbidities. Kamal and Peppercorn (2013) and Visser, Hadley and Wee (2015) point out several challenges of efficacy studies in this specialist area, including the unlikelihood of determining a homogenous group of single morbidity. Coupled with poor attrition rates, where patients are simply unable to complete the study because of their deteriorating health, obtaining adequate numbers of participants and sufficient data to achieve statistical significance is virtually impossible. Added to which, subject burden and reduced compliance collectively leads to inadequate follow-up and reduced efficacy of the intervention being evaluated. Consequently, palliative care researchers are moving to the other end of the research continuum towards effectiveness studies.

Effectiveness studies

At this end of the research spectrum, Kamal and Peppercorn (2013) and Visser *et al.* (2015) report a broader level of inclusivity, where patients with multiple health issues are invited to receive interventions which closely resemble the 'real world'. The limited inclusion criteria allow for heterogeneous groups which are also open to patients with co-morbidities. Effectiveness studies take a more pragmatic approach, allowing for concurrent medications, tailoring to the individual's needs, as well as incorporating minimal restrictions on dose regimes, modifications and co-therapies.

How does this translate into aromatherapy research within palliative care?

Clearly, evaluating aromatherapy interventions within the palliative care setting does not lend itself to the rigid framework of an efficacy study. The dramatic differences of an intervention in patients with life-limiting illness may go undetected because their health is progressively deteriorating. Furthermore, we risk losing the patient's values and the holistic principles of our practice to bureaucracy. As such, aromatherapists are faced with the conundrum of sustaining aromatherapy interventions while working within the full remit of evidence-based practice.

The answer lies in the original report *Complementary Therapies in Cancer Care* (Kohn 1999), where the patient's perspective informed clinical guidelines and practice. Few studies have since considered why patients with life-limiting illness engage in complementary therapies such as aromatherapy, their experiences and the perceived benefits. One qualitative synthesis evaluated a variety of complementary therapies in patients with cancer, reporting that patients experience improved physical and psychosocial well-being, empowerment and a connection with the therapist (Smithson *et al.* 2012).

More recently, Armstrong *et al.* (2019b), focused specifically on qualitative studies evaluating aromatherapy, massage and reflexology in patients with advanced forms of cancer. This well-designed, qualitative synthesis identified three consistent themes to explore the patient's experience in more depth:

- Experience during the therapy
- Beyond the complementary therapy session
- The process of delivery of aromatherapy in palliative care

The findings of Armstrong *et al.*'s (2019b) analytical review are invaluable to clinical practice, as all participants, across all five studies, reported the positive effects of complementary therapy. Of importance is the emphasis placed by patients on personal autonomy and self-worth. It includes the freedom to choose whether they would like to receive complementary therapy or not, and involvement in choosing the essential oils and the area to be massaged. Patients highly value these small, considered details.

Emphasis is also placed on the relaxed and inviting environment that contributes to patients experiencing a feeling of safety and trust. Moreover, they emphasize the special connection with a therapist experienced in palliative care, who understands their specific situation. Most notable is how therapists focus on the present moment, which is a preference the patients said helped relieve the anxiety about their disease, their situation and the future. Collectively, this contributed to their psychosocial and physical well-being beyond the complementary therapy session, with patients relating how this imparted a sense of hope for the future.

Unquestionably, the richness of data retrieved from this qualitative approach provides valuable insight into the patient's experience of complementary therapy. The immediate benefits of respite from their process of dying to provide hope for their future are experiences and outcomes which are impossible to capture through quantitative research methods. How can a person's 'feeling of peace' or experience of 'floating away', 'altering time' or 'relief from suffering' be accurately measured? As yet, there are no quality of life measurement scales which are sufficiently sensitive and responsive to reflect all the aspects which patients with life-limiting illness consider important (McCaffrey *et al.* 2016). In truth, only the patients' own words can accurately convey these outcomes.

Future research initiatives

The consensus among qualitative researchers is for palliative care services to continue offering complementary therapies, specifically, aromatherapy, massage and reflexology, as part of a patient's holistic care until more robust research is undertaken (Armstrong *et al.* 2019a;

Armstrong *et al.* 2019b; Candy *et al.* 2020). However, the paradox arises when it comes to evidence-based practice because conventional health-care professionals are resolute in applying quantitative measures. These are unrealistic for the patient with life-limiting illness because they miss the vital part of understanding the inter-connectedness of being human. In order to fulfil the remit of evidence-based practice in the healthcare setting we need to consider the following areas.

Clinical case studies

A valuable starting point for any aromatherapist, clinical case studies ensure accurate and detailed documentation of patient sessions. The specifics of the presenting issue, the aim of the therapeutic intervention, the botanical products used, methods of application and evaluation of the overall effectiveness are important. Clinical case studies are often catalysts for the creation of pragmatic and realistic research questions. Furthermore, published case studies or sharing with the International Case Study Collaboration (2022) assist clinical practice, particularly in less common situations, for example the patient with malignant wounds.

Research methodology

Qualitative research methods, involving the patient's perspective, are highly appropriate for evaluating aromatherapy intervention within palliative care. Such approaches bring us closer to the patient's actual experience. Themes can be determined which can guide and enhance patient-centred clinical practice. Additionally, formulating relevant research questions from the patient's perspective is important. The Macmillan Listening study's findings (Wright *et al.* 2007) are an excel-lent example since they identified patients' clinical research priorities. Interestingly, the wide-ranging impact of cancer on everyday life and the need for support to self-manage ranked as the highest priorities of patients, above research into new treatments or basic understanding of their disease.

Mixed-method designs with varying integration of qualitative and quantitative methods are useful to generate how interventions are deliv-ered in the clinical setting and perceived by patients, families, caregivers and funding stakeholders (Fàbriques *et al.* 2020). In an Editorial Review published in *Palliative Medicine*, researchers are urged to 'proactively consider research design and any innovations to maximize the impact of their research', the aim being to minimize small, single-site trials and studies lacking sufficient methodological rigour (van der Steen, Bloomer and Pereira 2020, p.2).

Aromatherapy education

Aromatherapy qualification needs to incorporate a curriculum research component whereby students can critically examine published research (beyond the abstract), determine the quality of the evidence and its relevance to our clinical practice, together with developing a basic appreciation of research methodology.

Inter-professional collaboration

Collaboration is crucial to the success of any research initiative. Aromatherapists are fundamental to clinical research teams evaluating the effectiveness of aromatherapy interventions. Our unique contribution rests with the specific knowledge of essential oils, botanical products and their appropriate application, including use of the correct botanical names and species. This alone enables future researchers to successfully replicate studies and compare effects in other populations. Furthermore, an aromatherapist's insight into the holistic needs of patients with life-limiting illness and the clinical experience of hosting therapy sessions with patients is paramount.

Working alongside researchers can facilitate trial design which is realistic and appropriate to the questions being evaluated. With the establishment of platforms such as the International Clinical Aromatherapy Network (ICAN) and a range of international aromatherapy conferences, including Botanica, Aromatica, Phyt'Arome and the Alliance of International Aromatherapists, qualified aromatherapists have the opportunity to globally network with clinical researchers, essential oil distributors and experts in their field of specialization, to generate new and exciting research initiatives, as well as to present and share clinical findings.

Palliative care researchers advocate qualitative approaches to evaluate complementary therapies such as aromatherapy interventions, in accordance with the key principles described by patients (Armstrong *et al.* 2019a; Armstrong *et al.* 2019b; Candy *et al.* 2020):

- Patient–therapist relationship
- Complementary therapy environment
- Patient choice
- Number of sessions

Additional to these recommendations are those highlighted throughout this book which are specific to the nature, intensity and duration of symptoms common to this patient group. Aromatherapists are well placed to collaboratively develop and evaluate outcome measures which capture the diversity and richness of the patient's aromatherapy experience. Such clarity guides evidence-based clinical practice and appropriate, patient-centred and relationship-centred service provision within palliative care.

Conclusion

At the heart of this book and every clinical encounter is the patient approaching their end-of-life journey, their family and caregivers. These final months, weeks and days are unique to the individual person, where their focus gradually tapers to the simple things in life that really matter to them. Being invited into this intimate space, where we enter their private world, is a privilege which deserves our utmost respect and mindfulness.

Interpreting the patient's uniqueness spiritually, emotionally, socially and physically, whilst simultaneously applying these same holistic principles to their presenting symptoms, is central to clinical aromatherapy intervention. As part of a MDT, qualified aromatherapists have the capacity to facilitate circumstances where the patient can contemplate their thoughts, perspectives, concerns, needs and wishes. Sensitive communication is crucial, listening is foremost, silences are valued and the patient's words become the shared vocabulary with which to enable deeper insight into their situation.

Integrating essential oils, botanical products and methods of application then develops into a collaborative experience that reflects the patient's priorities of concern and strives to restore human wholeness. The emphasis of such aromatherapy intervention is to bring the person to the present moment, provide respite from their process of dying and in doing so, impart a sense of peacefulness and acceptance.

References

Abdel-Aziz, H., Windeck, T., Ploch, M. & Verspohl, E. (2006) Mode of action of gingerols and shogaols on 5HT3 receptors: Binding studies, cation uptake by the receptor channel and contraction of guinea-pig ileum. *European Journal of Pharmacology 530*, 1-2, 136-143.

Abdelghfar, S., Elsebae, S., Elhadry, S. & Haasan, A. (2017) Effect of aromatherapy among patients undergoing hemodialysis. *IOSR Journal of Nursing and Health Science 6*, 2, 22-30.

Abernethy, A., McDonald, C., Frith, P., Clark, K. *et al.* (2010) Effect of palliative oxygen versus room air in relief of breathlessness in patients with refractory dyspnoea: A double-blind, randomised controlled trial. *The Lancet 376*, 784-793.

Abernethy, A. & Wheeler, J. (2008) Total dyspnoea. *Current Opinion in Supportive Palliative Care 2*, 2, 110-113.

Adam, M. & Jewell, A. (2007) The use of complementary and alternative medicine by cancer patients. *International Seminars in Surgical Oncology 4*, 10, 1-7.

Agar, M., Currow, D., Plummer, J., Seidel, R., Carnahan, R. & Abernethy, A. (2009) Changes in anticholinergic load from regular prescribed medications in palliative care as death approaches. *Palliative Medicine 23*, 3, 257-265.

Agra, G., Ferreira, T., Oliveira, D., Nogueira, W. *et al.* (2017) Neoplastic wounds: Controlling pain, exudate, odor and bleeding. *International Archives of Medicine: Oncology 10*, 118, 1-11. doi: 10.3823/2388.

Ahlberg, K., Ekman, T., Gaston-Johansson, F. & Mock, V. (2003) Assessment and management of cancer-related fatigue in adults. *The Lancet 362*, 640-650.

Ahles, T., Tope, D., Pinkson, B., Walch, S. *et al.* (1999) Massage therapy for patients undergoing autologous bone marrow transplantation. *Journal of Pain and Symptom Management 18*, 3, 157-163.

Alcorn, S., Balboni, M., Prigerson, H., Reynolds, A. *et al.* (2010) 'If God wanted me yesterday, I wouldn't be here today': Religious and spiritual themes in patients' experiences of advanced cancer. *Journal of Palliative Medicine 13*, 5, 581-588.

Alexander, S. (2010) An intense and unforgettable experience: The lived experience of malignant wounds from the perspectives of patients, caregivers and nurses. *International Journal of Wound Care 7*, 6, 456-465.

Allan, J. & Gray, L. (2017) Aromatherapy interventions for a fungating breast tumour: Case study. *International Journal of Clinical Aromatherapy 12*, 2, 25-29.

Alshammary, S., Duraisamy, B. & Alsuhail, A. (2017) Review of management of pruritus in palliative care. *Journal of Health Specialties (review article)*, 1P 37.216.233.146.

Alves, A., Gonçalves, J., Cruz, J. & Araújo, D. (2010) Evaluation of the sesquiterpene (-)-alpha-bisabolol as a novel peripheral nervous blocker. *Neuroscience Letters 472*, 1, 11-5.

Alves, M., Jardim, M. & Gomes, B. (2017) Effect of massage therapy in cancer patients in palliative situation. *Universal Journal of Public Health 5*, 4, 164-171.

American Thoracic Society. (1999) Dyspnea: Mechanisms, assessment and management: A consensus statement. *American Journal of Respiratory and Critical Care 159*, 321-340.

Ames, D. (2006) Aromatic wound care in a healthcare system: A report from the United States. *International Journal of Clinical Aromatherapy 3*, 2b, 3-8.

Anh, N. & Son, H. (2016) Potentials of plant oils in pruritus alleviation. *Journal of Advances in Medical and Pharmaceutical Sciences 11*, 2, 1–14.

Aoshima, H. & Hamamoto, K. (1999) Potentiation of GABAA receptors expressed in Xenopus oocytes by perfume and phytoncide. *Bioscience, Biotechnology and Biochemistry 63*, 743–748.

Araujo, T., Jarrin, D., Leanza, Y. & Morin, C. (2017) Qualitative studies of insomnia: Current state of knowledge in the field. *Sleep Medicine Review 31*, 58–69.

Aresi, G., Rayner, H., Hassan, L., Burton, J. *et al.* (2019) Reasons for under-reporting of uraemic pruritus in people with chronic kidney disease: A qualitative study. *Journal of Pain and Symptom Management 58*, 4, 578–586.

Aretin, M. (2021) Obstipation and diarrhoea in palliative care – a pharmacist's view. *Magazine of European Medical Oncology 14*, 44–47.

Armstrong, M., Flemming, K., Kupeli, N., Stone, P., Wilkinson, S. & Candy, B. (2019a) Aromatherapy, massage and reflexology: A systematic review and thematic synthesis of the perspectives from people with palliative care needs. *Palliative Medicine 33*, 7, 757–769.

Armstrong, M., Kupeli, N., Flemming, K., Stone, P., Wilkinson, S. & Candy, B. (2019b) Complementary therapy in palliative care: A synthesis of qualitative and quantitative systematic reviews. *Palliative Medicine 34*, 10, 1332–1339.

Austen, P., Macleod, R., Siddall, P., McSherry, W. & Egan, R. (2016) The ability of hospital staff to recognise and meet patients' spiritual needs: A pilot study. *Journal for the Study of Spirituality 6*, 1, 20–37.

Avila, C., Massick, S., Kaffenberger, B., Kwatra, S. & Bechtel, M. (2020) Cannabinoids for the treatment of chronic pruritus: A review. *Journal of the American Academy of Dermatology 82*, 5, 1205–1212.

Bagetta, G., Morrone, L., Rombolà, L., Amantea, D. *et al.* (2010) Neuropharmacology of the essential oil of bergamot. *Fitoterapia 81*, 6, 453–461.

Bahraini, S. (2011) The effect of aromatherapy massage on the fatigue severity in women with multiple sclerosis. *Journal of Sabzevar University of Medical Sciences 18*, 3, 172–178.

Balaban, C. & Yates, B. (2017) What is nausea? A historical analysis of changing views. *Autonomic Neuroscience 202*, 5–17.

Balboni, T., Paulk, M., Balboni, M., Phelps, A. *et al.* (2009) Provision of spiritual care to patients with advanced cancer: Associations with medical care and quality of life near death. *American Society of Clinical Oncology 28*, 3, 445–452.

Balboni, T., Vanderwerker, L., Block, S., Paulk, M. *et al.* (2007) Religiousness and spiritual support among advanced cancer patients and associations with end-of-life treatment preferences and quality of life. *Journal of Clinical Oncology 25*, 5, 555–560.

Baldwin, J. & Cox, J. (2016) Treating dyspnea: Is oxygen therapy the best option for all patients? *The Medical Clinics of North America 100*, 5, 1123–1130.

Balkstra, C. (2010) 'Dyspnea.' In M. Matzo & D. Sherman (eds) *Palliative Care Nursing: Quality of Life to the End (third edition).* New York, NY: Springer Publishing.

Bardia, A., Barton, D., Prokop, L., Bauer, B. & Moynihan, T. (2006) Efficacy of complementary and alternative medicine therapies in relieving cancer pain: A systematic review. *Journal of Clinical Oncology 24*, 34, 5457–5464.

Barton, D., Soori, G., Bauer, B., Sloan, J., Johnson, P., Fiqueras C. *et al.* (2009) Pilot study of Panax quinquefolius (American ginseng) to improve cancer-related fatigue: A randomised, double-blind, dose-finding evaluation: NCCTG trial NO3CA. *Supportive Cancer Care 18*, 179–187.

Battaglia, S. (2018) *The Complete Guide to Aromatherapy: Volume 1 Foundations and Materia Medica (third edition).* Australia: Black Pepper Creativity.

Baudoux, D. (2007) Aromatology for respiratory pathologies. *International Journal of Clinical Aromatherapy 4*, 1, 34–39.

Baudoux, D., Blanchard, J. & Malotaux, A. (2006) *Les Cahiers ratiques d'aromathérapie selon l'école française: soins palliatifs (vol. 4).* Belgium: Lannoo.

Bausewein, C., Schunk, M., Schumacher, P., Dittmer, J., Bolzani, A. & Booth, S. (2018) Breathlessness services as a new model of support for patients with respiratory disease. *Chronic Respiratory Disease 15*, 1, 48–59.

Bauters, T., Schandevyl, G. & Laureys, G. (2016) Safety in the use of Vaseline during oxygen therapy: The pharmacist's perspective. *International Journal of Clinical Pharmacy 38*, 1032–1034.

Benavides, J. (2021) Sensing, feeling, repairing: Aromatic suggestions for anxiety and mild depression. *International Clinical Aromatherapy Network: Deep Dive Aroma Series* (7 Oct 2021).

Benson, J., Oliver, D., Demiris, G. & Washington, K. (2019) Accounts of family conflict in home hospice care: The central role of autonomy for informal caregiver resilience. *Journal of Family Nursing 25*, 2, 190–218.

Bensouilah, J. & Buck, P. (2006) *Aromadermatology.* Oxford: Radcliffe Publishing.

Berger, L., Tavares, M. & Berger, B. (2013) A Canadian experience of integrating complementary therapy in a hospital palliative care unit. *Journal of Palliative Medicine 16*, 10, 1294–1298.

Bethann, M., Scarborough, M., Cardinale, B. & Smith, M. (2018) Optimal pain management for patients with cancer in the modern era. *CA: A Cancer Journal for Clinicians 68*, 182–196.

Billhut, A., Bergbom, I. & Stenes-Victorin, E. (2007) Massage relieves nausea in women with breast cancer who are undergoing chemotherapy. *Journal of Alternative and Complementary Therapy 13*, 1, 53–57.

Boehm, K., Büssing, A. & Ostermann, T. (2012) Aromatherapy as an adjuvant treatment in cancer care – A descriptive systematic review. *African Journal of Traditional, Complementary and Alternative Medicine 9*, 4, 503–518.

Bonanno, G., Westphal, M. & Mancini, A. (2011) Resilience to loss and potential trauma. *Annual Review of Clinical Psychology.* doi: 10.1146/annurev-clinpsy-032210-104526.

Bossi, P., Antonuzzo, A., Cherny, N., Rosengarten, O. *et al.* (2018) Diarrhoea in adult cancer patients: ESMO clinical practice guidelines. *Annals of Oncology 29*, suppl 4, iv126–iv142.

Bouya, S., Ahmadidarehsima, S., Badakhsh, M. & Balouchi, A. (2018) Effect of aromatherapy interventions on haemodialysis complications: A systematic review. *Complementary Therapies in Clinical Practice 32*, 130–138.

Bowles, E. (2003) *The Chemistry of Aromatherapeutic Oils (third edition).* Crows Nest, New South Wales, Australia: Allen & Unwin.

BPJ. (2012) Managing breathlessness in palliative care. *Best Practice Journal New Zealand 47*, 23–27.

Bredin, M., Corner, J., Krishnasamy, M., Plant, H., Bailey, C. & A'Hern, R. (1999) Multicentre randomised controlled trial of nursing intervention for breathlessness in patients with lung cancer. *British Medical Journal 318*, 901–904.

Breidenbach, C., Heidkamp, P., Hiltrop, K., Pfaff, H. *et al.* (2022) Prevalence and determinants of anxiety and depression in long-term breast cancer survivors. *BMC Psychiatry 22*, 101.

Bremault-Phillips, S., Parmar, J., Johnson, M., Huhn, A. *et al.* (2016) The voices of family caregivers of seniors with chronic conditions: A window into their experience using a qualitative design. *Springer Plus 5*, 620. doi: 10.1186/s40064-016-2244-z.

Brennan, F. (2016) The pathophysiology of pruritus – A review for clinicians. *Progress in Palliative Care 24*, 3, 133–144.

Brown, M. & Farquhar-Smith, P. (2018) Cannabinoids and cancer pain: A new hope or a false dawn? *European Journal of Internal Medicine 49*, 30–36.

Buckle, J. (2015) *Clinical Aromatherapy: Essential Oils in Healthcare (third edition).* St. Louis, MO: Elsevier.

Burrow, A., Eccles, R. & Jones, A. (2009) The effects of camphor, eucalyptus and menthol vapour on nasal resistance to airflow and nasal sensation. *Acta Oto-Laryngolica 96*, 1–2, 157–161.

Butow, P., Price, M., Shaw, J., Turner, J. *et al.* (2015) Clinical pathway for the screening, assessment and management of anxiety and depression in adult cancer patients: Australian guidelines. *Psychooncology 24*, 987–1001.

Cabo, J., Crespo, M., Jimenez, J. & Navarro, C. (1986) The spasmolytic activity of various aromatic plants from the province of Granada. The activity of the major components of their essential oils. *Plantes Medicinales et Phytotherapy 20*, 5, 213–218.

Calenda, E. (2006) Massage therapy for cancer pain. *Current Pain Headache Reports 10*, 4, 270–274.

Campelo, L., de Almeida, A., de Freitas, M., Cerqueira, G. *et al.* (2011) Antioxidant and antinociceptive effects of *citrus limon* essential oil in mice. *Journal of Biomedical and Biotechnology*. doi: 10.1155/2011/678673.

Can, G. (2013) 'Integrating Non-Pharmacological Therapies with Western Medicine in Cancer Treatment.' In *Evidence-Based Non-Pharmacological Therapies for Palliative Cancer Care*. Dordrecht: Springer.

Cancer Research UK. (2022) Causes of sweating. Retrieved from: www.cancerresearchuk.org/about-cancer/coping/physically/skin-problems/dealing-with-sweating/causes.

Candy, B., Armstrong, M., Flemming, K., Kupeli, N. *et al.* (2020) The effectiveness of aromatherapy, massage and reflexology in people with palliative care needs: A systematic review. *Palliative Medicine 34*, 2, 179–194.

Candy, B., Jones, L., Goodman, M., Drake, R. & Tookman, A. (2011) Laxatives or methylnaltrexone for the management of constipation in palliative patients. *Cochrane Database of Systematic Reviews 1*, Art No: CD003448.

Candy, B., Jones, L., Larkin, P., Vickerstaff, V., Tookman, A. & Stone, P. (2015) Laxatives for the management of constipation in people receiving palliative care. *Cochrane Database of Systematic Reviews 5*, Art No: CD003448.

Caraceni, A., Hanks, G., Kaasa, S., Bennett, M. *et al.* (2012) Use of opioid analgesics in the treatment of cancer pain: Evidence-based recommendations from the EAPC. *The Lancet Oncology 12*, 2, e58–e68.

Carlile, M. (2016) *The Death Talker*. London: New Holland Publishers.

Carr, C., Vertelney, H., Fronk, J. & Trieu, S. (2019) Dronabinol for the treatment of paraneoplastic night sweats in cancer patients: A report of five cases. *Journal of Palliative Medicine 22*, 10, 1221–1223.

Carr, F. (2022) Nursing Touch: an adjunct to massage. Personal communication.

Carson, C. & Riley, T. (1995) Antimicrobial activity of the major components of the essential oil of *Melaleuca alternifolia*. *Journal of Applied Microbiology 78*, 3, 264–269.

Carter, A. & Mackereth, P. (2017) *Aromatherapy, Massage and Relaxation in Cancer Care*. London: Singing Dragon.

Caruso, R., Nanni, M., Riba, M., Sabato, S. *et al.* (2017) Depressive spectrum disorders in cancer: Diagnostic issues and intervention: A critical review. *Current Psychiatry Reports 19*, 33, 146–155.

Cassileth, B. & Keefe, F. (2010) Integrative and behavioural approaches to the treatment of cancer-related neuropathic pain. *The Oncologist 15*, suppl 2, 19–23.

Cassileth, B. & Vickers, A. (2004) Massage therapy for symptom control: Outcome study at a major cancer centre. *Journal of Pain and Symptom Management 28*, 3, 244–249.

Catty, S. (2001) *Hydrosols: The Next Aromatherapy*. Vermont: Healing Arts Press.

Cavanagh, H. & Wilkinson, J. (2002) Biological activities of lavender essential oil. *Phytotherapy Research 16*, 301–308.

Ceccarelli, I., Lariviere, W., Fiorenzani, P., Sacerdote, P. & Aloisi, A. (2004) Effects of long-term exposure to lemon essential oil odour on behavioural, hormonal and neuronal parameters in male and female rats. *Brain Research 1001*, 78–86.

Chang, S. (2008) Effects of aroma hand massage on pain, state anxiety and depression in hospice patients with terminal cancer. *Taehan Kanho Hakhoe Chi (Journal of Korean Academy of Nursing) 38*, 4, 493–502.

Charalambous, A., Giannakopoulou, M., Bozas, E., Marcou, Y., Kitsios, P. & Paikousis, L. (2016) Guided imagery and progressive muscle relaxation as a cluster of symptoms management intervention in patients receiving chemotherapy: A randomised controlled trial. *PLoS ONE 11*, 6, e0156911. doi: 10.1371/journal.pone.0156911.

Chen, C., Yan, S., Yen, M., Wu, P. *et al.* (2016) Investigations of kanuka and manuka essential oils for in-vitro treatment of disease and cellular inflammation caused by infectious organisms. *Journal of Microbiology, Immunology and Infection 49*, 104–111.

Chen, N., Sun, G., Yuan, X., Hou, J. *et al.* (2014) Inhibition of lung inflammatory responses by bornyl acetate is correlated with regulation of myeloperoxidase activity. *Journal of Surgical Research 186*, 1, 436–445.

Chen, X. & Kistler, C. (2015) Oral health care for older adults with serious illness: When and how? *Journal of the American Geriatric Society 63*, 375–378.

Cherney, N. (2008) Evaluation and management of treatment-related diarrhoea in patients with advanced cancer: A review. *Journal of Pain and Symptom Management 36*, 4, 413–423.

Chochinov, H. & Cann, B. (2005) Interventions to enhance the spiritual aspects of dying. *Journal of Palliative Medicine 8*, suppl 1, S103–S115.

Chochinov, H., Hack, T., McClement, S., Kristjanson, L. & Harlos, M. (2002) Dignity in the terminally ill: A developing empirical model. *Social Science and Medicine 54*, 3, 433–443.

Choi, H., Song, H., Ukeda, H. & Sawamura, M. (2000) Radical-scavenging activities of citrus essential oils and their components: Detection using 1.1-diphenyl-2-picrylhydrazyl. *Journal of Agriculture Food Chemistry 4*, 4156–4161.

Chwistek, M. (2017) Recent advances in understanding and managing cancer pain. *F1000 Research 6*, F1000 Faculty Review, 945.

Cimprich, B. (1992a) Attentional fatigue following breast cancer surgery. *Research in Nursing and Health 15*, 199–207.

Cimprich, B. (1992b) Pre-treatment symptom distress in women newly diagnosed with breast cancer. *Cancer Nursing 22*, 185–194.

Clinton, A. & Carter, T. (2015) Chronic wound biofilms: Pathogenesis and potential therapies. *Laboratory Medicine 46*, 4, 277–284.

Coelho, A., de Brito, M. & Barbosa, A. (2018) Caregiver anticipatory grief: Phenomenology, assessment and clinical interventions. *Current Opinion in Supportive and Palliative Care 12*, 1, 52–57.

Cohen, L., Kahn, J. & Gutsgell, K. (2015) Nonpharmacologic symptom management. Palliative Care in Oncology Symposium (breakout session).

Cohen, S., Mount, B., Tomas, J. & Mount, L. (1996) Existential well-being is an important determinant of quality of life: Evidence from the McGill Quality of Life Questionnaire. *Cancer 77*, 576–586.

Conrad, P. (2019) *Women's Health Aromatherapy*. London: Singing Dragon.

Corner, J., Cawley, N. & Hildebrand, S. (1995a) An evaluation of the use of massage and essential oils in the well-being of cancer patients. *International Journal of Palliative Nursing 1*, 2, 67–73.

Corner, J., Plant, H. & Warner, I. (1995b) Developing a nursing approach to manage dyspnoea in lung cancer. *International Journal of Palliative Nursing 1*, 5–10.

Cornwell, P. & Barry, B. (1994) Sesquiterpene component of volatile oils as skin penetration enhancers for the hydrophilic permeant 5-fluorouracil. *Journal of Pharmacy and Pharmacology 46*, 4, 261–269.

Costa, C., Cury, T., Cassertari, B., Takahira, R., Florio, J. & Costa, M. (2013) *Citrus aurantium L* essential oil exhibits anxiolytic-like activity mediated by 5-HT1A-receptors and reduces cholesterol after repeated oral treatment. *BMC Complementary Alternative Medicine 13*, 42. doi: org/10.1186/1472-6882-13-42.

Cronfalk, B., Strang, P., Ternestedt, B. & Friedrichsen, M. (2009) The existential experiences of receiving soft tissue massage in palliative home care – an intervention. *Supportive Care in Cancer 17*, 1203–1211.

Cruceriu, D., Balacescu, O. & Rakosy, E. (2018) *Calendula officinalis*: Potential roles in cancer treatment and palliative care. *Integrative Cancer Therapies 17*, 4, 1068–1078.

Curcani, M. & Tan, M. (2014) The effects of aromatherapy on haemodialysis patients' pruritus. *Journal of Clinical Nursing 23*, 23–24, 3356–3365.

Curt, G., Breibart, W., Cella, D., Groopman, J. *et al.* (2000) Impact of cancer-related fatigue on the lives of patients: New findings from the Fatigue Coalition. *The Oncologist 5*, 353–360.

da Costa Santos, C., Pimenta, C. & Nobre, M. (2010) A systematic review of topical treatments to control the odor of malignant fungating wounds. *Journal of Pain and Symptom Management 39*, 6, 1065–1076.

Davidson, J., Feldman-Stewart, D., Brennenstuhl, S. & Ram, S. (2007) How to provide insomnia interventions to people with cancer: Insights from patients. *Psychooncology 16*, 1028–1038.

Davidson, J., MacLean, A., Brundage, M. & Schulze, K. (2002) Sleep disturbance in cancer patients. *Social Science and Medicine 54*, 1309–1321.

Delgado-Guay, M., Hui, D., Parsons, H., Govan, K. *et al.* (2011) Spirituality, religiosity and spiritual pain in advanced cancer patients. *Journal of Pain and Symptom Management 41*, 6, 986–994.

Denda, M., Tsuchiya, T., Shoji, K. & Tanida, M. (2000) Odorant inhalation affects skin barrier homeostasis in mice and humans. *British Journal of Dermatology 142*, 1007–1010.

Deng, G. & Cassileth, B. (2005) Integrative oncology: Complementary therapies for pain, anxiety, and mood disturbance. *CA: A Journal for Clinicians 55*, 2, 109–116.

Detering, K., Hancock, A., Reade, M. & Silvester, W. (2010) The impact of advance care planning on end-of-life care in elderly patients: Randomised controlled trial. *British Medical Journal 340*, c1345.

Dhifi, W., Bellili, S., Jazi, S., Bahloul, N. & Mnif, W. (2016) Essential oils' chemical characterization and investigation of some biological activities: A critical review. *Medicines (Basel) 3*, 4, 25.

Dhingra, L., Shulk, E., Grossman, B., Strada, A. *et al.* (2013) A qualitative study to explore psychological distress and illness burden associated with opioid induced constipation in cancer patients with advanced disease. *Palliative Medicine 27*, 5, 447–456.

Didwaniya, N., Tanco, K., Cruz, M. & Bruera, E. (2015) The need for a multidisciplinary approach to pain management in advanced cancer: A clinical case. *Palliative and Supportive Care 13*, 2, 889–394.

DiMatteo, M., Lepper, H. & Croghan, T. (2000) Depression is a risk factor for noncompliance with medical treatment. *Archives of Internal Medicine 160*, 2101–2107.

Dobetsberger, C. & Buchbauer, G. (2011) Actions of essential oils on the central nervous system: An updated review. *Flavour and Fragrance Journal 26*, 300–316.

Dobler, D., Runkel, F. & Schmidts, T. (2020) Effect of essential oils on oral halitosis treatment: A review. *European Journal of Oral Sciences 128*, 476–486.

Dosoky, N. & Setzer, W. (2018) Biological activities and safety of *Citrus* spp. essential oils. *International Journal of Molecular Sciences 19*, 1966. doi: 10.3390/ijms19071966.

Dropsmart Essential Oil Database. www.dropsmart.io.

Dudgeon, D., Kristjanson, L., Sloan, J., Lertzman, M. & Clement, K. (2001) Dyspnea in cancer patients: Prevalence and associated factors. *Journal of Pain and Symptom Management 21*, 2, 95–102.

Dunwoody, L., Smyth, A. & Davidson, R. (2002) Cancer patients' experiences and evaluations of aromatherapy massage in palliative care. *International Journal of Palliative Nursing 8*, 10, 497–504.

Dyer, J., Ashley, S. & Shaw, C. (2008) A study to look at the effects of a hydrolat spray on hot flushes in women being treated for breast cancer. *Complementary Therapies in Clinical Practice 14*, 4, 273–279.

Dyer, J., Cleary, L., McNeill, S., Ragsdale-Lowe, M. & Osland, C. (2016) The use of aromasticks to help sleep problems: A patient experience survey. *Complementary Therapies in Clinical Practice 22*, 51–58.

Edwards, A., Pang, N., Shiu, V. & Chan, C. (2010) The understanding of spirituality and the potential role of spiritual care in end-of-life and palliative care: A meta-study of qualitative research. *Palliative Medicine 24*, 8, 1–18.

Edwards-Jones, V. (2018) Microbiology and malodorous wounds. *Wounds UK 14*, 4, 72–75.

Eicher, M., Matzka, M., Dubey, C. & White, K. (2015) Resilience in adult cancer care: An integrative literature review. *Oncology Nursing Forum 42*, 1, E3–16. doi: 10.1188/15.ONF. E3-E16.

Elmariah, S. & Lerner, E. (2011) Topical therapies for pruritus. *Seminars in Cutaneous Medicine and Surgery 30*, 2, 118–126.

ElSohly, M. & Slade, D. (2005) Chemical constituents of marijuana: The complex mixture of natural cannabinoids. *Life Science 78*, 539–548.

Engstrom, C., Strohl, R., Rose, L., Lewandowski, L. & Stefanek, M. (1999) Sleep alterations in cancer patients. *Cancer Nursing 22*, 2, 143–148.

Epstein-Peterson, Z., Sullivan, A., Enzinger, A., Trevino, K. *et al.* (2015) Examining forms of spiritual care provided in the advanced cancer setting. *American Journal of Hospital Palliative Care 32*, 7, 750–757.

Ernst, E. & Pittler, M. (2000) Efficacy of ginger for nausea and vomiting: A systematic review of randomised clinical trials. *British Journal of Anaesthesia 84*, 3, 367–371.

Essential Therapeutics. *Professional Reference Guide*. Victoria, Australia.

European Oncology Nursing Society. (2015) *Recommendations for the Care of Patients with Malignant Fungating Wounds*. London: Harris DPI.

European Pressure Ulcer Advisory Panel, National Pressure Injury Advisory Panel & Pan Pacific Pressure Injury Alliance. (2019) *Prevention and Treatment of Pressure Ulcers/ Injuries: Quick Reference Guide (third edition)*. Ed. Emily Haesler. EPUAP/NPIAP/PPPIA.

Ezzo, J., Vickers, A., Richardson, M., Allen, C. *et al.* (2005) Acupuncture-point stimulation for chemotherapy-induced nausea and vomiting. *Journal of Clinical Oncology 23*, 28, 7188–7198.

Fàbriques, S., Hong, Q., Escalante-Barrios, E., Guetterman, T., Meneses, J. & Fetters, M. (2020) A methodological review of mixed methods research in palliative and end-of-life care (2014–2019). *International Journal of Environmental Research and Public Health 17*, 11, 3853.

Fellowes, D., Barnes, K. & Wilkinson, S. (2004) Aromatherapy and massage for symptom relief in patients with cancer. *The Cochrane Library 2*. Chichester: John Wiley & Sons.

Ferreira-da-Silva, F., da Silva-Alves, K., Alves-Fernandes, T., Coelho-de-Souza, A. & Leal-Cardoso, J. (2015) Effects of 1,8-cineole on Na(+) currents of superior cervical ganglia neurons. *Neuroscience Letters 595*, 45–49.

Ferrell, B. & Kravitz, K. (2017) Cancer care: Supporting underserved and financially burdened family caregivers. *Journal of Advanced Practice Oncology 8*, 5, 494–500.

Ferris, A., Price, A. & Harding, K. (2019) Pressure ulcers in patients receiving palliative care: A systematic review. *Palliative Medicine 33*, 7, 770–782.

Fine, E., Carrington-Reid, M. & Adelman, R. (2010). Directly observed patient–physician discussions in palliative and end-of-life care: A systematic review of the literature. *Journal of Palliative Medicine 13*, 5, 595–603.

Finnegan-John, J., Molassiotis, A., Richardson, A. & Ream, E. (2013) A systematic review of complementary and alternative medicine interventions for the management of cancer-related fatigue. *Integrative Cancer Therapies 12*, 4, 276–290.

Fiorentino, L. & Ancoli-Israel, S. (2007) Sleep dysfunction in patients with cancer. *Current Treatment Options in Neurology 9*, 5, 337–346.

Fischer, D., Epstein, J., Yao, Y. & Wilkie, D. (2014) Oral health conditions affecting functional and social activities of terminally ill cancer patients. *Support Care Cancer 22*, 3, 803–810.

Fischer-Rizzi, S. (1990) *Complete Aromatherapy Handbook*. New York, NY: Sterling Publishing.

Fleming, M., Craigs, C. & Bennett, M. (2020) Palliative care assessment of dry mouth: What matters most to patients with advanced disease? *Supportive Care in Cancer 28*, 1121–1129.

Flynn, K., Shelby, R., Mitchell, S., Fawzy, M. *et al.* (2010) Sleep–wake functioning along the cancer continuum: Focus group results from the patient-reported outcomes measurement information system (PROMIS). *Psychooncology 19*, 10, 1086–1093.

Frankl, V. (1984) *Man's Search for Meaning: An Introduction to Logotherapy*. New York, NY: Simon and Schuster. (Original work published in 1946).

Fringer, A., Hechinger, M. & Schnepp, W. (2018) Transitions as experienced by persons in palliative care circumstances and their families – a qualitative meta-synthesis. *BioMed Central Palliative Care 17*, Art No: 22.

Garland, S., Johnson, J., Savard, J., Gerhman, P. *et al.* (2014) Sleeping well with cancer: A systematic review of cognitive behavioural therapy for insomnia in cancer patients. *Neuropsychiatric Disease and Treatment 10*, 1113–1124.

Geiger, J. (2005) The essential oil of ginger, *Zingiber officinale*, and anaesthesia. *The International Journal of Aromatherapy 15*, 7–14.

Gethin, G., McIntosh, C. & Probst, S. (2016) Complementary and alternative therapies for management of odour in malignant fungating wounds: A critical review. *Chronic Wound Care Management and Research 3*, 51–57.

Gibbins, J., Bhatia, R., Forbes, K. & Reid, C. (2014) What do patients with advanced incurable cancer want from the management of their pain? A qualitative study. *Palliative Medicine 28*, 1, 71–78.

Gilligan, N. (2005) The palliation of nausea in hospice and palliative care patients with essential oils of *Pimpinella anisum* (aniseed), *Foeniculum vulgare var. dulce* (sweet fennel), *Anthemis nobilis* (roman chamomile), and *Mentha x piperita* (peppermint). *International Journal of Aromatherapy 15*, 4, 163–167.

Glare, P., Miller, J., Nikolova, T. & Tickoo, R. (2011) Treating nausea and vomiting in palliative care: A review. *Clinical Interventions in Aging 6*, 243–259.

Glaser, R. & Kiecolt-Glaser, J. (2005) Stress-induced immune dysfunction: Implications for health. *Nature Reviews Immunology 5*, 243–51.

Glaus, A. (1993) Assessment of fatigue in cancer and non-cancer patients and in healthy individuals. *Supportive Care Cancer 1*, 305–315.

Glick, M., Williams, D., Kleinman, D., Vujicic, M., Watt, R. & Weyant, R. (2016) A new definition for oral health developed by the FDI World Dental Federation opens the door to a universal definition of oral health. *International Dental Journal 66*, 6, 322–324.

Gomes, B. & Higginson, I. (2006) Factors influencing death at home in terminally ill patients with cancer: Systematic review. *British Medical Journal 332*, 7540, 515–521. doi: 10.1136/bmj.38740.614954.55.

Graham, P., Browne, L., Cox, H. & Graham, J. (2003) Inhalation aromatherapy during radiotherapy: Results of a placebo-controlled double-blind randomised trial. *Journal of Clinical Oncology 21*, 12, 2372–2376.

Graham, T., Grocott, P., Probst, S., Wanklyn, S. *et al.* (2013) How are topical opioids used to manage painful cutaneous lesions in palliative care? A Critical review. *Pain 154*, 10, 1920–1928.

Grassi, L., Spiegel, D. & Riba, M. (2017) Advancing psychosocial care in cancer patients. *F1000 Research 6*, F1000 Faculty Review, 2083.

Grealish, L., Lomasney, A. & Whiteman, B. (2000) Foot massage. A nursing intervention to modify the distressing symptoms of pain and nausea in patients hospitalised with cancer. *Cancer Nursing 23*, 3, 237–243.

Greer, S. (2002) Psychological intervention: The gap between research and practice. *Acta Oncologica 41*, 3, 238–243.

Grocott, P. (2000) The palliative management of fungating malignant wounds. *Journal of Wound Care 9*, 1, 4–9.

Gutsgell, K., Schluchter, M., Margevicius, S., DeGolia, P. *et al.* (2013) Music therapy reduces pain in palliative care patients: A randomised controlled trial. *Journal of Pain and Symptom Management 45*, 5, 822–831.

Gysels, M. & Higginson, I. (2011) The lived experience of breathlessness and its implications for care: A qualitative comparison in cancer, COPD, heart failure and MND. *Biomed Central Palliative Care 10*, 15. doi.org/10.1186/1472-684X-10-15.

Hackett, J., Godfrey, M. & Bennett, M. (2016) Patient and caregiver perspectives on managing pain in advanced cancer: A qualitative longitudinal study. *Palliative Medicine 30*, 8, 711–719.

Hadfield, N. (2001) The role of aromatherapy massage in reducing anxiety in patients with malignant brain tumours. *International Journal of Palliative Nursing 7*, 279–285.

Hadji-Minaglou, F. & Maeda, K. (2007) Mucus in the bronchi: Its nature, control and treatment with traditional Chinese medicine and phytotherapy. *International Journal of Clinical Aromatherapy 1*, 2, 22–30.

Hallam, C. & Whale, C. (2003) Acupuncture for the treatment of sweating associated with malignancy. *Acupuncture in Medicine: Journal of the British Medical Acupuncture Society 21*, 4, 155–156.

Hamamura, K., Katsuyama, S., Komatsu, T., Scuteri, D. *et al.* (2020) Behavioural effects of continuously administered bergamot essential oil on mice with partial sciatic nerve ligation. *Frontiers in Pharmacology 11.* doi: 10.3389/fphar.2020.01310.

Hanchanale, S., Adkinson, L., Daniel, S., Fleming, M. & Oxberry, S. (2015) Systematic literature review: Xerostomia in advanced cancer patients. *Supportive Cancer Care 23*, 881–888.

Hansel, A., Hong, S., Camara, R. & von Kanel, R. (2010) Inflammation as a psychophysiological biomarker in chronic psychosocial stress. *Neuroscience and Biobehavioural Reviews 35*, 115–21.

Harding, R., Higginson, I. & Donaldson, N. (2003) The relationships between patient characteristics and carer psychological status in home palliative care. *Support Cancer Care 11*, 638–643.

Hardy, J., Randall, C., Pinkerton, E., Flatley, C., Gibbons, K. & Allan, S. (2016) A randomised, double-blind controlled trial of intranasal midazolam for the palliation of dyspnoea in patients with life-limiting disease. *Supportive Care in Cancer 24*, 7, 3069–3076.

Harman, A. (2010) Healing waters: A spotlight on anti-inflammatory hydrolats. *International Journal of Clinical Aromatherapy 7*, 2, 7–10.

Harris, B. (2007) 1,8-cineole – a component of choice for respiratory pathologies. *International Journal of Clinical Aromatherapy 4*, 1, 3–8.

Harris, D. (2010) Nausea and vomiting in advanced cancer. *British Medical Bulletin 96*, 175–185.

Harris, R. (2004) Aromatic approaches to end-of-life care. *International Journal of Clinical Aromatherapy 1*, 2, 10–20.

Harris, R. (2012) Making a difference in cancer and palliative care: A spotlight on key interventions and essential oils in cancer and palliative care settings. *Journal of Japanese Society of Aromatherapy 11*, suppl, 48–54.

Harris, R. (2016) *Advanced Clinical Aromatherapy (Level 2).* Course notes of residential programme. France.

Hashemi, S., Hajbagheri, A. & Aghajani, M. (2015) The effect of massage with lavender oil on restless leg syndrome in haemodialysis patients: A randomised controlled trial. *Nursing Midwifery Student 4*, 4, 1–5.

Hasson, F., Muldrew, D., Carduff, E., Finucane, A. *et al.* (2019) 'Take more laxatives was their answer to everything': A qualitative exploration of the patient, carer and healthcare professional experience of constipation in specialist palliative care. *Palliative Medicine 34*, 8, 1057–1066.

Heimes, K., Hauk, F. & Verspohl, E. (2011) Mode of action of peppermint oil and (-)-menthol with respect to 5-HT3 receptor subtypes: Binding studies, cation uptake by receptor channels and contraction of isolated rat ileus. *Phytotherapy Research 25*, 5, 702–708.

Higginson, I., Wade, A. & McCarthy, M. (1990) Palliative care: Views of patients and their families. *British Medical Journal 301*, 277–281.

Hines, S., Steels, E., Chang, A. & Gibbons, K. (2018) Aromatherapy for treatment of post-operative nausea and vomiting (review). *Cochrane Database of Systematic Reviews 3*, Art No: CD007598.

Hodge, N., McCarthy, M. & Pierce, R. (2014) A prospective randomised study of the effectiveness of aromatherapy for relief of postoperative nausea and vomiting. *Journal of Peri Anesthesia Nursing 29*, 1, 5–11.

Hofman, M., Ryan, J., Figuero-Moseley, C., Jean-Pierre, P. & Morrow, G. (2007) Cancer-related fatigue: The scale of the problem. *The Oncologist 12*, suppl 1, 4–10.

Hökkä, M., Kaakinen, P. & Pölkki, T. (2014) A systematic review: Non-pharmacological interventions in treating pain in patients with advanced cancer. *Journal of Advanced Nursing 70*, 9, 1954–1969.

Holmes, P. (2016) *Aromatica: A Clinical Guide to Essential Oil Therapeutics (Volume 1).* London: Singing Dragon.

Holmes, P. (2019) *Aromatica: A Clinical Guide to Essential Oil Therapeutics (Volume 2).* London: Singing Dragon.

Hone, L. (2017) *Resilient Grieving.* New York, NY: The Experiment.

Hongratanaworakit, T. & Buchbauer, G. (2004) Evaluation of the harmonising effects of ylang-ylang oil on humans after inhalation. *Planta Medica 70*, 632–636.

Horvath, G. & Acs, K. (2015) Essential oils in the treatment of respiratory tract diseases highlighting their role in bacterial infections and their anti-inflammatory action: A review. *Flavour and Fragrance Journal 30*, 331–341.

Hosseini, M., Tirgari, B., Forouzi, M. & Jahani, Y. (2016) Guided imagery effects on chemotherapy induced nausea and vomiting in Iranian breast cancer patients. *Complementary Therapies in Clinical Practice 25*, 8–12.

Hou, X., Chen, D., Cheng, T., Wang, D. *et al.* (2021) Acupuncture treatment for nausea and vomiting after chemotherapy: A protocol for systematic review. *Medicine Case Reports and Study Protocols, 2*, 5, 1–4.

Howell, D., Oliver, T., Keller-Olaman, S., Davidson, J. *et al.* (2014) Sleep disturbance in adults with cancer: A systematic review of evidence for best practices in assessment and management for clinical practice. *Annals of Oncology 24*, 4, 791–800.

Hugel, H., Ellershaw, J., Cook, L., Skinner, J. & Irvine, C. (2004) The prevalence, key causes and management of insomnia in palliative care patients. *Journal of Pain and Symptom Management 27*, 4, 316–321.

Hunt, R., Dienemann, J., Norton, J., Hartley, W. *et al.* (2013) Aromatherapy as a treatment for postoperative nausea: A randomised trial. *Anaesthesia and Analgesia 117*, 3, 597–604.

Hur, M., Yang, Y. & Lee, M. (2006) Aromatherapy massage affects menopausal symptoms in Korean climacteric women: A pilot-controlled clinical trial. *Evidence-Based Complementary and Alternative Medicine 5*. doi.org/10.1093/ecam/nem027.

Hwang, I., Kim, Y., Lee, Y., Choi, Y. *et al.* (2018) Factors associated with caregivers' resilience in a terminal cancer care setting. *American Journal of Hospice and Palliative Care 35*, 677–683.

Ikeda, H., Taksu, S. & Murase, K. (2014) Contribution of anterior cingulate cortex and descending pain inhibitory system to analgesic effect of lemon odour in mice. *Molecular Pain 10*, 14. doi.org/10.1186/1744-8069-10-14.

Imanishi, J., Kuriyama, H., Shigemori, I., Watanabe, S. *et al.* (2009) Anxiolytic effect of aromatherapy massage in patients with breast cancer. *eCAM 6*, 1, 123–128.

Inouye, S., Takahashi, M. & Abe, S. (2008) A comparative study of forty-four hydrosols and their essential oils. *The International Journal of Essential Oil Therapeutics 2*, 89–104.

International Case Study Collaboration. (2022) *Educators Round Table Botanica 2022*. Retrieved from: www.ijpha.com/case-study-collaborative.

International Organization for Standardization. (2022) *Terms and definitions: 3.1 Essential Oil*. Retrieved from: www.iso.org/obp/ui#iso:std:iso:tr:23199:ed-1:v1:en:term:3.1.

Ishaque, S., Johnson, J. & Vohra, S. (2019) Individualised health-related quality of life instrument Measure Yourself Medical Outcome Profile (MYMOP) and its adaptations: A critical appraisal. *Quality of Life Research 28*, 879–893.

Jane, S., Chen, S., Wilkie, D., Lin, Y. *et al.* (2011) Effects of massage on pain, mood status, relaxation and sleep in Taiwanese patients with metastatic bone pain: A randomised clinical trial. *Pain 152*, 2432–2442.

Jobbins, J., Bagg, J., Finlay, I., Addy, M. & Newcombe, R. (1992) Oral and dental disease in terminally ill cancer patients. *British Medical Journal 304*, 6842, 1612.

Johnson, S., Rodriguez, D. & Allred, K. (2020) A systematic review of essential oils and the endocannabinoid system: A connection worthy of further exploration. *Evidence-Based Complementary and Alternative Medicine,* Art No: 8035301.

Joung, D., Song, C., Ikei, H., Okuda, T. *et al.* (2014) Physiological and psychological effects of olfactory stimulation with d-limonene. *Advances in Horticultural Science 28*, 2, 90–94.

Juergens, U. (2014) Anti-inflammatory properties of the monoterpene 1,8-cineole: Current evidence for co-medication in inflammatory airway diseases. *Drug Research 64*, 12, 638–646.

Kamal, A., Maguire, J., Wheeler, J., Currow, D. & Abernethy, A. (2011) Dyspnea review for palliative care professional: Assessment, burdens, and etiologies. *Journal of Palliative Medicine 14*, 10, 1167–1172.

Kamal, A., Maguire, J., Wheeler, J., Currow, D. & Abernethy, A. (2012) Dyspnea review for the palliative care professional: Treatment goals and therapeutic options. *Journal of Palliative Medicine 15*, 1, 106–114.

Kamal, A. & Peppercorn, J. (2013) The generalisability of paradox within palliative care clinical trials. *Palliative Medicine 2*, 2, 101–104.

Kamudoni, P., Mueller, B., Halford, J., Schouveller, A., Stacey, B. & Salek, M. (2017) The impact of hyperhidrosis on patients' daily life and quality of life: A qualitative investigation. *Health and Quality of Life Outcomes 15*, 121.

Kang, H., Na, S. & Kim, Y. (2010) Effects of oral care with essential oil on improvement in oral health status of hospice patients. *Journal of Korean Academy of Nursing 40*, 4, 473–481.

Kang, S. & Kim, N. (2008) The effects of aroma hand massage on pruritis, fatigue and stress of haemodialysis patients. *Korean Journal of Adult Nursing 20*, 883–894.

Kantor, R., Dalai, P., Cella, D. & Silverberg, J. (2016) Research letter: Impact of pruritus on quality of life – a systematic review. *Journal of the American Academy of Dermatology 75*, 5, 885–886.

Karnell, A. & Smith, L. (2016) Attitudes towards use of benzodiazepines among US hospice clinicians: Survey and review of the literature. *Journal of Palliative Medicine 19*, 5, 516–522.

Katsuyama, S., Towa, A., Amio, S., Ato, K. *et al.* (2015) Effect of plantar subcutaneous administration of bergamot essential oil and linalool on formalin-induced nociceptive behaviour in mice. *Biomedical Research 36*, 47–54.

Kawagoshi, A., Shibata, K., Sugawara, K., Takahashi, H. *et al.* (2018) The effects of a warmed steam inhalation on patients with chronic obstructive pulmonary disease: A cross-sectional, controlled study. *Journal of Pulmonary and Respiratory Medicine 8*, 4. doi: 10.4172/2161-105X.1000471.

Kazemzadeh, R., Nikjou, R., Rostamnegad, M. & Norouzi, H. (2016) Effect of lavender aromatherapy on menopause hot flushing: A crossover randomised clinical trial. *Journal of the Chinese Medical Association 79*, 489–492.

Keating, A. & Chez, R. (2002) Ginger syrup as an anti-emetic in early pregnancy. *Alternative Therapies in Health & Medicine 8*, 89–91.

Keefe, F., Abernethy, A. & Campbell, L. (2005) Psychological approaches to understanding and treating disease-related pain. *Annual Review of Psychology 56*, 601–630.

Kerkhof, M. (2018) *CO_2 Extracts in Aromatherapy*. Wernhout, Netherlands: Kicozo.

Kerkhof-Knapp Hayes, M. (2015) *Complementary Nursing in End-of-Life Care*. Wernhout, Netherlands: Kicozo.

Khemlani, M. (2008) Insomnia in palliative care. *Palliative Medicine Grand Round – HKSPM Newsletter 2*, 20–25.

Khodabakhsh, P., Shafaroodi, H. & Asgarpanah, J. (2015) Analgesic and anti-inflammatory activities of citrus aurantium L. blossoms essential oil (neroli): Involvement of the nitric oxide/cyclic-guanosine monophosphate pathway. *Journal of Natural Medicine 69*, 324–331.

Kiberd, M., Clarke, S., Chorney, J., d'Eon, B. & Wright, S. (2016) Aromatherapy for the treatment of PONV in children: A pilot RCT. *BMC Complementary and Alternative Medicine 16*, 450. doi: 10.1186/s12906-016-1441-1.

Kim, I. & Kim, N. (2009) Effects of aroma massage on pain, activities of daily living and fatigue in patients with knee osteoarthritis. *Journal of Muscle and Joint Health 16*, 145–153.

Kim, M., Sakong, J., Kim, E., Kim, E. & Kim, E. (2005) Effect of aromatherapy massage for the relief of constipation in the elderly. *Journal of Korean Academy of Nursing 35*, 1, 56–64.

Kirk, P., Kirk, I. & Kristjanson, L. (2004) What do patients receiving palliative care for cancer and their families want to be told? A Canadian and Australian qualitative study. *British Medical Journal 5*, 328, 7452:1343. doi: 10.1136/bmj.38103.423576.55.

Kite, S., Maher, E., Anderson, K., Young, T. *et al.* (1998) Development of an aromatherapy service at a Cancer Centre. *Palliative Medicine 12*, 171–180.

Kitta, A., Hagin, A., Unseld, M., Adamidis, F. *et al.* (2021) The silent transition from curative to palliative treatment: A qualitative study about cancer patients' perceptions of end-of-life discussions with oncologists. *Supportive Care in Cancer 29*, 2405–2413.

Klasson, C., Helde-Frankling, M., Lundh-Hagelin, C. & Björkhem-Bergman, L. (2021) Fatigue in cancer patients in palliative care – a review on pharmacological interventions. *Cancers 13*, 985.

Kohara, H., Miyauchi, T., Suehiro, Y., Ueoka, H., Takeyama, H. & Morita, T. (2004) Combined modality treatment of aromatherapy, footsoak and reflexology relieves fatigue in patients with cancer. *Journal of Palliative Medicine 7*, 6, 791–6.

Kohn, M. (1999) *Complementary Therapies in Cancer Care*. London: Macmillan.

Kotronoulas, G., Wengström, Y. & Kearney, N. (2012) A critical review of women's sleep-wake patterns in the context of neo-/adjuvant chemotherapy for early-stage breast cancer. *Breast 21*, 2, 128–141.

Kouwenhoven, T., van de Kerkof, P. & Kamsteeg, M. (2017) Use of oral anti-depressants in patients with chronic pruritus: A systematic review. *Journal of the American Academy of Dermatology 77*, 6, 1068–1073.

Kovač, M. (2017) Aroma-oral care in palliative care: A pilot study. *International Journal of Clinical Aromatherapy 12*, 1, 26–35.

Krishnasamy, M. (2008) 'Pain.' In J. Corner & C. Bailey (eds) *Cancer Nursing Care in Context (second edition)*. Oxford: Blackwell Publishing.

Kübler-Ross, E. (1969) *On Death and Dying*. New York, NY: Macmillan.

Kutner, J., Smith, M., Corbin, L., Hemphill, L. *et al.* (2008) Massage therapy versus simple touch to improve pain and mood in patients with advanced cancer. *Annals of Internal Medicine 149*, 369–379.

Kuttan, R., Sudheeran, P. & Joseph, C. (1987) Tumeric and curcumin as topical agents in cancer therapy. *Tumori 73*, 1, 29–31.

Kuwahata, H., Komatsu, T., Katsuyama, S., Corasaniti, M. *et al.* (2013) Peripherally injected linalool and bergamot essential oil attenuate mechanical allodynia via inhibiting spinal ERK phosphorylation. *Pharmacology, Biochemistry and Behaviour 103*, 4, 735–741.

Kvalheim, S., Strand, G., Husebø, B. & Marthinussen, M. (2016) End-of-life palliative oral care in Norwegian health institutions. An exploratory study. *Gerodontology 33*, 4, 522–529.

Kyle, G. (2006) Evaluating the effectiveness of aromatherapy in reducing levels of anxiety in palliative care patients: Results of a pilot study. *Complementary Therapy Clinical Practice 12*, 148–155.

Lagman, R., Davis, M., LeGrand, S., Walsh, D. *et al.* (2017) Single-dose fluconazole therapy for oral thrush in hospice and palliative medicine patients. *The American Journal of Hospice and Palliative Care 34*, 645–649.

Lai, T., Cheung, M., Lo, C., Ng, K. *et al.* (2011) Effectiveness of aroma massage on advanced cancer patients with constipation: A pilot study. *Complementary Therapies in Clinical Practice 17*, 1, 37–43.

Laird, B., Boyd, A., Calvin, L. & Fallon, M. (2009) Are cancer pain and depression interdependent? A systematic review. *Psychooncology 18*, 459–464.

Lakhan, S., Sheafer, H. & Tepper, D. (2016) The effectiveness of aromatherapy in reducing pain: A systematic review and meta-analysis. *Pain Research and Treatment,* Art No: 8158693. doi: 10.1155/2016/8158693.

Lane, I. (2005) Managing cancer-related fatigue in palliative care. *Nursing Times 101*, 18, 38–41.

Langemo, D. (2005) When the goal is palliative care. *Advances in Skin and Wound Care 19*, 3, 148–154.

Langemo, D. & Brown, G. (2006) Skin fails too: Acute, chronic and end-stage skin failure. *Advances in Skin and Wound Care 19*, 4, 206211.

Langford, D., Lee, K. & Miaskowski, C. (2012) Sleep disturbance interventions in oncology patients and family caregivers: A comprehensive review and meta-analysis. *Sleep Medicine Reviews 16*, 397–414.

Langmore, S., Grillone, G., Elackattu, A. & Walsh, M. (2009) Disorders of swallowing: Palliative care. *Otolaryngologic Clinics of North America 42*, 87–105.

Larkin, P., Cherny, N., La Carpia, D., Guglielmo, M. *et al.* (2018) Diagnosis, assessment and management of constipation in advanced cancer: ESMO clinical practice guidelines. *Annals of Oncology 29*, 4, iv111–iv125.

Lauro, F., Ilari, S., Giancotti, L., Morabito, C. *et al.* (2016) The protective role of bergamot polyphenolic fraction on several animal models of pain. *Pharmanutrition 4*, S35–S40.

Lee, E. & Frazier, S. (2011) The efficacy of acupressure for symptom management: A systematic review. *Journal of Pain and Symptom Management 42*, 4, 589–602.

Lee, S. (2004) Effects of aromatherapy inhalation on fatigue and sleep quality of post-partum mothers. *Korean Journal of Women's Health in Nursing 10*, 3, 235–243.

Lee, Y., Wu, Y., Tsan, H., Leung, A. & Cheung, W. (2011) A systematic review on the anxiolytic effects of aromatherapy in people with anxiety symptoms. *The Journal of Alternative and Complementary Medicine 17*, 2, 101–108.

Leung, L. (2012) From ladder to platform: A new concept for pain management. *Journal of Primary Healthcare 4*, 3, 254–258.

Lewis, R. (2015) Aroma-psychology in clinical care: Evidence and applications. Workshop discussion: Aromatica Conference. Gold Coast, Australia.

Lewis, R. (2018) Clinical aromatherapy spotlight: Acute procedural anxiety in cancer care. *International Journal of Clinical Aromatherapy 13*, 1, 19–31.

Li, M., Yang, Y., Liu, L. & Wang, L. (2016) Effects of social support, hope and resilience on quality of life among Chinese bladder cancer patients: A cross-sectional study. *Health Quality of Life Outcomes 14*, 73. doi: 10.1186/s12955-016-0481-z.

Lim, M. (2018) Basic oral care for patients with dysphagia. *Journal of Clinical Practice in Speech-Language Pathology 20*, 3, 142–149.

Limardi, S., Stievano, A., Rocco, G., Vellone, E. & Alvaro, R. (2015) Caregiver resilience in palliative care: A research protocol. *Journal of Advanced Nursing 72*, 2, 421–433.

Linck, V., da Silva, A., Figueiró, M., Caramão, E., Moreno, P. & Elisabetsky, E. (2010) Effects of inhaled linalool in anxiety, social interaction and aggressive behaviour in mice. *Phytomedicine 17*, 8–9, 679–683.

Lis-Balchin, M. & Hart, S. (1999) Studies on the mode of action of the essential oil of lavender (*Lavandula angustifolia*). *Phytotherapy Research 13*, 6, 540–542.

López-Sendín, N., Alburquerque-Sendín, F., Cleland, J. & Fernández-de-las-Peñas, C. (2012) Effects of physical therapy on pain and mood in patients with terminal cancer: A pilot randomised clinical trial. *The Journal of Alternative and Complementary Medicine 18*, 5, 480–486.

Louis, M. & Kowalski, S. (2002) Use of aromatherapy with hospice patients to decrease pain, anxiety and depression and to promote an increased sense of well-being. *The American Journal of Hospice and Palliative Care 19*, 6, 381–386.

Lua, P., Salihah, N. & Mazlan, N. (2015) Effects of inhaled ginger aromatherapy on chemotherapy-induced nausea and vomiting and health-related quality of life in women with breast cancer. *Complementary Therapies in Medicine 23*, 3, 396–404.

Lund-Nielsen, B., Adamsen, L., Kolmos, H., Rorth, M., Tolver, A. & Gottrup, H. (2011). The effect of honey-coated bandages compared with silver-coated bandages on treatment of malignant wounds: A randomised study. *Wound Repair Regeneration 19*, 6, 664–670.

MacDonald, G. (2007) *Medicine Hands: Massage Therapy for People with Cancer*. Forres: Findhorn Press.

Mackereth, P. & Maycock, P. (2017) 'Aromatherapy: The Symptom Model.' In A. Carter & P. Mackereth (eds) *Aromatherapy, Massage and Relaxation in Cancer Care*. London: Singing Dragon.

Mackereth, P., Maycock, P. & Tomlinson, L. (2017) 'Easing the Breathing Body.' In A. Carter & P. Mackereth (eds) *Aromatherapy, Massage and Relaxation in Cancer Care*. London: Singing Dragon.

Mackereth, P. & Tomlinson, L. (2014) Procedure-related anxiety and needle phobia: Rapid techniques to calm. *Nursing in Practice 80*, 55–57.

MacLeod, R. & Macfarlane, S. (2019) *The Palliative Care Handbook (ninth edition)*. Sydney, New South Wales HammondCare Media.

Macmillan Cancer Relief. (2002) *Directory of Complementary Therapy Services in UK Cancer Care: Public and Voluntary Sectors*. London: Macmillan.

Maddocks-Jennings, W., Wilkinson, J., Cavanagh, M. & Shillington, D. (2009) Evaluation of the effects of essential oils of *Leptospermum scoparium* (manuka) and *Kunzea ericoides* (kanuka) on radiotherapy-induced mucositis: A randomised, placebo-controlled feasibility study. *European Journal of Oncology Nursing 13*, 2, 87–93.

Maida, V., Alexander, S., Case, A. & Fakhraei, P. (2016) Malignant wound management. *Public Health and Emergency 1*, 12. https://doi.org/doi:10.21037/phe.2016.06.15.

Maida, V., Ennis, M., Kuziemsky, C. & Trozzolo, L. (2009) Symptoms associated with malignant wounds: A prospective case series. *Journal of Pain and Symptom Management 37*, 2, 206–211.

Manne, S., Myers-Virtue, S., Kashy, D., Ozga, M. *et al.* (2015) Resilience, positive coping, and quality of life among women newly diagnosed with gynaecological cancers. *Cancer Nursing 38*, 5, 375–82.

Mannix, K. (2006) Palliation of nausea and vomiting in malignancy. *Clinical Medicine 6*, 2, 144–147.

Mannix, K. (2017) *With the End in Mind*. London: William Collins.

Mannix, K. (2021) *Listen: How to Find Words for Tender Conversations*. London: William Collins.

Marx, W., Ried, K., McCarthy, A., Vitetta, L. *et al.* (2017) Ginger – mechanism of action in chemotherapy-induced nausea and vomiting: A review. *Critical Reviews in Food Science and Nutrition 57*, 1, 141–146.

Maver, T., Kureck, M., Smorke, D., Kleinschek, K. & Maver, U. (2018) 'Plant-centred Medicines with Potential Use in Wound Treatment.' In P. Builders (ed.) *Herbal Medicine*. http://dx.doi.org/10.5772/intechopen.72813.

McCaffrey, N., Bradley, S., Ratcliffe, J. & Currow, D. (2016) What aspects of quality of life are important from palliative care patients' perspectives? *Journal of Pain & Symptom Management 52*, 2, 318–328.

McClurg, D. & Lowe-Strong, A. (2011) Does abdominal massage relieve constipation? *Nursing Times 107*, 12, 20–22.

McParlin, C., O'Donnell, A., Robson, S., Beyer, F. *et al.* (2016) Treatments for hyperemesis gravidarum and nausea and vomiting in pregnancy. *The Journal of the American Medical Association 316*, 1392–1401.

Melzack, R. (1999) From the gate to the neuromatrix. *International Association for the Study of Pain*, Pain supplement 6, s121–s126.

Melzack, R. & Wall, P. (1965) Pain mechanisms: A new theory. *Science 150*, 971–979.

Menanti, L., Tansinda, P. & Vaglio, A. (2009) Uraemic pruritus. *Drugs 69*, 251–263.

Mercadante, S., Porzio, G., Valle, A., Fusco, F. *et al.* (2013) Orphan symptoms in advanced cancer patients followed at home. *Supportive Care in Cancer 21*, 3525–3528.

Mercier, D. & Knevitt, A. (2005) Using topical aromatherapy for the management of fungating wounds in a palliative care unit. *Journal of Wound Care 14*, 497–501.

Miaskowski, C., Lee, K., Dunn, L., Dodd, M. *et al.* (2011) Sleep–wake circadian activity rhythm parameters and fatigue in oncology patients before the initiation of radiotherapy. *Cancer Nursing 34*, 4, 255–268.

Mills, S. (1991) *The Essential Book of Herbal Medicine*. London: Arkana Penguin Books.

Miranzadeh, S., Adib-Hajbaghery, M., Soleymanpoor, L. & Ehansi, M. (2015) Effect of adding the herb *Achillea millefolium* on mouthwash chemotherapy induced oral mucositis in cancer patients: A double-blind randomised controlled trial. *European Journal of Oncology Nursing 19*, 207–213.

Mitchell, A., Chan, M., Bhatti, H., Halton, M. *et al.* (2011) Prevalence of depression, anxiety and adjustment disorder in oncological, haematological and palliative-care settings: A meta-analysis of 94 interview-based studies. *The Lancet 12*, 160–174.

Mitchell, S. (2010) Cancer-related fatigue: State of the science. *American Academy of Physical Medicine and Rehabilitation 2*, 364–383.

Moharam, B., Jantan, I., Ahmed, F. & Jalil, J. (2010) Antiplatelet aggregation and platelet activity factor (PAF) receptor antagonistic activities of the essential oils of five *Goniothalamus* species. *Molecules 15*, 8, 5124–5138.

Mojay, G. (1997) *Aromatherapy for Healing the Spirit*. Rochester, VT: Healing Arts Press.

Molassiotis, A., Yung, H., Yam, B., Chan, F. & Mok, T. (2002) The effectiveness of progressive muscle relaxation training in managing chemotherapy-induced nausea and vomiting in Chinese breast cancer patients: A randomised controlled trial. *Support Cancer Care 10*, 237–246.

Molina, Y., Yi, J., Martinez-Gutierrez, J., Reding, K., Yi-Frazier, J. & Rosenberg, A. (2014) Resilience among patients across the cancer continuum: Diverse perspectives. *Clinical Journal of Oncological Nursing 18*, 1, 93–101.

Monroe, B. & Oliviere, D. (2009) *Resilience in Palliative Care – Achievement in Adversity (second edition)*. New York, NY: Oxford University Press.

Montgomery, G., Bovbjerg, D., Schnur, J., David, D. *et al.* (2007) A randomised clinical trial of brief hypnosis intervention to control side effects in breast surgery patients. *Journal of National Cancer Institution 99*, 1304–1312.

Morice, A., Marshall, A., Higgins, K. & Grattan, T. (1994) Effect of inhaled menthol on citric-acid induced cough in normal subjects. *Thorax 49*, 10, 1024–1026.

Muldrew, D., Hasson, F., Carduff, E., Clarke, M. *et al.* (2018) Assessment and management of constipation for patients receiving palliative care in specialist palliative care settings: A systematic review of the literature. *Palliative Medicine 32*, 5, 930–938.

Mustian, K., Morrow, G., Carroll, J., Figuero-Moseley, C., Jean-Pierre, P. & Williams, G. (2007) Integrative nonpharmacological behavioural interventions for the management of cancer-related fatigue. *The Oncologist 12*, suppl 1, 52–67.

Muthia, R., Wahyu, W. & Dachriyanus. (2013) Effect of ginger infusion on chemotherapy-in-duced nausea and vomiting in breast cancer patients. *Journal of Biology, Agriculture and Healthcare 3*, 13, 42–46.

Mystakidou, K., Parpa, E., Tsilika, E., Gennatas, C., Galanos, A. & Vlahos, L. (2009) How is sleep quality affected by the psychological and symptom distress of advanced cancer patients? *Palliative Medicine 23*, 1, 46–53.

Nakajima, N. (2017) Characteristics of oral problems and effects of oral care in terminally ill patients with cancer. *The American Journal of Hospice and Palliative Medicine 34*, 430–434.

Nakayama, M., Okizaki, A. & Takahashi, K. (2016) A randomised controlled trial for effec-tiveness of aromatherapy in decreasing salivary gland damage following radioactive iodine therapy for differentiated thyroid cancer. *BioMed Research International*, Art ID: 9509810. doi.org/10.1155/2016/9509810.

Nardi, A., Freire, R. & Zin, W. (2009) Panic disorder and control of breathing. *Respiratory Physiology and Neurobiology 167*, 1, 133–143.

National Comprehensive Cancer Network. (2010) Clinical practice guidelines in oncology: Cancer-related fatigue. Retrieved from: www.nccn.org/professionals/physician_gls/f_guidelines.asp.

National Sleep Foundation. (2017) What is insomnia? Retrieved from: https://sleepfounda-tion.org/insomnia/content/what-is-insomnia.

Naylor, W. (2005) A guide to wound management in palliative care. *International Journal of Palliative Nursing 11*, 11, 572–579.

Nazzaro, F., Fratianni, F., Coppola, R. & De Feo, V. (2017) Essential oils and anti-fungal activity. *Pharmaceuticals 10*, 86. doi: 10.3390/ph10040086.

Negut, I., Grumezescu, V. & Grumezescu, A. (2018) Treatment strategies for infected wounds. *Molecules 23*, 2392. doi: 10.3390/molecules23092392.

Noorani, N. & Montagnini, M. (2007) Recognising depression in palliative care patients. *Journal of Palliative Medicine 10*, 2, 458–464.

North Haven Hospice. (2020) *Primary Palliative Care Guidelines (third edition)*. Whangarei, New Zealand: North Haven Hospice.

Nowak, D. & Yeung, J. (2017) Diagnosis and treatment of pruritus. *Canadian Family Physician 63*, 918–924.

O'Connor, M., White, K., Kristjanson, L., Cousins, K. & Wilkes, L. (2010) The prevalence of anxiety and depression in palliative care patients with cancer in Western Australia and New South Wales. *The Medical Journal of Australia 193*, 5, S44–S47.

Oechsle, K. (2019) Current advances in palliative & hospice care: Problems and needs of rel-atives and family caregivers during palliative and hospice care – an overview of current literature. *Medical Sciences 7*, 43. doi: 10.3390/medsci7030043.

Oechsle, K., Goerth, K., Bokemeyer, C. & Mehnert, A. (2013) Anxiety and depression in care-givers of terminally ill cancer patients: Impact on their perspectives of the patient's symptoms burden. *Journal of Palliative Medicine 16*, 1095–1101.

Ohayon, M. (2002) Epidemiology of insomnia: What we know and what we still need to learn. *Sleep Medicine Reviews 6*, 2, 97–111.

Olofsson, J. (2014) Time to smell: A cascade model of human olfactory perception based on response-time (RT) measurement. *Frontiers in Psychology 5*, 33. doi.org/10.3389/fpsyg.2014.00033.

Olver, I. (2011) *The MASCC Textbook of Cancer Supportive Care and Survivorship*. New York, NY: Springer.

Oxberry, S. & Edwards, A. (2005) Guidelines on the management of sweating. Retrieved from: www.palliativedrugs.com/download/Final%20GuidelinessweatingDEC05.pdf.

Page, M., Berger, A. & Johnson, L. (2006) Putting evidence into practice: Evidence-based interventions for sleep–wake disturbances. *Clinical Journal of Oncological Nursing 10*, 6, 753–767.

Palesh, O., Collie, K., Batiuchok, D., Tilston, J. *et al.* (2007) A longitudinal study of depression, pain, and stress as predictors of sleep disturbance among women with metastatic breast cancer. *Biological Psychology 75*, 37–44.

Palesh, O., Roscoe, J., Mustian, K., Roth, T. *et al.* (2010) Prevalence, demographics, and psychological associations of sleep disruption in patients with cancer: University of Rochester Cancer Center–Community Clinical Oncology Program. *Journal of Clinical Oncology 28*, 2, 292–298.

Park, H., Chun, Y. & Kwak, S. (2016) The effects of aromatherapy hand massage on fatigue and sleeping among hospice patients. *Open Journal of Nursing 6*, 515–523.

Parker, S. (2014) *Power of the Seed*. Port Townsend, WA: Process Media.

Payne, S. (2009) 'Resilient Carers and Caregivers.' In B. Monroe & D. Oliviere (eds) *Resilience in Palliative Care – Achievement in Adversity*. New York, NY: Oxford University Press.

Pearce, S. & Richardson, A. (1996) Fatigue in cancer: A phenomenological perspective. *European Journal of Cancer Care 5*, 111–115.

Pénoël, D. & Franchomme, P. (1990) *L'Aromathérapie Exactement*. Limoges: Roger Jollois.

Perdue, C. (2016) Management of pruritus in palliative care. *Nursing Times 112*, 24, 20–23.

Perdue, C. (2019) Neuropathic pain in advanced cancer: Causes and management. *Nursing Times (online) 115*, 11, 50–54.

Pergolizzi, J., Taylor, R., LeQuang, J. & Raffa, R. (2017) The role and mechanism of action of menthol in topical analgesic products. *Journal of Clinical Pharmacy and Therapeutics 43*, 313–319.

Perry, N. & Perry, E. (2006) Aromatherapy in the management of psychiatric disorders. *CNS Drugs 20*, 4, 257–280.

Pertz, H., Lehmann, J., Roth-Ehrang, R. & Elz, S. (2011) Effects of ginger constituents on the gastrointestinal tract: Role of cholinergic M3 and serotonergic 5-HT3 and 5-HT4 receptors. *Planta Medicine 77*, 973–978.

Piggin, C. & Jones, V. (2007) Malignant fungating wounds: An analysis of the lived experience. *International Journal of Palliative Nursing 13*, 8, 384–391.

Plevkova, J., Kollarik, M., Poliacek, I., Brozmanova, M. *et al.* (2013) The role of trigeminal nasal TRPM8-expressing afferent neurons in the antitussive effects of menthol. *Journal of Applied Physiology 115*, 2, 268–274.

Pollard, A. & Krishnasamy, M. (2008) 'Anxiety and Depression.' In J. Corner & C. Bailey (eds) *Cancer Nursing: Care in Context*. Oxford: Blackwell Publishing.

Post-White, J., Kinney, M., Savik, K., Gau, J., Wilcox, C. & Lerner, I. (2003) Therapeutic massage and healing touch improve symptoms in cancer. *Integrative Cancer Therapies 2*, 322–344.

Potter, J. (2004) Fatigue experience in advanced cancer: A phenomenological approach. *International Journal of Palliative Nursing 10*, 1, 15–23.

Praptiwi, A. (2017) The potentials of honey in managing breast cancer wounds: A literature review. *Asian Journal of Pharmaceutical and Clinical Research*. https://doi.org/10.22159/ajpcr.2017.v10s2.19500.

Preece, J. (2002) Introducing abdominal massage in palliative care for the relief of constipation. *Complementary Therapies in Nursing and Midwifery 8*, 2, 101–105.

Price, L. & Price, S. (2004) *Understanding Hydrolats: The Specific Hydrosols for Aromatherapy.* Edinburgh: Elsevier.

Price, L. & Price, S. (2014) *Carrier Oils for Aromatherapy and Massage (fourth edition).* New York, NY: Riverhead Publishing.

Price, S. & Price, L. (2012) *Aromatherapy for Healthcare Professionals (fourth edition).* London: Elsevier.

Pringle, J., Johnson, B. & Buchanan, D. (2015) Dignity and patient-centred care for people with palliative care needs in the acute hospital setting: A systematic review. *Palliative Medicine 29*, 8, 675–694.

Probst, S. (2010) Evidence-based management of fungating wounds. *Palliative Wound Care Supplement,* 7–11. Wounds UK.

Probst, S., Arber, A. & Faithfull, S. (2013a) Coping with an exulcerated breast carcinoma: An interpretative phenomenological study. *Journal of Wound Care 22*, 7, 352–360.

Probst, S., Arber, A. & Faithfull, S. (2013b) Malignant fungating wounds – the meaning of life in an unbounded body. *European Journal of Clinical Oncology 17*, 1, 38–45.

Puchalski, C. (2012) Spirituality in the cancer trajectory. *Annals of Oncology 23*, suppl 3, iii49–iii55.

Rabow, M., Kvale, E., Barbour, L., Cassel, J. *et al.* (2013) Moving upstream: A review of the evidence of the impact of outpatient palliative care. *Palliative Medicine 16*, 12, 1540–1549.

Raharivelomanana, P., Ansel, J., Lupo, E., Mijouin, L. *et al.* (2018) Tamanu oil and skin active properties: From traditional to modern cosmetic uses. *Oilseeds & Fats, Crops and Lipids 25*, 5. doi.org/10.1051/ocl/2018048.

Rajesvari, R. & Lakshmi, T. (2013) Lemongrass oil for improvement of oral health. *Dental Hypotheses 4*, 4, 115–117.

Ramasamy, V. & Taylor, J. (2017) Using acupuncture to treat hot flashes and night sweating for patients with breast cancer. *BMJ Supportive and Palliative Care 7*, suppl 2, A68.

Ramasubbu, D., Smith, V., Hayden, F. & Cronin, P. (2017) Systemic antibiotics for treating malignant wounds. *Cochrane Database of Systemic Reviews 8*, Art No: CD011609. doi: 10.1002/14651858.CD011609.pub2.

Rea, H., McAuley, S., Jayaram, L., Garrett, J. & Hockey, H. (2010) The clinical utility of long-term humidification therapy in chronic airway disease. *Respiratory Medicine 104*, 525–533.

Reynolds, H. & Gethin, G. (2015) The psychological effects of malignant fungating wounds. *European Wound Management Association Journal 15*, 29–32.

Rhind, J. P. (2012) *Essential Oils: A Handbook for Aromatherapy Practice (second edition).* London: Singing Dragon.

Rhind, J. P. (2014) *Fragrance and Wellbeing.* London: Singing Dragon.

Richardson, P. (2014) Spirituality, religion and palliative care. *Annals of Palliative Medicine 3*, 3, 150–159.

Ripamonti, C., Santini, D., Maranzano, E., Berti, M. & Roila, F. (2012) Management of cancer pain: ESMO clinical practice guidelines. *Annals of Clinical Oncology 23*, 7, vii139–vii154.

Rivas da Silva, A., Lopes, P., Barros de Azevedo, M., Costa, D., Alviano, C. & Alviano, D. (2012) Biological activities of α-pinene and β-pinene enantiomers. *Molecules 17*, 6, 6305–6316.

Ro, Y., Ha, H., Kim, C. & Yeom, H. (2002) The effects of aromatherapy on pruritus in patients undergoing haemodialysis. *Dermatology Nursing 14*, 4, 231–256.

Roen, I., Stifoss-Hanssen, H., Grande, G., Brenne, A. *et al.* (2018) Resilience for family carers of advanced cancer patients – how can health care providers contribute? A qualitative interview study with carers. *Palliative Medicine 32*, 8, 1410–1418.

Rohr, Y., Adams, J. & Young, L. (2010) Oral discomfort in palliative care: Results of an exploratory study of the experience of terminally ill patients. *International Journal of Palliative Nursing 16*, 9, 439–444.

Rombolà, L., Amantea, D., Russo, R., Adornetto, A. *et al.* (2016) Rational basis for the use of bergamot essential oil in complementary medicine to treat chronic pain. *Mini-reviews in Medicinal Chemistry 16*, 721–728.

Rosenblatt, P. (2017) Researching grief: Cultural, relational and individual possibilities. *Journal of Loss and Trauma 22*, 617–630.

Rothman, S. (1941) Physiology of itching. *Physiological Reviews 21*, 2, 357–381.

Rousseau, P. (2000a) Spirituality and the dying patient. *Journal of Clinical Oncology 18*, 2000–2002.

Rousseau, P. (2000b) The meaning of hope. *Western Journal of Medicine 173*, 2, 117–118.

Running, A. & Seright, T. (2012) Integrative oncology: Managing cancer pain with complementary and alternative therapies. *Current Pain and Headache Reports 16*, 325–331.

Ryan, J., Heckler, C., Roscoe, J., Dakhill, S. *et al.* (2012) Ginger (*Zingiber officinale*) reduces acute chemotherapy-induced nausea: A URCC CCOP study of 576 patients. *Supportive Cancer Care 20*, 7, 1479–1489.

Saiki, J., Cao, H., Wassenhove, D., Viswanathan, V. *et al.* (2018) Aldehyde dehydrogenase 3A1 activation prevents radiation-induced xerostomia by protecting salivary stem cells from toxic aldehydes. *Proceeds of the National Academy of Sciences of the USA 115*, 24, 6279–6284.

Saiyudthong, S. & Mekseepralard, C. (2011) Acute effects of bergamot oil on anxiety-related behaviour and corticosterone level in rats. *Phytotherapy Research 25*, 6, 858–862.

Sakurada, T., Mizoguchi, H., Kuwahata, H., Katsuyama, S. *et al.* (2011) Intraplantar injection of bergamot essential oil induces peripheral antinociception mediated by opioid mechanism. *Pharmacology Biochemistry Behaviour 97*, 436–443.

Sampson, C., Finlay, I., Byrne, A., Snow, V. & Nelson, A. (2014) The practice of palliative care from the perspective of patients and carers. *British Medical Journal 4*, 291–298.

Sanchez-Vidana, D., Ngai, S., He, W., Chow, J., Lau, B. & Tsang, H. (2017) The effectiveness of aromatherapy for depressive symptoms: A systematic review. *Evidence-Based Complementary and Alternative Medicine*, Art. ID: 5869315. https://doi.org/10.1155/2017/5869315.

Sand, L., Olsson, M. & Strang, P. (2009) Coping strategies in the presence of one's own impending death from cancer. *Journal of Pain and Symptom Management 37*, 1, 13–22.

Sanger, G. & Andrews, P. (2018) A history of drug discovery for treatment of nausea and vomiting and the implications for future research. *Frontiers in Pharmacology 9*, Art 913.

Santucci, N. (2020) Functional nausea, gut brain or both? *The Journal of Paediatrics 225*, 8–9.

Sapeta, A. & Simoes, A. (2018) Silences in palliative care – the primacy of human presence. *Hospice and Palliative Medicine International Journal 2*, 3, 161–164.

Saria, M., Courchesne, N., Evangelista, L., Carter, J. *et al.* (2017) Cognitive dysfunction in patients with brain metastases: Influences on caregiver resilience and coping. *Supportive Cancer Care 25*, 1247–1256.

Satija, A. & Bhatnagar, S. (2017) Complementary therapies for symptom management in cancer patients. *Indian Journal of Palliative Care 23*, 4, 468–479.

Saunders, C. (1964) The symptomatic treatment of incurable malignant disease. *Prescribers' Journal 4*, 4, 68–73.

Saunders, C. (1967) *The Management of Terminal Illness*. London: Hospital Medical Publications.

Savard, J. & Morin, C. (2001) Insomnia in the context of cancer: A review of a neglected problem. *Journal of Clinical Oncology 19*, 895–908.

Savard, J., Simard, S., Blanchet, J., Ivers, H. & Morin, C. (2001) Prevalence, clinical characteristics, and risk factors for insomnia in the context of breast cancer. *Sleep 24*, 5, 583–590.

Savvidis, C. & Koutsilieris, M. (2012) Circadian rhythm disruption in cancer biology. *Molecular Medicine 18*, 1249–1260.

Schelz, Z., Hohmann, J. & Molnar, J. (2010) 'Recent Advances in Research of Antimicrobial Effects of Essential Oils and Plant Derived Compounds on Bacteria.' In C. Debprasad (ed.) *Ethnomedicine: A Source of Complementary Therapeutics*. Kerala, India: Research Signpost.

Schnaubelt, K. (1998) *Advanced Aromatherapy*. Rochester, VT: Healing Arts Press.

Schneider, R. (2016) There is something in the air: Testing the efficacy of a new olfactory stress relief method (Aromastick®). *Stress Health 32*, 4, 411–426.

Schneider, R. (2017) From pain to pleasure: A newly developed essential oil inhaler (Aromastick®) alters pain dynamics and increases well-being. Results from two randomised controlled documentation studies. *Current Psychopharmacology 6*, 136–147.

Schneider, R., Singer, N. & Singer, R. (2018) Medical aromatherapy revisited – basic mechanisms, critique and a new development. *Human Psychopharmacology: Clinical and Experimental 34*, e2683. doi.org/10.1002/hup.2683.

Schroedl, C., Yount, S., Szmuilowicz, E., Hutchison, P., Rosenberg, S. & Kalhan, R. (2014) A qualitative study of unmet healthcare needs in chronic obstructive pulmonary disease: A potential role for specialist palliative care? *Annals of the American Thoracic Society 11*, 9, 1433–1438.

Schwan, R. & Ash, P. (2004) Integrative palliative aromatherapy care program at San Diego Hospice and palliative care. *International Journal of Clinical Aromatherapy 1*, 2, 5–9.

Scuteri, D., Hamamura, K., Sakurada, T., Watanabe, C. *et al.* (2021) Efficacy of essential oils in pain: A systematic review and meta-analysis of preclinical evidence. *Frontiers in Pharmacology 12*, Art 640128, 1–18.

Seale, M. (2012) The use of peppermint oil to reduce nausea of the Palliative Care and Hospice patient. *Nursing Theses and Capstone Projects 143*. Retrieved from: https://digitalcommons.gardner-webb.edu/nursing_etd/143.

Seiler, A. & Jenewein, J. (2019) Resilience in cancer patients. *Frontiers in Psychiatry 10*, 208, 1–31.

Seiler, A., von Känel, R. & Slavich, G. (2020) The psychobiology of bereavement and health: A conceptual review from the perspective of social signal transduction theory of depression. *Frontiers in Psychiatry 11*. doi.org/10.3389/fpsyt.2020.565239.

Sepulveda, C., Marlin, A., Yoshida, T. & Ullrich, A. (2002) Palliative care: The World Health Organization's global perspective. *Journal of Pain and Symptom Management 24*, 2, 91–96.

Serfaty, M., Wilkinson, S., Freeman, C., Mannix, K. & King, M. (2012) Helping with touch or talk: A pilot randomised controlled trial to examine the clinical effectiveness of aromatherapy massage versus cognitive behavioural therapy for emotional distress in patients in cancer and palliative care. *Psychoncology 21*, 5, 563–569.

Setzer, W. (2009) Essential oils and anxiolytic aromatherapy. *Natural Product Communications 4*, 9, 1305–1316.

Shahgolian, N., Dehghan, M., Mortazavi, M., Gholami, F. & Valiani, M. (2010) Effects of aromatherapy on pruritus relief in haemodialysis patients. *Iranian Journal of Nursing and Midwifery Research 15*, 4, 240–244.

Sharp, D., Lorenc, A., Little, P., Stewart, M. *et al.* (2018) Complementary medicine and the NHS: Experiences of integration with UK primary care. *European Journal of Integrative Medicine 24*, 8–16.

Sheehan, C., Clark, K., Lam, L. & Chye, R. (2011) A retrospective analysis of primary diagnosis, comorbidities, anticholinergic load, and other factors on treatment for noisy respiratory secretions at the end of life. *Palliative Medicine 14*, 11, 1211–1216.

Shin, E., Lee, S., Seo, K., Park, Y. & Nguyen, T. (2016) Aromatherapy massage for symptom relief in patients with cancer. *Cochrane Database of Systematic Reviews 6*, Art No: CD009873.

Siemens, W., Xander, C., Meerpohl, J., Buroh, S. *et al.* (2016) Pharmacological interventions for pruritus in adult palliative care patients. *Cochrane Database of Systematic Reviews 11*. doi: 10.1002/14651858.CD008320.pub3.

Simon, S., Higginson, I., Booth, S., Harding, R., Weingärtner, V. & Bausewein, C. (2010) Benzodiazepines for the relief of breathlessness in advanced malignant and non-malignant diseases in adults. *Cochrane Database of Systematic Reviews 1*. doi: 10.1002/14651858.CD007354.pub2.

Sinclair, M. (2011) The use of abdominal massage to treat chronic constipation. *Journal of Bodywork and Movement Therapies 15*, 4, 436–445.

Singh, P., Yoon, S. & Kuo, B. (2016) Nausea: A review of pathophysiology and therapeutics. *Therapeutic Advances in Gastroenterology 9*, 1, 98–112.

Skorpen-Tarberg, A., Kvangarsnes, M., Hole, T., Thronaes, M., Madssen, T. & Lanstad, B. (2019) Silent voices: Family caregivers' narratives of involvement in palliative care. *Nursing Open 6*, 1446–1454.

Smith, H. (2015) Depression in cancer patients: Pathogenesis, implications and treatment (review). *Oncology Letters 9*, 1509–1514.

Smith, H., Smith, E. & Smith, A. (2012) Pathophysiology of nausea and vomiting in palliative medicine. *Annals of Palliative Medicine 1*, 2, 87–93.

Smithson, J., Britten, N., Paterson, C., Lewith, G. & Evans, M. (2012) The experience of using complementary therapies after a diagnosis of cancer: A qualitative synthesis. *Health 16*, 1, 19–39.

Soden, K., Vincent, K., Craske, S., Lucas, C. & Ashley, S. (2004) A randomised controlled trial of aromatherapy massage in a hospice setting. *Palliative Medicine 18*, 2, 87–92.

Somasundaram, R. & Devamani, K. (2016) A comparative study on resilience, perceived social support and hopelessness among cancer patients treated with curative and palliative care. *Indian Journal of Palliative Care 22*, 2, 135–40.

Sood, A., Barton, D., Bauer, B. & Loprinzi, C. (2007) A critical review of complementary therapies for cancer-related fatigue. *Integrative Cancer Therapies 6*, 1, 8–13.

Soysa, N., Samaranayake, L. & Ellepola, A. (2004) Cytotoxic drugs, radiotherapy and oral candidiasis. *Oral Oncology 40*, 10, 971–978.

Speck, P. (2011) 'Spiritual/Religious Issues in Care of the Dying.' In J. Ellershaw & S. Wilkinson (eds) *Care of the Dying: A Pathway to Excellence*. Oxford: Oxford University Press.

Steinhorn, D., Din, J. & Johnson, A. (2017) Healing, spirituality and integrative medicine. *Annals of Palliative Medicine 6*, 3, 237–247.

Stern, R., Koch, K. & Andrews, P. (2011) *Nausea: Mechanisms and Management*. New York, NY: Oxford University Press.

Stringer, J. (2017) Why are essential oils helpful for fungating malignant wounds? *International Journal of Clinical Aromatherapy 12*, 1, 19–25.

Stringer, J. & Donald, G. (2011) Aromasticks® in cancer care: An innovation not to be sniffed at. *Complementary Therapies in Clinical Practice 17*, 2, 116–21.

Stringer, J., Donald, G., Knowles, R. & Warn, P. (2014) The symptom management of fungating malignant wounds using a novel essential oil cream. *Wounds UK 10*, 3, 54–59.

Stringer, J., Swindell, R. & Dennis, M. (2008) Massage in patients undergoing intensive chemotherapy reduces serum cortisol and prolactin. *Psychooncology 17*, 1024–1031.

Stroebe, M. & Schut, H. (1999) The dual process model of coping with bereavement: Rationale and description. *Death Studies 23*, 3, 197–224.

Tanen, D., Danish, D., Reardon, J., Chisholm, C., Matteucci, M. & Riffenburgh, R. (2008) Comparison of oral aspirin versus topical applied methyl salicylate for platelet inhibition. *The Annals of Pharmacotherapy 42*, 1396–1401.

Tavares, M. (2003) *National Guidelines for the Use of Complementary Therapies in Supportive and Palliative Care*. London: The Prince of Wales Foundation for Integrated Health.

Tavares, M. (2011) *Integrating Clinical Aromatherapy in Specialist Palliative Care*. Toronto, Canada: Viveka Group.

Taylor, C. (2011) Malignant fungating wounds: A review of the patient and nurse experience. *British Journal of Community Nursing 16*, suppl 12, S16–S22. doi: 10.12968/bjcn.2011.16.Sup12.S16.

Taylor, J. (2007) The non-pharmacological management of breathlessness. *End of Life Care 1*, 1, 20–27.

Teno, J., Gruneir, A., Schwartz, Z., Nanda, A. & Wetle, T. (2007) Association between advance directives and quality end-of-life care: A national study. *Journal of American Geriatric Society 55*, 2, 189–194.

Theno, M. (2022) Bioesse® aromapatches. Personal communication, April.

Tisserand Institute. (2022) What to do in case of adverse reaction. Retrieved from: https://tisserandinstitute.org/safety/what-to-do-when-experiencing-an-adverse-reaction.

Tisserand, M. (2015) *Aromatherapy vs MRSA*. London: Singing Dragon.

Tisserand, R. & Young, R. (2014) *Essential Oil Safety (second edition)*. Edinburgh: Churchill Livingstone.

Tomic, M., Popovic, V., Petrovic, S., Stepanovic-Petrovic, R. *et al.* (2014) Antihyperalgesic and antiedematous activities of bisabolol-oxides-rich matricaria oil in a rat model of inflammation. *Phytotherapy Research 28*, 759–766.

Tornoe, K., Danbolt, L., Kvigne, K. & Sorlie, V. (2014) The power of consoling presence – hospice nurses' lived experience with spiritual and existential care for the dying. *BioMed Central Nursing 13*, 25. doi: 10.1186/1472-6955-13-25.

Tóth, K., Ádám, D., Bíró, T. & Oláh, A. (2019) Cannabinoid signalling in the skin: Therapeutic potential of the 'C(ut)annabinoid' system. *Molecules 24*, 5, 918. doi: 10.3390/molecules24050918.

Tugade, M., Fredrickson, B. & Barrett, L. (2004) Psychological resilience and positive emotional granularity: Examining the benefits of positive emotions on coping and health. *Journal of Personality 72*, 6, 1161–90.

Turland, N., Wiersema, J., Barrie, F., Greuter, W. *et al.* (2018) *International Code for Nomenclature for Algae, Fungi and Plants (Shenzhen Code adopted by the Nineteenth International Botanical Congress Shenzhen, China 2017).* Regnum Vegetabile 159. Glashütten, Germany: Koeltz Botanical Books.

Twycross, R., Wilcock, A., Charlesworth, S. & Dickman, A. (2002) *Palliative Care Formulary (second edition).* Oxford: Radcliffe Medical Press.

Vadivelu, M., Kai, A., Kodumudi, G., Babayan, K., Fontes, M. & Burg, M. (2017) Pain and psychology – a reciprocal relationship. *Oschsner Journal 17*, 173–180.

Van den Beuken-van Everdingen, M., Hochstenbach, L., Joosten, E., Tjan-Heijnen, V. & Janssen, D. (2016) Update on prevalence of pain in patients with cancer: Systematic review and meta-analysis. *Journal of Pain and Symptom Management 51*, 6, 1070–1090.

van der Steen, J., Bloomer, M. & Pereira, S. (2020) The importance of methodology to palliative care research: A new article type for Palliative Medicine. *Palliative Medicine 36*, 1, 4–6.

Venkatasalu, M., Murang, Z., Ramasamy, D. & Dhaliwal, J. (2020) Oral health problems among palliative and terminally ill patients: An integrated systematic review. *BMC Oral Health 20*, 79. https://doi.org/10.1186/s12903-020-01075-w.

Visser, C., Hadley, G. & Wee, B. (2015) Reality of evidence-based practice in palliative care. *Cancer Biological Medicine 12*, 193–200.

Walsh, D., Davis, M., Ripamonti, C., Bruera, E., Davies, A. & Molassiotis, A. (2017) 2016 Updated MASCC/ESMO consensus recommendations: Management of nausea and vomiting in advanced cancer. *Supportive Cancer Care 25*, 1, 333–340.

Wang, H., Kroenke, K., Wu, J., Tu, W., Theobald, D. & Rawl, S. (2011) Cancer-related pain and disability: A longitudinal study. *Journal of Pain and Symptom Management 42*, 813–821.

Wang, P., Hsu, C., Lui, C., Lai, T., Tzeng, F. & Huang, C. (2019) Effect of acupressure on constipation in patients with advanced cancer. *Supportive Care in Cancer 27*, 3473–3478.

Wang, X. & Yin, J. (2015) Complementary and alternative therapies for chronic constipation. *Evidence-Based Complementary and Alternative Medicine*, Art ID: 396396.

Wang, Z. & Heinbockel, T. (2018) Essential oils and their constituents targeting the GABAergic system and sodium channels as treatment of neurological diseases. *Molecules 23*, 1061. doi: 10.3390/molecules23051061.

Warner, F. (2013) *The Soul Midwives Handbook.* London: Hay House.

Warner, F. (2018) *Sacred Oils.* London: Hay House.

Warnke, P., Sherry, E., Russo, P., Acil, Y. *et al.* (2006) Antibacterial essential oils in malodorous cancer patients: Clinical observations in 30 patients. *Phytomedicine 13*, 7, 463–467.

Warnke, P., Terheyden, H., Ac, Y., Springer, I. *et al.* (2004) Tumour smell reduction with antibacterial essential oils. *International Journal of Clinical Aromatherapy 1*, 2, 21–22.

Wells, M. (2008) 'The Impact of Cancer.' In J. Corner & C. Bailey (eds) *Cancer Nursing: Care in Context.* Oxford: Blackwell Publishing.

Wickham, R. (2017) Managing constipation in patients with cancer. *Journal of the Advanced Practitioner in Oncology 8*, 2, 149–161.

Wiffen, P., Wee, B., Derry, S. & Moore, R. (2017) Opioids for cancer pain – an overview of Cochrane reviews (Review). *Cochrane Database of Systematic Reviews 7*, Art No: CD012592.

Wilkinson, J., Codipilly, D. & Wilfahrt, R. (2021) Dysphagia: Evaluation and collaborative management. *American Family Physician 103*, 2, 97–106.

Wilkinson, S., Aldridge, J., Salmon, I., Cain, E. & Wilson, B. (1999) An evaluation of aromatherapy massage in palliative care. *Palliative Medicine 13*, 5, 409–417.

Wilkinson, S., Love, S., Westcombe, A., Gambles, M. *et al.* (2007) Effectiveness of aroma-therapy massage in the management of anxiety and depression in patients with cancer: A multicentre randomised controlled trial. *American Journal of Clinical Oncology 25*, 5, 532–539.

Williams, A. & Barry, B. (1991) Terpenes and the lipid-protein-partitioning theory of skin penetration enhancement. *Pharmacological Research 8*, 1, 17–24.

Williams, A., Wang, L. & Kitchen, P. (2014) Differential impacts of care-giving across three caregiver groups in Canada: End-of-life care, long-term care and short-term care. *Health and Social Care in the Community 22*, 187–196.

Winardi, A. & Irwan, A. (2019) Topical treatment for controlling malignant wound odour: A systematic review. *Journal of the European Wound Management Association 20*, 2, 7–17.

Woo, K., Santos, V. & Alam, T. (2018) Optimising quality of life for people with non-healing wounds. *Wounds International 9*, 3, s–14.

Woo, K. & Sibbald, R. (2010) Local wound care for malignant and palliative wounds. *Advanced Skin Wound Care 23*, 9, 417–428.

Worden, W. (2009) *Grief Counselling and Grief Therapy: A Handbook for the Mental Health Practitioner (fourth edition)*. New York, NY: Springer Publishing.

World Health Organization. (1996) *Cancer Pain Relief (second edition)*. Geneva, Switzerland.

World Health Organization. (2020) *Definition of Palliative Care*. Retrieved from: www.who.int/cancer/palliative/definition/en.

Wright, D., Corner, J., Hopkinson, J. & Foster, C. (2007) The case for user involvement in research: The research priorities of cancer patients. *Breast Cancer Research 9*, suppl 2. doi: 10.1186/bcr1801.

Xu, L., Zhang, H., Liu, J. & Chen, X. (2013) Investigation of the oral infections and manifestations seen in patients with advanced cancer. *Pakistan Journal of Medical Sciences 29*, 5, 1112–1115.

Yaghoobi, R., Kazerouni, A. & Kazerouni, O. (2013) Evidence for the clinical use of honey in wound healing as an antibacterial, anti-inflammatory, antioxidant and antiviral agent: A review. *Jundishapur Journal of Natural Pharmaceutical Products 8*, 3, 100–104.

Yennurajalingam, S., Tannir, N., Williams, J., Lu, Z. *et al.* (2017) A double-blind, randomized, placebo-controlled trial of *Panax ginseng* for cancer-related fatigue in patients with advanced cancer. *Journal of the National Comprehensive Cancer Network 15*, 1111–1120.

Yildirim, D., Can, G. & Talu, G. (2019) The efficacy of abdominal massage in managing opioid-induced constipation. *European Journal of Oncology Nursing 41*, 110–119.

Yoong, J. & Poon, P. (2018) Principles of cancer pain management. *Australian Journal of General Practice 47*, 11, 758–762.

Yoshimoto-Furuie, K., Yoshimoto, K., Tanaka, T., Saima, S. *et al.* (1999) Effects of oral supplementation with evening primrose oil for six weeks on plasma essential fatty acids and uremic skin symptoms in haemodialysis patients. *Nephron 81*, 151–159.

Yosipovitch, G. & Bernhard, J. (2013) Clinical practice – chronic pruritus. *New England Journal of Medicine 368*, 1625–1634.

Yosipovitch, G., Greaves, M. & Schmelz, M. (2003) Itch. *The Lancet 361*, 9354, 690–694.

Yosipovitch, G. & Samuel, L. (2008) Neuropathic and psychogenic itch. *Dermatology Therapy 21*, 1, 32–41.

Young, T. (2017) Caring for patients with malignant and end-of-life wounds. *Wounds UK EWMA Special*, 20–26.

Youngson, R. (2012) *Time to Care*. Raglan, New Zealand: Rebelheart Publishers.

Yu, D., Wang, J., Shao, X., Xu, F. & Wang, H. (2015) Antifungal modes of action of tea tree oil and its two characteristic components against *Botrytis cinerea*. *Journal of Applied Microbiology 119*, 5, 1253–1262.

Zaza, C. & Baine, N. (2002) Cancer pain and psychosocial factors: A critical review of the literature. *Journal of Pain and Symptom Management 24*, 526–542.

Zeck, R. (2014) *The Blossoming Heart (third edition)*. East Ivanhoe, Victoria: BPA Print Group.

Zelman, D., Smith, M., Hoffman, D., Edwards, L. *et al.* (2004) Acceptable, manageable and tolerable days: Patient daily goals for medication management of persistent pain. *Journal of Pain and Symptom Management 28*, 5, 474–487.

Zhang, N., Zhang, L., Feng, L. & Yao, L. (2016) The anxiolytic effect of essential oil *Cananga odorata* exposure on mice and determination of its major constituents. *Phytomedicine* 23, 14, 1727–1734.

Zimmermann, C., Swami, N., Krzyzanowska, M., Hannon, B. *et al.* (2014) Early palliative care for patients with advanced cancer: A cluster-randomised controlled trial. *The Lancet* 383, 1721–1730.

Zimmermann, C., Swami, N., Krzyzanowska, M., Leighi, N. *et al.* (2016) Perceptions of palliative care among patients with advanced cancer and their caregivers. *Canadian Medical Association Journal* 188, 10, E217–E227.

Zimmermann, F., Burrell, B. & Jordan, J. (2018) The acceptability and potential benefits of mindfulness-based interventions in improving psychological well-being for adults with advanced cancer: A systematic review. *Complementary Therapies in Clinical Practice 30*, 68–78.

Subject Index

Author Index

Hildebrand, S. 53
Hines, S. *et al.* 174
Hodge, N. 174
Hofman, M. *et al.* 100
Hohmann, J. 218
Hökkä, M. 124, 128, 133
Holmes, P. 23–4, 27, 31, 52, 96,
    131–2, 166, 209, 242
Hone, L. 257–8
Hongratanaworakit, T. 92
Horvath, G. 32, 146
Hosseini, M. *et al.* 173
Howell, D. *et al.* 110–12, 115
Hugel, H. *et al.* 109, 115
Hunt, R. *et al.* 174
Hur, M. 208
Hwang, I. *et al.* 234

Ikeda, H. 126
Imanishi, J. *et al.* 89, 133
Inouye, S. 202
International Organization
    for Standardization 23
Irwan, A. 215, 217
Ishaque, S. 267

Jane, S. *et al.* 133
Jardim, M. 173
Jenewein, J. 61–4, 66, 234, 237
Jewell, A. 54, 73
Jobbins, J. *et al.* 159
Johnson, A. 21
Johnson, B. 245
Johnson, J. 267
Johnson, L. 111–12
Johnson, S. 34
Johnson, S. *et al.* 125, 127, 131
Jones, A. 32
Jones, V. 213
Jordan, J. 88
Joseph, C. 217
Joung, D. *et al.* 30
Juergens, U. 33

Kaakinen, P. 124, 128, 133
Kahn, J. 124
Kamal, A. 268–9
Kamal, A. *et al.* 140–1, 143–5
Kamsteeg, M. 195

Kamudoni, P. *et al.* 209
Kang, H. 165
Kang, S. 102–4
Kantor, R. *et al.* 194
Karnell, A. 111
Katsuyama, S. *et al.* 127
Kawagoshi, A. *et al.* 153
Kazemzadeh, R. *et al.* 208
Kazerouni, A. 217
Kazerouni, O. 217
Kearney, N. 108
Keating, A. 173
Keefe, F. 120, 124
Keicolt-Glaser, J. 259
Kerhof, M. 232
Kerkhof-Knapp Hayes, M. 18,
    57, 74, 77, 92, 105, 117, 132,
    166–7, 187, 203–4, 209, 259
Kerkhof, M. 28, 177
Khemlani, M. 111
Khodabakhsh, P. *et al.* 126–7
Kiberd, M. *et al.* 174
Kim, I. 102, 104
Kim, M. *et al.* 187
Kim, N. 102–4
Kim, Y. 165
Kirk, I. 90
Kirk, P. 90
Kistler, C. 159
Kitchen, P. 233–4
Kite, S. *et al.* 53, 74
Kitta, A. *et al.* 244–5
Klasson, C. *et al.* 101
Knevitt, A. 219, 222
Koch, K. 169
Kohara, H. *et al.* 58, 79, 102, 104
Kohn, M. 18, 264, 269
Kotronoulas, G. 108
Koutsilieris, M. 109
Kouwenhoven, T. 195
Kovač, M. 167
Kowalski, S. 89
Kravitz, A. 236
Krishnasamy, M. 86–7, 119, 128
Kristjanson, L. 90
Kübler-Ross, E. 98, 256
Kuo, B. 169, 171
Kutner, J. *et al.* 133
Kuttan, R. 217
Kuwahata, H. *et al.* 126